Clinical Trial
Methodology

Chapman & Hall/CRC Biostatistics Series

Editor-in-Chief

Shein-Chung Chow, Ph.D.
Professor
Department of Biostatistics and Bioinformatics
Duke University School of Medicine
Durham, North Carolina, U.S.A.

Series Editors

Byron Jones
Senior Director
Statistical Research and Consulting Centre
(IPC 193)
Pfizer Global Research and Development
Sandwich, Kent, U.K.

Jen-pei Liu
Professor
Division of Biometry
Department of Agronomy
National Taiwan University
Taipei, Taiwan

Karl E. Peace
Georgia Cancer Coalition
Distinguished Cancer Scholar
Senior Research Scientist and
Professor of Biostatistics
Jiann-Ping Hsu College of Public Health
Georgia Southern University
Statesboro, Georgia

Bruce W. Turnbull
Professor
School of Operations Research
and Industrial Engineering
Cornell University
Ithaca, New York

Chapman & Hall/CRC Biostatistics Series

Published Titles

Chapman & Hall/CRC Biostatistics Series

Clinical Trial Methodology

Karl E. Peace

Jiann-Ping Hsu College of Public Health
Georgia Southern University
Statesboro, Georgia, U.S.A.

Ding-Geng (Din) Chen

Jiann-Ping Hsu College of Public Health
Georgia Southern University
Statesboro, Georgia, U.S.A.

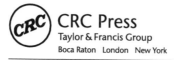

CRC Press
Taylor & Francis Group
Boca Raton London New York

CRC Press is an imprint of the
Taylor & Francis Group, an **informa** business

A CHAPMAN & HALL BOOK

Chapman & Hall/CRC
Taylor & Francis Group
6000 Broken Sound Parkway NW, Suite 300
Boca Raton, FL 33487-2742

First issued in paperback 2020

© 2011 by Taylor and Francis Group, LLC
Chapman & Hall/CRC is an imprint of Taylor & Francis Group, an Informa business

---

Library of Congress Cataloging-in-Publication Data

Peace, Karl E., 1941-
    Clinical trial methodology / Karl E. Peace, Ding-Geng (Din) Chen.
        p. ; cm. -- (Chapman & Hall/CRC biostatistics series ; 35)
    Includes bibliographical references and index.
    Summary: "Now viewed as its own scientific discipline, clinical trial methodology encompasses the methods required for the protection of participants in a clinical trial and the methods necessary to provide a valid inference about the objective of the trial. Drawing from the authors courses on the subject as well as the first authors more than 30 years working in the pharmaceutical industry, Clinical Trial Methodology emphasizes the importance of statistical thinking in clinical research and presents the methodology as a key component of clinical research. From ethical issues and sample size considerations to adaptive design procedures and statistical analysis, the book first covers the methodology that spans every clinical trial regardless of the area of application. Crucial to the generic drug industry, bioequivalence clinical trials are then discussed. The authors describe a parallel bioequivalence clinical trial of six formulations incorporating group sequential procedures that permit sample size re-estimation. The final chapters incorporate real-world case studies of clinical trials from the authors own experiences. These examples include a landmark Phase III clinical trial involving the treatment of duodenal ulcers and Phase III clinical trials that contributed to the first drug approved for the treatment of Alzheimers disease. Aided by the U.S. FDA, the U.S. National Institutes of Health, the pharmaceutical industry, and academia, the area of clinical trial methodology has evolved over the last six decades into a scientific discipline. This guide explores the processes essential for developing and conducting a quality clinical trial protocol and providing quality data collection, biostatistical analyses, and a clinical study report, all while maintaining the highest standards of ethics and excellence"--Provided by publisher.
        ISBN 978-1-58488-917-5 (hardcover : alk. paper)
        1. Clinical trials. 2. Drugs--Testing. I. Chen, Ding-Geng. II. Title. III. Series: Chapman & Hall/CRC biostatistics series ; 35.
        [DNLM: 1. Clinical Trials as Topic--methods. 2. Drug Approval--methods. 3. Drug Evaluation--methods. 4. Meta-Analysis as Topic. QV 771 P355c 2011]
    R853.C55P43 2011
    615.5072'4--dc22   2010021864

Visit the Taylor & Francis Web site at
http://www.taylorandfrancis.com

and the CRC Press Web site at
http://www.crcpress.com

To the memory of my late mother, Elsie Mae Cloud Peace; my late wife,

Jiann-Ping Hsu; my son, Christopher K. Peace; granddaughter, Camden Peace;

and daughter-in-law, Ashley Hopkins Peace.

Karl E. Peace

To my wife, Ke He; my son, John D. Chen; and my daughter, Jenny K. Chen.

Ding-Geng (Din) Chen

Contents

Preface

This book is the result of teaching a course in clinical trial methodology, developed by Karl E. Peace, in the Jiann-Ping Hsu College of Public Health at Georgia Southern University, Statesboro, Georgia, from the fall of 2004 through the fall of 2009. The course is a requirement for students who enroll in the master's of public health (MPH) biostatistics degree program. Many of the graduates have gone on to become biostatisticians in the pharmaceutical industry, contract research organizations, public health departments, and government agencies.

The Jiann-Ping Hsu College of Public Health is relatively young, having been approved as the first school of public health at the University System of Georgia in January 2004. Therefore, many of the students who enrolled in the MPH biostatistics degree program early on did not have a strong background in mathematical sciences. The clinical trial methodology course was therefore taught without placing much emphasis on complicated mathematical statistics. Rather, emphasis was placed on clinical trial methodology as a component of clinical research as a scientific discipline, and on the importance of statistical thinking in clinical research. Thus, this book should appeal not only to statisticians and biostatisticians, but also to anyone responsible for the design, conduct, and analysis of clinical trials.

The content of the course is largely based on Karl E. Peace's experience from working in and providing consultation to the pharmaceutical industry for over 30 years. Chapter 1 sets the stage for the reader to begin thinking about what comprises clinical trial methodology. Chapter 2 provides an overview of the drug development process and the regulation of clinical trials, and recognizes the importance of federal regulations on the design, conduct, analysis, and reporting of clinical trials. It is essential for practicing biostatisticians, especially in the pharmaceutical industry, to have an understanding of how regulation affects their work. Chapter 3 provides a summary of important milestones in the evolution of clinical trial ethics as well as ethical considerations in the design, conduct, analysis, and reporting of clinical trials.

Sample size considerations in the design of clinical trials are presented in Chapter 4, and recommendations are given for sample sizes of clinical trials in all phases of clinical drug development. Chapter 5 is devoted to statistical methods useful in the monitoring of clinical trials: sequential, group-sequential, stochastic curtailment, and adaptive design procedures.

The importance of quality clinical trial protocol development and biostatistical aspects of the protocol are stressed in Chapter 6. Chapter 7 presents the framework for, and an example of, the statistical analysis plan. The importance of careful attention to the pooling of data from multicenter clinical trials is the focus of Chapter 8. Requisites for the validity of statistical inferences from clinical trials are addressed in Chapter 9.

Chapter 10 focuses on the importance of bioequivalence clinical trials. Such trials are essential if the formulation of an approved drug or the site of manufacturing is changed, and are of great importance to the generic drug industry. Chapter 10 includes an example of a parallel bioequivalence clinical trial of six formulations that incorporated group-sequential procedures to allow sample size reestimation, and an example of a two-by-two crossover bioequivalence trial of two formulations of an antibiotic.

Chapters 11 through 16 reflect clinical trials from Karl E. Peace's experience and are presented as case studies. The flow of the material in these chapters reflects sound scientific and statistical principles. Chapter 11 summarizes the use of response surface methodology in the determination of dose and frequency of dosing in Phase II clinical trials of stress test–induced angina. Chapter 12 is a case study of a landmark Phase III clinical trial that confirmed the clinically optimal dosing of an H_2-receptor antagonist drug in the treatment of duodenal ulcer.

Design, monitoring, regulatory interaction, and analysis of Phase III clinical trials that led to the approval of the first drug (a synthetic prostaglandin inhibitor) for the prevention of NANSAID-induced gastric ulceration are presented in Chapter 13. A very detailed account of the design, analysis, and interpretation of Phase III clinical trials in the treatment of Alzheimer's disease based on enrichment designs is provided in Chapter 14. These trials contributed to the approval of the first drug for the treatment of Alzheimer's disease.

Chapter 15 summarizes the design, analysis, and interpretation of a landmark clinical trial that led to the approval of the first drug for reducing the risk of coronary heart disease. The design, analysis, and interpretation of pivotal proof-of-efficacy clinical trials that led to the approval of a benzodiazepine for the treatment of panic disorder are detailed in Chapter 16.

Establishing the effectiveness of a combination product of two drugs and estimating the contribution each drug makes to the effectiveness of the combination is the focus of Chapter 17. This chapter contains, as an example, a summary of the clinical trial that was required to establish the efficacy of a combination product for the treatment of seasonal allergic rhinitis. Chapter 18 presents methods for monitoring the accumulating safety data, particularly adverse events, in clinical trials based on one-sided, per-group confidence intervals.

We would like to express our gratitude to many individuals. First, thanks to David Grubbs from Taylor & Francis for his interest in the book and to Marsha Pronin for her editorial assistance. Thanks also extend to the Georgia Cancer Coalition whose grant in selecting the first author as one of their Distinguished Cancer Scholars supported, in part, his time in developing the book. Finally, from the Jiann-Ping Hsu College of Public Health at Georgia Southern University, thanks are merited to Ruth Whitworth for her IT support and contributions to the development of Chapter 2; to Benjamin Maligalig,

Macaulay Okwakenye, and Yan Wang, my graduate assistants, for assistance in proofing the format of the chapters and development of graphs and tables; to Hanni Samawi for reviewing Chapter 8; to Dean Charlie Hardy for his support and encouragement to finish the project; and to Lee T. Mitchell for her jocularity and good cheer that brighten our entire college.

Karl E. Peace
Georgia Southern University
Statesboro, Georgia

Ding-Geng (Din) Chen
Georgia Southern University
Statesboro, Georgia

1

Overview of Clinical Trial Methodology

1.1 Clinical Trials

A clinical trial is a research study conducted to assess the utility of an intervention in volunteers. Interventions may be diagnostic, preventative, or therapeutic in nature and may include drugs, biologics, medical devices, or methods of screening. Interventions may also include procedures whose aim is to improve the quality of life or to better understand how the intervention works in volunteers.

Most textbooks on clinical trial methodology include a chapter or section on the history of clinical trials. This one does not, at least not explicitly, although there is some history in Chapters 2 and 9. The history of clinical trials up through the early 1950s is chronicled by Bull [1]. A more recent history of the evolution of clinical trials is found in the excellent textbooks by Meinert and Tonascia [2], Bulpitt [3], Everitt and Pickles [4], Green et al. [5], Chow and Liu [6], and the chapter by Day and Ederer [7].

1.2 Clinical Trial Methodology

Clinical trial methodology comprises all methods required for the protection of participants in a clinical trial and all methods necessary to provide a valid inference (see Chapter 9) about the objective of the trial. Clinical trial methodology has evolved over the last six decades into a scientific discipline with the U.S. Food and Drug Administration (FDA), the National Institutes of Health (NIH), the pharmaceutical industry, and academia being major contributors to the evolution.

1.2.1 Randomization and Control

Two very important clinical trial methods are (1) randomization of participants to intervention groups and (2) selecting an appropriate control group against which a particular intervention can be compared. It is widely held that the first randomized controlled clinical trial was conducted by the MRC Tuberculosis Research Unit [8–10] and that the randomization and control design aspects of the trial were the brainchildren of Sir Austin Bradford Hill, Director of the MRC Statistical Research Unit [11,12].

The 1962 Kefauver–Harris (K–F) Amendments [13] to the Food, Drug, and Cosmetics (FD&C) Act of 1938 represented a watershed event in the evolution of evidence to support drug claims and laid the groundwork for much clinical trial methodology that followed (see Chapter 2). This landmark legislation required that all drugs thereafter be proven effective prior to market approval by the U.S. FDA and recognized that effectiveness must be demonstrated by substantial evidence from adequate and well-controlled clinical trials.

1.2.2 Kefauver–Harris Amendment and Its Impact on Clinical Trial Methodology

From the 1962 Amendments to the FD&C Act, one notes that substantial evidence consists of adequate and well-controlled clinical investigations (see Section 2.4) conducted by experts qualified by scientific training and experience to evaluate effectiveness of a drug. These investigations form the basis for such experts to fairly and responsibly conclude that a drug has the effect it purports or is represented to have under the conditions of use prescribed, recommended, or suggested in the labeling. Many authorities, including Dr. Maxwell Finland from Harvard Medical School, Dr. Louis Lasagna, Head of the Division of Clinical Pharmacology at Johns Hopkins, and Dr. Charles May, Professor of Pediatrics at New York University Medical School, gave testimony insisting that evidence of the effectiveness of drugs could only derive from controlled clinical trials. They noted that a careful scientific experiment requires (1) careful biostatistical preparation and analysis; (2) randomized selection of similar patients into groups that are to receive the drug being tested and the placebo (control); (3) careful efforts to withholding of knowledge from the patient as to whether he or she is being given an active drug or placebo; and (4) careful efforts to withhold from the investigator the identity of the drug (if the experiment is to be, by definition, of a double-blind character). They recognized that care must be taken to eliminate bias (whether overt or subtle) of any kind—including that arising from patients or investigators having knowledge of the drug to which the patient is assigned. In fact, Dr. May held the opinion that efficacy was unlikely to be determined unless a drug was tested by a systematic, scientific evaluation according to the best modern procedures.

The 1962 Amendments to the FD&C Act not only required clinical trials to be randomized and controlled, but also to be **double blinded** (a third most important clinical trial method) and be carefully **biostatistically prepared and analyzed**. Therefore, design and biostatistical analyses are clinical trial methods.

The 1962 Amendments delineated 10 scientific principles necessary for adequate and well-controlled clinical investigations and are recognized by the scientific, medical, statistical, and regulatory communities.

1. There has to be a protocol or study plan.
2. The protocol must have a clear statement of objectives.
3. The protocol must use a method for selecting participants that provides adequate confirmation of the presence of the disease state.
4. The protocol has to include a method for assigning patients to interventions being studied without bias.
5. The protocol should include an outline of the methods of quantification and of observations on the participants in the trial.
6. The protocol must include a description of the steps taken to document comparability of data collected prior to assignment to study medications.
7. The protocol must include a description of the methods for recording and analyzing patient response variables studied.
8. The protocol must contain a description of methods or steps taken to minimize bias in the observations.
9. The protocol should include a precise statement of the nature of the control group against which the effects of the new drug treatment can be compared.
10. The protocol should include a survey of statistical methods to be used in the analysis of the data derived from the patients.

At present, a survey of statistical methods stated in # 10 above is interpreted as the statistical analysis section (see Chapter 6) of the clinical trial protocol and the attendant statistical analysis plan (see Chapter 7). A more thorough discussion of the 10 principles may be found in Section 2.4.

1.2.3 Categorization of Clinical Trial Methodology

This book takes a broad view of what comprises clinical trial methodology. As previously indicated, clinical trial methodology includes all methods required for the protection of participants in a clinical trial and all methods necessary to provide a valid inference about the objective of the trial. Many categorizations of clinical trial methodology are possible. For example, one could categorize clinical trial methodology as being primarily clinical, primarily biostatistical, primarily data management, or primarily administrative (or operations management) in nature. Diagnostic and medical treatment procedures are primarily clinical in nature, but may require biostatistical methods for validation. Experimental design and statistical analysis procedures are primarily biostatistical in nature. Computerization and quality assurance of the data collected in a clinical trial and the creation of analysis data sets are primarily data management in nature. All other procedures related to the conduct of a clinical trial may be lumped into an administrative category.

Implicit in the excellent book by Chow and Liu [6] is the recognition that clinical trial methodology includes randomization and blinding, and design aspects—including sample size determination and statistical analyses of clinical trials. In another excellent textbook by Piantadosi [14], one surmises that clinical trial methodology includes not only the three categories identified above from Chow and Liu [6], but also recognition of procedures or steps to minimize bias, identify the population to be studied, specify the objective and endpoints, report results, and ensure ethics, as clinical trial methods.

Clinical trial methodology may also be categorized according to methods inherent in the development of the protocol—those that are operative in the conduct of the protocol and those that are utilized in the analysis and reporting of the data collected. It is indeed difficult to categorize clinical trial methods into mutually exclusive categories. Biostatistical design and analysis methods are described in the protocol, but some, such as statistical monitoring plans, are utilized during the conduct of the clinical trial, while others are utilized in the analysis of the data collected.

1.3 Summary of Clinical Trial Methodology

Clinical trial methods are summarized in Table 1.1 in a reasonably chronological order (top to bottom), with the admission that management spans all aspects of the clinical trial—from protocol development to completion of the clinical study report. In summary, clinical trial methodology consists of all methods necessary to develop and conduct a quality clinical trial protocol and to provide quality data collection, biostatistical analyzes, and a clinical study report while maintaining the highest standards of ethics and excellence.

Chapters 2 through 9 present clinical trial methodology that spans all clinical trials regardless of area of application. Chapter 2 provides an overview of the drug development process and the regulation of clinical trials and recognizes the importance of federal regulations on the design, conduct, analysis, and reporting of clinical trials. Ethical considerations in the design, conduct, analysis, and reporting of clinical trials appear in Chapter 3. Sample size considerations in the design of clinical trials are presented in Chapter 4, and recommendations are given for sample sizes of clinical trials in all phases

TABLE 1.1

Summary of Clinical Trial Methodology

Clinical trial objectives
   Unambiguous and clearly stated
   Translated into statistical questions
Basis for sample size clearly presented
   Endpoints identified and appropriate for objective
   Mean and variance estimates of endpoint
   Type I error is specified
   Adequate power is specified
   δ is specified and is consistent with the objective
   Sidedness is specified and is consistent with the objective
Trial population clearly defined
   Inclusion criteria
   Exclusion criteria
   Appropriate diagnostic workup
   Concurrent/concomitant medication use
   Treatments/interventions, including dosing regimens clearly defined
Methods for eliminating or minimizing bias
   Method of assigning subjects to interventions
   Randomization schedule
   Procedures for blinding
   Data measurement process
   Procedures for reducing extraneous sources of variation
Monitoring procedures
   For adherence to protocol, good clinical practice guidelines, and other regulations
   For patient safety and intervention as necessary
   For data clarity, quality, and consistency
   Methods for assessing medication compliance
Database management procedures
   Permit flow of data collection forms to minimize lag time between field completion
     and data entry
   Appropriate and adequate validation of entry
   Appropriate and adequate validation of database
   Appropriate and adequate validation of analysis datasets
Biostatistical analysis methods
   Analysis methods stated in protocol
   Appropriate for design and data collected
   Underlying assumptions validated
   Integrity of Type I error
   Adequate handling of missing values
   Validation of analysis software programming
   Robustness of inference

(continued)

TABLE 1.1 (continued)

Summary of Clinical Trial Methodology

Management structure
   Informed consent document
   IRB review and approval
   Investigator meetings for multicenter trials
   Data safety monitoring committee
   Endpoint verification committee
   Site monitoring
   Documentation procedures
   Auditing procedures including compliance with regulations and protocol
   Procedures for problem management and resolution
Clinical trial study report
   Summarizes what was to be done, what was done, and how differences might affect inferences
   Sufficient detail to permit thorough review
   Inferences appropriate for objective, the data, and analysis methods

of clinical drug development. Chapter 5 is devoted to statistical methods useful in the monitoring of clinical trials: sequential, group sequential, stochastic curtailment, and adaptive design procedures. The importance of biostatistical aspects of the clinical trial protocol is stressed in Chapter 6. Chapter 7 presents the framework for, and an example of, the statistical analysis plan (SAP). The importance of careful attention to the pooling of data from multicenter clinical trials is the focus of Chapter 8. Requisites for the validity of statistical inferences from clinical trials are addressed in Chapter 9.

Chapter 10 focuses attention on the importance of bioequivalence clinical trials. Such trials are essential if the formulation of an approved drug or the site of manufacturing is changed, and are of great importance to the generic drug industry. A parallel bioequivalence clinical trial of six formulations incorporating group sequential procedures permitting sample size reestimation is discussed in Chapter 10.

Chapters 11 through 18 reflect clinical trials from the authors' own experience and are presented as case studies. The flow of the material in these chapters reflects sound scientific and statistical principles. Chapter 11 summarizes the use of response surface methodology in the determination of dose and frequency of dosing in Phase II clinical trials of stress test–induced angina. Chapter 12 is a case study of a landmark Phase III clinical trial that confirmed the clinically optimal dosing of an H_2-receptor antagonist drug in the treatment of duodenal ulcer. Design, monitoring, regulatory interaction, and analysis of Phase III clinical trials that led to the approval of the first drug (a synthetic prostaglandin inhibitor) for the prevention of NSAID-induced gastric ulceration are presented in Chapter 13. A very detailed account of the design, analysis, and interpretation of Phase III clinical trials in the treatment of Alzheimer's disease based upon enrichment designs is provided in Chapter 14. These trials contributed to the approval of the first drug for the treatment of Alzheimer's disease. Chapter 15 summarizes the design, analysis, and interpretation of a landmark clinical trial that led to the approval of the first drug for the reduction of coronary heart disease risk. Design, analysis, and interpretation of pivotal proof of efficacy clinical trials that led to approval of a benzodiazepine for the treatment of panic disorder are detailed in Chapter 16. Establishing the effectiveness of a combination product of two drugs and estimating the contribution each drug makes to the effectiveness of the combination is the focus of Chapter 17. Chapter 17 contains as an example, a summary of the clinical trial that was required to establish the efficacy of a combination product for the treatment of seasonal allergic rhinitis. Chapter 18 presents methods for monitoring accumulating safety data, particularly adverse events, in clinical trials.

The material presented in this book forms the basis of a master's level course in clinical trial methodology that the authors have taught several times. Instructors who use this book to teach a course in clinical trial methodology should as an exercise have students identify clinical trial methods used in Chapters 10 through 18.

References

1. Bull JP (1959): The historical development of clinical therapeutic trials. *Journal of Chronic Diseases*; **10**: 218–248.
2. Meinert CL, Tonascia S (1986): *Clinical Trials: Design, Conduct and Analysis*, Oxford University Press, New York.
3. Bulpitt CJ (1996): *Randomised Controlled Clinical Trials*, 2nd edn., Kluwer Academic Publishers, London, U.K.
4. Everitt B, Pickles A (1999): *Statistical Aspects of the Design and Analysis of Clinical Trials*, Imperial College Press, London, U.K.
5. Green S, Benedetti J, Crowley J (2003): *Clinical Trials in Oncology*, Chapman and Hall/CRC, Boca Raton, FL.
6. Chow SC, Liu JP (2004): *Design and Analysis of Clinical Trials: Concepts and Methodologies*, 2nd edn., John Wiley & Sons, New York.
7. Day S, Ederer F (2004): Brief history of clinical trials. In: *Textbook of Clinical Trials*, Machin, D, Day, S, Green, S (eds.), John Wiley & Sons, Ltd, Chichester, U.K.
8. MRC Streptomycin in Tuberculosis Trials Committee (1948): Streptomycin treatment of pulmonary tuberculosis. *British Medical Journal*; **ii**: 769–783.
9. Landsborough TA (1975): *Half a Century of Medical Research*, Her Majesty's Stationary Office, London, U.K., pp. 238–239.
10. Sutherland I (1998): Medical research council streptomycin trial. In: *Encyclopedia of Biostatistics*, Wiley, Chichester, U.K., pp. 2559–2566.

11. Bradford Hill A (1990): Memories of the British streptomycin trial in tuberculosis. *Controlled Clinical Trials*; **11**: 77–90.
12. Armitage P (1992): Bradford Hill and the randomised controlled trial. *Pharmaceutical Medicine*; **6**: 23–37.
13. Bren L (2007): The advancement of controlled clinical trials. *FDA Consumer Magazine*, http://www.fda.gov/fdac/features/2007/207_trials.html
14. Piantadosi S (1997): *Clinical Trials: A Methodological Perspective*, John Wiley & Sons, New York.

2

Overview of the Drug Development Process and Regulation of Clinical Trials

2.1 Introduction

The primary aims of this chapter are to provide an overview of the pharmaceutical clinical development process and federal regulations governing clinical trial conduct in the United States. We begin with a summary of the drug development process. This includes activities both pre- and post-investigational new drug (IND) application. Post-IND activities include an overview of the phases of clinical trials, an overview of the new drug application (NDA), and post-NDA review activities. Next, a brief history of legislation and Food and Drug Administration (FDA) guidances pertinent to the regulation of drugs is presented. Regulations and guidances cited are primarily those that have some impact on the role of the biostatistician supporting clinical drug development. Then guiding principles of adequate and well-controlled investigations follow.

Next, the content and format of an IND application and a NDA are summarized. We pay particular attention to the clinical and statistical sections of an NDA because of their importance in the activities of the biostatistician, particularly the integrated summaries of efficacy, safety, and benefit to risk. Then the reader is familiarized with the organizational structure of the FDA, the FDA review process, and the content of the product label and the package insert.

Pharmaceutical research and clinical drug development is highly regulated [1]. It is helpful for the biostatistician supporting pharmaceutical research and clinical development to have a broad overview of the FDA, particularly how this giant organization that is charged with protecting the nation's health (in terms of not allowing ineffective or unsafe drugs to reach the market) does its business. Penultimately, the role of the biostatistician within the context of a pharmaceutical company is discussed. The chapter concludes with some final remarks.

2.2 The Drug Development Process

This chapter focuses on drugs (chemical entities) rather than biologics or medical devices. However, much of what is covered applies to the development of biological products and medical device products as well. Information on regulations pertinent to the clinical development of biologics and medical devices is presented in some sections.

2.2.1 Pre-Investigational New Drug Exemption Application

The drug development process begins with the discovery of a new chemical or biological compound. The compound undergoes testing both *in vivo* and *in vitro* to determine whether it has sufficient activity to warrant continuing research. If the decision is to continue, additional studies in animals are conducted. These are specific as well as comprehensive animal pharmacology studies, and some initial toxicology studies.

Work also begins to assess whether the compound may be formulated (tablet, capsule, etc.) with characteristics (stability properties, taste, solubility, etc.) that would warrant its use in the clinical development program and eventual marketing. Chemists begin developing the formulation long before the start of the first clinical trial. At the start of the clinical development program there should be a sufficient supply of the specific formulation to permit enrollment of the numbers of patients required by the clinical development plan.

2.2.2 Investigational New Drug Exemption Application

If the decision is made to clinically develop the compound, the company develops an IND exemption application and files it with the FDA. Parenthetically, although the use of the acronym IND is widespread, the more correct acronym is INDE. From a legal perspective [2] the utility of the IND application is to permit a non-approved drug to be shipped cross state lines—which will be necessary in the conduct of clinical trials in the clinical development program. It also alerts the FDA of the sponsor's intention to conduct clinical trials with an investigational (non-approved) drug, and provides the basis for its commercial clinical development.

The FDA provides written notification to the sponsor of the date the IND application was received. The IND goes into effect 30 days after the FDA receives the application—unless the sponsor is notified by the FDA of a clinical hold [3]. If the pharmaceutical sponsor has not heard back from the FDA within this 30-day period, they may begin the first clinical trial in humans.

The IND application [4] is a huge document containing several sections. There is an introductory statement that identifies the drug, drug class, route, and formulation as well as the objectives of the drug development program. The general clinical investigational or drug development plan, including the protocols for clinical trials to be conducted, is included. Technical information about the chemistry of the drug as well as its pharmacology and toxicology in animals is also included. The investigator brochure (IB) of the drug is included.

The IB [5] is an important document as it becomes the blueprint or source documentation as to what is known about the drug at this particular point in time. It therefore serves as "labeling" during the investigational phase of clinical trials. Among the information included are summaries of pharmacology, pharmacokinetics, previous clinical studies (the IB is updated periodically as more information becomes known), and the possible risks or side effects of the drug.

Specifics of the content and format of the IND application are reviewed in Section 2.5.

2.2.3 Phases of Clinical Trials

The clinical development plan identifies clinical trials that are conducted in phases: Phase I, Phase II, and Phase III. Phase I trials generally include single-dose tolerance studies; multiple-dose tolerance studies; studies to assess pharmacokinetic characteristics such as absorption, distribution, metabolism, and excretion; more detailed pharmacokinetic studies; and pharmacology studies in humans.

Phase I studies are rarely conducted in patients. They are usually conducted in normal, healthy volunteers. The main objective of Phase I clinical trials is to identify a range of tolerable doses so that patients participating in future studies with doses in the tolerance range would not be expected to suffer severe adverse events (AEs). Additional objectives are as follows: to understand what happens to the drug once it gets into the human circulatory system, and to reveal the mechanism of action of the drug.

Phase II clinical trials represent the first introduction of the drug into patients that have the disease for which the drug is being developed. These trials are aimed at defining the regimen (dose and frequency of dosing) needed to successfully treat patients. They are initial efficacy studies since patients with the disease in question are being treated to provide some evidence of effectiveness. More detailed pharmacokinetic studies as well as more extensive pharmacology studies in patients may also be conducted as Phase II clinical trials. In order to proceed to Phase III, the drug must be deemed effective at some dose and frequency in Phase II. At this stage, effectiveness has been indicated, but not confirmed.

Phase III clinical trials represent definitive proof-of-efficacy or confirmatory-efficacy trials of the treatment regimen determined as optimal in Phase II.

The primary objectives of the Phase III program are to confirm the effectiveness of the drug in a more heterogeneous population, and to collect more and longer term safety data. Information from Phase II provides pilot data for the purpose of sample size determination in Phase III.

For the purpose of obtaining more safety data under conditions that better approximate the anticipated clinical use of the drug, relatively large, uncontrolled, noncomparative trials may also be conducted in Phase III. If the drug is approved for marketing, it may be used in various subpopulations; e.g., diabetics, the renally impaired, etc. Since no or inadequate numbers of such patients may be enrolled in other trials, studies in special populations may also be conducted in Phase III.

More specifics of the phases of clinical trials appear in Chapter 4. Figure 2.1 may also be viewed for more information regarding the phases of clinical trials. An electronic version of Figure 2.1 may be accessed [6] to obtain more detailed information.

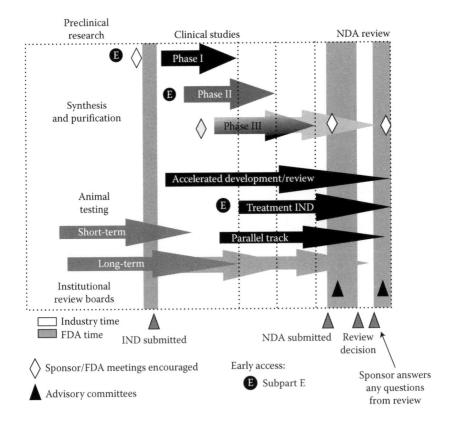

FIGURE 2.1
The new drug development process: steps from test tube to NDA review. (Courtesy of www.fda.gov/cder/handbook/Develop.gif)

2.2.4 The New Drug Application

Drug research activities conducted up to filing the IND typically require about six and one-half years. Clinical development activities conducted thereafter (Phases I, II, and III) up through filing the NDA typically require another 32 months. So the total time for research and development on average is just over 9 years. Drugs for some indications may require longer. For example, the Helsinki Heart Study (HHS) specified a 10-year treatment period [7]. The first 5 years were double blinded. The last 5 years were open label. Before the NDA (actually a supplemental new drug application [SNDA] as the drug was already marketed for lowering triglycerides) could be filed, results of the double blind Phase had to be analyzed and included. So that particular NDA Phase required more than 5 years. Parenthetically, the HHS was a landmark clinical trial that led to the validation of the lipid hypothesis: elevating HDL and lowering LDL lead to a reduced risk of coronary heart disease (CHD). It also formed the basis for FDA approval of gemfibrozil (Lopid) as the first drug to be marketed for the reduction in CHD risk. The research and development of drugs is not only time consuming, it is a very expensive process as well. Average development costs range from one-half to just under a billion dollars (per drug).

The NDA is a huge document or dossier [8] that contains several sections or layers: an overall summary (that goes to all FDA reviewers), several technical sections, and a complete copy for archival purposes. The overall summary [8] should be written so that readers may gain a good understanding of the data and information contained in the application. The level of details is expected to be consistent with the requirements of refereed scientific and medical journals. If the NDA is approved, the overall summary document may be used to draft the Summary Basis of Approval (SBA) [9] and will be accessible by the public via FOI (freedom of information).

The **overall summary** must include: (1) the proposed labeling; (2) identification of the pharmacologic class and scientific rationale for use and potential clinical benefits; (3) any marketing history outside the United States; (4) a summary of chemistry, manufacturing, and controls; (5) a summary of the nonclinical pharmacology and toxicology; (6) a summary of human pharmacokinetics and bioavailability; (7) a summary of the microbiology (for anti-infective drugs); (8) a summary of the clinical data section—including the results of statistical analyses of the clinical trials; and (9) a discussion that summarizes benefit and risk considerations related to the drug, including general plans for any proposed additional studies, surveillance and risk management strategy the sponsor plans to conduct post-approval.

The NDA must contain **technical sections** that include data and information sufficient to enable the FDA to make a knowledgeable judgment as to whether the NDA should be approved. These [8] are (1) the chemistry, manufacturing, and controls section; (2) the nonclinical pharmacology and toxicology section; (3) the human pharmacokinetics and bioavailability section; (4) the microbiology section for an anti-infective drug; (5) the clinical data section (that includes integrated summaries of efficacy, safety and benefit to risk); and (6) the statistical section.

More specifics of the content and format of the NDA are reviewed in Sections 2.6 and 2.8. Figure 2.1 may also be viewed regarding the NDA and how the entire drug development process including how the NDA and the FDA review of the NDA interrelate.

2.2.5 Post-FDA NDA Review Activities

Following its review of the NDA, the FDA may conclude that the NDA is not approvable, may enlist the review and input from an advisory committee [10] prior to making a decision as to approvability, or may conclude that the NDA is approvable based on the content submitted, or may conclude that the NDA is approvable subject to the sponsor conducting additional studies. Clinical trials conducted post-FDA review are typically considered as Phase IV trials.

Some Phase IV trials may be conducted to better quantitate efficacy, particularly within some subpopulations with respect to the original indication. Usually requests for additional clinical trials after FDA review of the NDA are intended to gather more information as to the safety of the drug, particularly among patients who are prescribed the drug by their physicians. Such post-approval clinical trials are referred to as post-marketing surveillance trials. Recently, the FDA began requiring the sponsor to file a risk management, post-marketing strategy for monitoring of safety [11,12].

It is acknowledged that once the NDA has been approved for the indication(s) sought, the pharmaceutical sponsor often expands the product line by conducting additional trials to gather evidence to support additional claims. Such trials may be thought of as pivotal proof-of-efficacy trials for the additional indications (such as the Helsinki Heart Study), and are usually the responsibility of the corporate side of the pharmaceutical company rather than the responsibility of research and development. If the company files applications for additional indications, the vehicle for doing so in the United States is the SNDA [13].

Figure 2.1 [6] provides an excellent overview of the drug development process, including FDA review. When one accesses the figure from the FDA Web site, one has the capability of clicking on various components of the figure to pull up screens laden with helpful information.

It is noted in passing that the acronyms PLA (product licensing application), BLA (biologics licensing application), or PMA (premarket approval application) are the counterparts of NDA if the pharmaceutical product is a biological derived compound or a medical device, respectively.

2.3 History of Drug Regulation

It's important that a course in clinical trial methodology reviews aspects of federal regulation pertinent to drug research and development, particularly clinical drug development. Drug research and clinical development are highly regulated. All biostatisticians providing supports to drug research and clinical development should be aware of the history of such regulations and of their relevance to the work of the pharmaceutical company, including the work of the biostatistician.

2.3.1 The Pure Food and Drugs Act—1906

The Pure Food and Drugs Act of 1906 [14] prohibited the misbranding and adulteration of foods, drinks, and drugs, and was enforced by the Bureau of Chemistry in the Department of Agriculture. There was no requirement to submit any information to the Bureau prior to marketing, and the law required only that drugs meet standards of strength and purity. Government bore the burden of proof to show that the labeling of a drug was false and misleading before it could be removed from the market.

2.3.2 The Sherley Amendment—1912

Six years after passage of the Pure Food and Drugs Act, the Sherley Amendment was passed in 1912 [15]. This amendment prohibited labeling medicines with false therapeutic claims intended to defraud the purchaser. The amendment was not ideal as the government had to prove that there was intention to defraud.

2.3.3 The Food and Drug Administration—1930

The FDA was created in 1930 [16]. All activities pertinent to the regulation of foods and drugs were removed from the Bureau of Chemistry in the Department of Agriculture and transitioned under the newly created FDA. The FDA remained under the Department of Agriculture until mid-June, 1940. It was not until 1955 that FDA became a part of the Public Health Service under the U.S. Department of Health, Education and Welfare (HEW).

2.3.4 The Food, Drug, and Cosmetic Act—1938

The Food, Drug, and Cosmetic Act of 1938 extended FDA's oversight from foods and drugs to also include cosmetics. It also required labeling of drugs for their safe use and required adequate factory inspections. Its passage also eliminated the Sherley Amendment [17].

2.3.5 The Durham–Humphrey Amendment Act—1951

The Durham–Humphrey Amendment act of 1951 [18] required that certain drugs be labeled for sale by prescription only.

2.3.6 The Kefauver–Harris Drug Amendments—1962

In 1962, the Kefauver–Harris Amendments to the Federal Food, Drug, and Cosmetics Act of 1938 were passed. This landmark legislation—often referred to tongue-in-cheek as the "Full Employment Act" of biostatisticians in the pharmaceutical industry—required that all drugs thereafter be proven effective in order to gain approval by the FDA for marketing in the United States. Prior to 1962, drugs were on the market, but their effectiveness had not necessarily been proven via evidence from clinical trials.

The 1962 Kefauver–Harris Amendments [19] represented a watershed event in the evolution of using evidence to support drug claims. Strengthening the evidence to support claims deriving from clinical investigations is the result of first recognizing the need for improvement and second, the collective desire to improve quality in all aspects of such. Improving the experimental design of the investigation is one aspect, and this includes ensuring an adequate number of participants. Improving the quality of reporting the investigation is a second important aspect of quality improvement in all aspects of clinical trials [20].

2.3.7 The Fair Packaging and Labeling Act—1966

The Fair Packaging and Labeling Act of 1966 [21] required that all consumer products in interstate commerce be honestly and informatively labeled and gave FDA jurisdiction to enforce the provisions on foods, drugs, cosmetics, and medical devices. The Act was substantially amended in 1992.

2.3.8 The DESI Review—1970

Following passage of the Kefauver–Harris Amendments, all drugs approved between 1938 and 1962 had to be reviewed for efficacy. The FDA contracted with the National Academy of Sciences/National Research Council (NAS/NRC) who set up a task force to perform a retrospective review. The review process was referred to as the Drug Efficacy Study Implementation (DESI). Parenthetically, a positive by-product of the DESI effort was the development of the abbreviated new drug application (ANDA). A sponsor could submit an ANDA for reviewed products that required only changes in existing labeling to be in compliance [22].

The NAS/NRC task force utilized information from three sources: manufacturers, FDA files, and the medical literature. Each indication was judged to be effective (evidence justified the claim); probably effective (more evidence needed); possibly effective (substantial research needed from adequate and well-controlled trials); ineffective as a single ingredient; or ineffective as a fixed combination [23].

The task force reviewed 3443 products reflecting more than 16,000 therapeutic claims. The last NAS/NRC report was submitted to FDA in 1969. The initial agency review of the NAS/NRC task force reports was completed in November 1970 [24]. By 1984, final action had been completed on over 3400 products; of these, 2225 were found to be effective, 1051 were found not to be effective, and 167 were still pending [24].

2.3.9 The FDA Package Insert Requirement—1970

In 1970, the FDA required for the first time that all drugs approved for marketing contain a package insert [25].

2.3.10 FDA Review of OTC Products—1972

FDA began reviewing OTC drugs for safety and efficacy in 1972 [26]. Oral contraceptives were required to contain information about their benefits and risks using language easily understood prior to this legislation.

2.3.11 The National Research Act—1974

In May 1974, regulations governing the protection of human subjects involved in research, development, and related activities supported or conducted by the Department of HEW through grants and contracts were published [27]. At that time it was indicated that notices of proposed rulemaking would be developed to provide additional protection for subjects in research studies. Two months later, the National Research Act [28] was signed into law. This law effectively created the National Commission for the Protection of Human Subjects of Biomedical and Behavioral Research.

The Commission was also charged to study the Institutional Review Board (IRB) mechanism, and to make recommendations to the Secretary of HEW as it deemed appropriate to assure that biomedical and behavioral research conducted or supported under programs administered by HEW met the Commission's requirements respecting informed consent [29].

2.3.12 The Medical Device Amendments—1976

In 1976, the medical device amendments were passed [30]. The requirements for a drug to be approved were in principle also required for a medical device to be approved, although in practice it is difficult if not impossible to blind device trials.

2.3.13 The Good Laboratory Practices—1978

Good laboratory practices (GLPs) for conducting nonclinical laboratory studies were published in 1978 via 43 FR 60013, amended in 1987 via 52 FR 33779 and amended again in 1999 via 64 FR 399 [31]. The GLPs apply to nonclinical studies conducted to support applications for research or marketing permits for products regulated by the FDA, including food and color additives, additives for animal food, drugs for use in animals or humans, medical devices for human use, biological products, and electronic products. Compliance with the GLPs is intended to assure the quality and integrity of the safety data filed with applications [32,33].

2.3.14 Good Clinical Practice Guidelines—1978

Following World War II, the Nuremburg Code of 1947 recognized the importance of the protection of human subjects in biomedical research. The World Medical Association developed the Declaration of Helsinki in 1964. The Declaration delineated ethical responsibilities of researchers in using human volunteers in their research. The FDA codified the Declaration of Helsinki's guidelines into Good Clinical Practice (GCP) guidelines in 1978. Then in 1995 the FDA led the International Conference on Harmonisation (ICH), in an effort to evolve international standards for conducting research, particularly in clinical trials assessing the safety and efficacy of new drugs [34].

GCP guidelines continue to evolve through the ICH effort today. GCP is an accepted term that collectively describes the responsibilities of sponsors, investigators, monitors, and IRBs in the conduct of clinical research and protection of human subjects [35].

GCP is regarded as the international ethical and quality "standard for the design, conduct, performance, monitoring, auditing, recording, analysis, and reporting of clinical trials that involve participation of human subjects" and defines the network of obligations that clinical trial sponsors and investigators use to design, conduct, analyze, and interpret data from clinical trials of the safety and efficacy of drugs. Following GCP guidelines aims to ensure that data collected in a clinical trial are accurate, verifiable, and reproducible—which are necessary in advancing scientific and medical knowledge. Compliance with GCP is the law, and helps to assure the public that the rights, safety and well-being, and confidentiality of participants in clinical trials are protected [36].

2.3.15 Protection of Human Subjects and IRB Standards—1981

The standards for the protection of human subjects and institutional review boards (IRBs) were strengthened in 1981. IRB membership consisted of scientists and nonscientists in hospitals and research institutions whose responsibility was to ensure the safety and well-being of human research volunteers [37].

2.3.16 The Federal Anti-Tampering Regulations—1983

The Federal Anti-Tampering Act was passed in 1983 and made it a crime for anyone to tamper with packaged consumer products [21]. This regulation was passed in response to seven people dying in Chicago after swallowing Tylenol capsules laced with Cyanide.

2.3.17 The Orphan Drug Act—1983

In January 1983 the Federal Food, Drug, and Cosmetic Act (FFDCA) was amended to permit development of "orphan drugs." The amendment provided guidance in the identification of orphan products (primarily drug and biological products) and the facilitation of their development. Congress subsequently amended the orphan drug act in 1984, 1985, and 1988. The term, orphan, did not actually appear in the text of the law. It has been adopted to refer to an area of drug development for treating rare ($\leq$200,000) diseases or conditions. Huntington's disease, ALS (or Lou Gehrig's disease), and Tourette syndrome are examples of "orphan" diseases. The objective of the orphan drug act was to make it financially attractive for drug development companies to develop drugs for treating rare disease (for which no effective treatments existed) by guaranteeing the developer 7 years of market exclusivity for the orphan drug following the approval of the drug by the FDA [38].

2.3.18 The Hatch–Waxman Act—1984

The Drug Price Competition and Patent Term Restoration Act of 1984, most often referred to as the Hatch–Waxman Act of 1984 [39], was passed in an effort to promote the development of generic drugs while not removing financial incentives for research and development. It permitted FDA to approve generic copies of the original formulation of a drug based on the submission of bioequivalence and dissolution studies—rather than go through the phases of more expensive clinical trials. It also granted a period of additional marketing exclusivity to make up for the time a patented pipeline drug remained in development. This extension could not exceed 5 years, and was in addition to the 20 years exclusivity granted at the issuance of the patent for the original formulation. The Office for Generic Drugs (in the Center for Drug Evaluation and Research [CDER]) was later established in 1989.

2.3.19 The IND/NDA Rewrite—1983–1987

In June 1983, the FDA proposed to revise its regulations governing the review of IND applications and the monitoring of the progress of investigational drug use. FDA took this action to improve the investigational drug development process while maintaining high standards of human subject protection. The improvements were intended to assist sponsors of clinical investigations to prepare and submit high quality applications, both in content and format, and to permit FDA to review them efficiently and with minimal delay. This action was one of a larger effort to review and improve all aspects of FDA's drug regulatory process [40].

The proposal was published in the federal register and provided a period for the public as well as the pharmaceutical industry to provide input. The FDA, particularly FDA Biometrics, participated in several professional sessions (e.g., under the umbrella of the Drug Information Association and the American Statistical Association) targeted to the impact on biostatistical support the IND/NDA rewrite regulations would have. These regulations were finalized and published in the federal register in 1987 [41].

This legislation provided specifics about content and format of the IND document as well as the NDA document. The IND/NDA rewrite is an example of an effort that recognized the need for better design and quality throughout drug research and development, particularly clinical development, coupled with the need for better summarization and presentation of results. This legislation introduced for the first time the dose comparison or clinical dose–response trial.

One impact of the IND/NDA rewrite was to serve notice to the pharmaceutical industry that it had to do a better job at identifying dose regimens for drugs to be marketed. It is widely held that Dr. Bob Temple at the FDA was of the opinion that the doses of drugs on the market prior to the IND/NDA rewrite were generally too high. This position is understandable in the absence of regulation requiring evidence of clinical dose–response. This had considerable impact on the design of clinical development programs. The IND/NDA rewrite also had an enormous impact on how data are organized and presented in NDAs to expedite FDA review.

2.3.20 Drugs for Life-Threatening Illnesses—1987

The treatment IND was proposed in 1982 to allow patients with life-threatening illnesses to participate in clinical trials of promising new drugs. It was finalized in 1987 [42].

2.3.21 Inclusion of Older Patients in Clinical Trials—1989

The FDA issued guidelines in 1989 for the inclusion of older patients in the clinical development trials [43,44]. The idea here is to gather data that can be analyzed to assess whether response to drug differs across age categories (young, middle age, and old age).

2.3.22 Accelerated Approval—1992

The FDA permitted the accelerated approval of new drugs in 1992 [45]. This type of drug approval applies to development of drugs to treat diseases that require a long period to observe the efficacy endpoint in individual patients given that a surrogate endpoint of the disease has been established. Accelerated approval is possible based on the surrogate endpoint conditional on the sponsor later verifying the actual clinical effectiveness.

2.3.23 The Prescription Drug User Fee Act—1992

In response to public criticism that the FDA approval process for new drugs took too much time, the FDA explored the establishment of user fees. The Prescription Drug User Fee Act (PDUFA) was passed in 1992 [46]. This Act required drug companies to pay user fees for the review of their applications. This would enable the FDA to add resources and speed up approval process, without compromising review standards.

2.3.24 MedWatch—1993

Data collected in the clinical development program provide a snapshot of the safety of the compound [47]. Consequently, it is not possible to predict all effects of the compound during the clinical development program. As patients have access to the compound following FDA approval, additional safety data is created. Such data, if reported to the sponsor and to the FDA, represent a valuable resource to additionally assess the safety of the compound under more general conditions of use. For years both sponsor and FDA have had in place a spontaneous reporting system for AEs. The FDA launched MedWatch in 1993. MedWatch is a voluntary system that makes it easier for doctors and consumers to report AEs. If significant new risks are discovered, they are added to the labeling of the compound and the public is informed. In some cases, the use of the compound may be substantially limited, if not withdrawn from the market [17].

2.3.25 The Food and Drug Modernization Act—1997

The Food and Drug Modernization Act (FDAMA) was enacted in 1997 [48]. It provided accelerated approval and an extra 6 months of marketing exclusivity to drug sponsors who conducted clinical trials in children—to better define use of drugs in children. The Act also called for FDA to work with other countries to harmonize drug regulatory requirements—which reaffirmed the ICH effort started by FDA in 1995 [49].

2.3.26 PDUFA Renewed—1997, 2002, and 2007

PDUFA was renewed under the Food and Drug Administration Modernization Act for 5 more years in 1997, 2002, and 2007.

2.3.27 The Gender Guideline—1993

The FDA issued the gender guideline in 1993, which required both male and females be entered into clinical development trials. In doing so, FDA revoked the 1977 guideline that excluded women of childbearing potential from early clinical trials. The guideline also required drug sponsors to assess whether the effects of drugs are consistent among males and females [17]. There are two ways of doing this. One is to stratify by sex and design the trial to have sufficient power to assess the effectiveness of the drug in each subpopulation. The other is stratified by sex to ensure balance, design the trial to assess effectiveness across subpopulations, and then assess generalizability of drug response across subpopulations using interaction tests [50].

2.3.28 The Demographic Rule—1998

The FDA required all applications (NDA, ANDA, and SNDA) analyze data on safety and effectiveness by age, gender, and race. This is known as the Demographic Rule [51]. Again there are two ways of doing this. One is to stratify by subpopulation and design the trial to have sufficient power to assess the effectiveness of the drug in each subpopulation. The other is to stratify by subpopulation to ensure balance, design the trial to assess effectiveness across subpopulations, and then assess generalizability of drug response across subpopulations using interaction tests [50].

2.3.29 Best Pharmaceuticals for Children Act—2002

The Best Pharmaceuticals for Children legislation was enacted in 2002. The objective of this Act was to improve efficacy and safety of drugs when taken by children. The Act continued (originally stipulated by the FDAMA of 1997) to provide six additional months of marketing exclusivity for drugs on which clinical trials were conducted in children.

2.3.30 Pediatric Research Equity Act—2003

The 2003 Pediatric Research Equity Act [52] gave FDA authority to require drug development companies to conduct clinical trials for pediatric applications of new drugs.

2.3.31 Drug Safety Oversight Board—2005

In order to improve the assessment of drug safety, the FDA created the Drug Safety Oversight Board in 2005 [53]. The function of the board was to advise the CDER on matters relevant to the safety of drugs. Members of the Board include FDA staff and representatives from both the National Institutes of Health (NIH) and the Veterans Administration (VA).

2.3.32 Other Regulations and Guidances

Current FDA regulations are found in 21 CFR 50 (Informed Consent), 21 CFR 56 (IRB Standards, 21 CFR 312 (Investigational New Drugs), and 21 CFR 812 and 813 (Medical Devices) [54]. The FDA CDER Web site [55] and the link [56] provide helpful access to additional regulations and additional detail on those cited in this chapter.

2.4 Principles of Adequate and Controlled Investigations

In reading the Kefauver–Harris Amendments one notices the introduction of the term "substantial evidence." Basically, substantial evidence to support drug efficacy derives from adequate and well-controlled clinical trials. There is quite a lengthy discussion on adequate and well-controlled trials, from the standpoint of determining what is adequate as well as interpreting or identifying what are controls in clinical trials [57].

It is inspiring to read the opinions of world renown medical, pharmacological, and other scientific researchers, such as Dr. Lewis Thomas, Dr. Louis Lasagna, and Dr. Al Feinstein, regarding the need for evidence from adequate and well-controlled clinical investigations to support drug claims. Dr. Lewis Thomas said so eloquently [58] *"From here on, as far ahead as one can see, medicine must be building as a central part of its scientific base a solid underpinning of biostatistical and epidemiological knowledge. Hunches and intuitive impressions are essential for getting the work started, but it is only through the* **quality of numbers at the end that the truth can be told.**" Surely Dr. Thomas understood the concept of statistical power. We would add *"No analysis of data can salvage a poorly designed or poorly conducted investigation."*

There are 10 scientific principles for adequate and well-controlled investigations.

First, there has to be a protocol or study plan.

Second, the protocol must have a clear statement of objectives.

Third, the protocol must use a method for selecting participants that provides adequate confirmation of the presence of the disease state including criteria for diagnosis and appropriate confirmatory laboratory tests; i.e., there must be assurance that the patients who enter the trial have the disease that is being studied.

Fourth, the protocol has to include a method for assigning patients to interventions being studied without bias. The method for doing this is randomization. On an historical note, Sir Bradford Hill is considered to be the father of randomized clinical trials. It is generally accepted that the Society for Safety and Medicine in the United Kingdom, in which he worked as a statistician, conducted the first controlled randomized clinical trial [20]. The objective of the trial was to evaluate the use of streptomycin in patients with tuberculosis.

Fifth, the protocol should include an outline of the methods of quantification and of observation of the patients in the trial. For example, if one is developing an antihypertensive medication, a multitude of blood pressure measurements could be taken. There are at least three different positions for taking blood pressure: standing, sitting, or supine. There are two types of blood pressure: systolic and diastolic. This leads to six possible blood pressure measurements (systolic or diastolic by position). In addition there are several ways of measuring blood pressure; e.g., with a sphygmomanometer or with a digital reader.

In any particular protocol one must be specific in stating how the measurements are to be obtained. In the blood pressure example there could potentially be different nurses seeing the same patient periodically in time. There is variability in the way nurses read blood pressure particularly, if they are using the sphygmomanometer. So, in designing a clinical trial all sources of variation should be minimized, other than the natural variation in the data reflecting the condition being studied. This goes to the heart of what experimental design is about.

Sixth, the protocol must include a description of the steps taken to document comparability of data collected prior to assignment to study medications. Examples of such data are age, sex, race or ethnicity, weight or body surface area (potentially important in hypertension trials), duration of disease, use of drugs other than those being studied, values of efficacy variables or safety variables (clinical laboratory or vital signs) just prior to randomization, etc.

To illustrate, suppose we design a clinical trial to assess the efficacy of a drug at a specified dose as compared to placebo. As patients come to the clinic and qualify for the protocol, certain data (as delineated above, called baseline data) are recorded prior to randomly assigning them, usually in a balanced fashion (each patient has a 50-50 chance of receiving the drug or the placebo) to the drug group or the placebo group. To preserve (double) blinding, medication (doses of drug and placebo) to be taken by patients assigned to the drug group or to the placebo group is packaged so that they are identical in appearance.

Neither patient, nor investigator, nor investigational site personnel knows whether the medication taken by each patient is drug or placebo. It is important to think of how to document that the random assignment of patients to treatment groups is successful in balancing the groups in terms of factors that may influence response variables reflecting protocol objectives.

To address this, one statistically compares (usually at the 0.05 level) the drug group to the placebo group in terms of the data collected prior to randomization using univariate statistical methods appropriate for the data. Although there may be a problem in multiple inference, it is reasonable to conclude that the randomization was successful if on average, not more than 1 in 20 comparisons yield a *P*-value <0.05. If based on the baseline data collected, one concludes that the randomization was successful in balancing the treatment groups, one has some assurance that the randomization balanced the treatment groups in terms of variables that could influence response not collected or not possible to collect.

So, randomization is a wonderful tool. It not only provides assurance of baseline balance, but also provides the basis for statistical inferences about the effectiveness and safety of the drugs being studied. In analyzing more than 500 randomized clinical trials, we do not recall ever seeing a randomization that was not successful. We have seen randomizations that were misapplied; e.g., where patients that were supposed to get the drug actually got the placebo and vice versa, but not an unsuccessful randomization.

Seventh, the protocol must include a description of the methods for recording and analyzing patient response variables studied. This indicates that the protocol must contain an appropriate and adequate statistical analysis section (see Chapter 6), which states how the data will be computerized and quality assured and statistically analyzed so that valid statistical inferences can be obtained.

Eighth, the protocol must contain a description of methods of steps taken to minimize bias in the observations. Any factor that distorts the true outcome of a trial, leading to overestimating or underestimating the efficacy or safety of the drug being developed represents bias. Bias would be introduced if an investigator interpreted results in one group more or less favorably than results in the other group, even if they were similar. Bias would also be introduced if an investigator used his or her knowledge of a patient's severity of the disease being studied to assign that patient to a specific intervention group. Randomization and blinding are methods that can be taken to minimize these types of bias [19,59]. But other types of bias are possible.

For example, in a blood pressure trial, although different blood pressure observers may be used, each patient should have the same observer throughout the trial. The tool (sphygmomanometer or digital reader) for obtaining blood pressure should be standardized for all patients. Accuracy and precision of the tool should be documented so that any bias in the observations is minimized.

Ninth, the protocol should include a precise statement of the nature of the control group against which the effects of the new drug treatment can be compared. If the control is a placebo, then the ingredients in the placebo should be the same as those in the drugs except for the amount of the drug. If one chooses as the control a drug that is already marketed, the dose of the marketed drug used in the trial must be the therapeutic dose stated in its labeling.

Tenth, the protocol should include a survey of statistical methods to be used in the analysis of the data derived from the patients. In general, the purpose of clinical trials of a drug is to distinguish the effect of the drug from other influences such as spontaneous change in the disease, a placebo effect, and biased observations. Randomization helps balance out, blinding helps reduce bias, and spontaneous change in disease is addressed by having a control, particularly by having a placebo control. Further, inferences from adequate and well-controlled trials represent the primary basis for determining whether there is substantial evidence to support claims of effectiveness.

Every clinical trial that is conducted should have a clinical study report that contains the findings from that study. Clinical study reports are the basic building blocks in an NDA. Such a report must contain sufficient details of the study design, study conduct, statistical analysis, and conclusions to allow critical evaluation of adequate and well-controlled characteristics. In general, the clinical study report should describe what was to be done, what was done, and how any differences impact conclusions. Today, almost all NDAs are filed with the FDA electronically. FDA biometricians will require the pharmaceutical company to supply data in specified format, including SAS data sets, so that they can conduct their own analysis to assess whether adequate and well-controlled characteristics are met.

2.5 Content and Format of the IND

There are several sections of an IND application. There is an introductory statement that identifies the drug, drug class, route and formulation, as well as the objectives of the drug development program. A section that describes in detail the pharmacological activity of the drug is required. Any previous human experience of the drug must be described and included in the application document (generally, only unapproved drugs in-licensed from outside the United States will have any human experience). The general clinical development plan, as it is known at the time of application, is required.

The IB must be included. The IB [5] is an important document as it becomes the blueprint or source documentation as to what is known about the drug at this particular point in its development. It therefore serves as "labeling" during the investigational phase of clinical trials. Among the information included are summaries of pharmacology, pharmacokinetics, previous clinical studies (the IB is updated periodically as more information becomes known), and the possible risks or side effects of the drug.

Copies of the protocols for the trials identified in the clinical development plan are included in a section. A section that provides technical details (chemistry, animal pharmacology, and toxicology) of the drug is also included. Key sections and a brief overview of their content are summarized below:

1. Introductory statement—identify drug/drug class/route and formulation/objectives
2. Detailed description of pharmacological activity
3. Summary of previous human experience/regulatory history in other countries
4. General investigational plan
5. Investigator brochure
   a. Serves as "labeling" during the investigational phase of clinical studies
   b. Summarizes toxicology, pharmacology, and pharmacokinetics
   c. Summarizes previous clinical studies
   d. Describes possible risks/side effects and precautions/special monitoring
6. Clinical protocols
   a. Statement of objective
   b. Name/address of investigators
   c. Name/address of the institutional review board (IRB)
   d. Inclusion/exclusion criteria
   e. Estimated number of patients
   f. Study design
   g. Method used to determine dose(s) and duration of treatment used in study
   h. Observations/measurements
   i. Clinical procedures/lab tests
7. Technical information
   a. Chemistry
   b. Animal pharmacology/toxicology
   c. Previous human experience

In the clinical protocols (see Chapter 6 for discussion of protocol development) section, information about the IRB must be included. The IRB is the body that basically reviews a protocol and gives its okay to conduct clinical trials in humans, provided that in doing so does not represent an undue safety risk to humans who participate in protocols. Investigator initiated or single investigator clinical trials usually use a local IRB at their affiliated hospital or medical university. Pharmaceutical companies conducting multi-center clinical trials most often employ a commercial IRB; e.g., the Western IRB. Commercial IRBs are in the business of reviewing protocols from an IRB regulatory standpoint and pharmaceutical companies pay them for their review of protocols. The company is not buying a sanction; rather they are paying the IRB for their work. If in the review of the protocol something is noted that is unsafe to the patient, or is deficient medically or scientifically, no IRB would approve the protocol—ethical considerations aside, the liability consequences would be too severe.

When the IND application document is submitted to the FDA, it goes to the Medical Review Division. There is documentation that has to be filed on the investigators. This documentation is facilitated through form 1572 [60]. The FDA keeps a blacklist of investigators. Over time they have created a list of investigators that are precluded from conducting research in humans, due to bad past practices. Before a company selects an investigator to participate in a protocol in their clinical development plan, it is to their benefit to consult with the FDA on this blacklist to ensure that the investigator has not been excluded.

The IND goes into effect 30 days after FDA receives application unless notified by the FDA of "clinical hold" [3]. If the pharmaceutical sponsor has not heard back from the FDA after 30 days the pharmaceutical company may begin the first study in humans.

FDA's aim in reviewing an IND application is to provide assurance that the safety and rights of participants in clinical trials of the drug are protected and that the quality of the proposed scientific evaluation of the drug is adequate. The IND application is facilitated by form 1571 [61]. The content and format of the IND application should follow those specified by the FDA in 21 CRD 312.23 [62] to foster an efficient review process.

2.6 Content and Format of the NDA

The NDA is a huge document or dossier [8] that contains several sections or layers: an overall summary (that goes to all FDA reviewers), several technical sections, and a complete copy for archival purposes. The overall summary [8] should be written so that a reader may gain a good understanding of the data and information contained in the application. The level of detail is expected to be consistent with the requirements of refereed scientific and medical journals. If the NDA is approved, the overall summary document may be used to draft the SBA, which is accessible by the public via FOI.

2.6.1 Overall Summary

The **overall summary** must contain the following:

1. Proposed labeling for the drug (from which the package insert may evolve)
2. Identity of the pharmacologic class of the drug and the scientific rationale for its intended use and its potential clinical benefits
3. Description of any marketing history of the drug outside the United States
4. Summary of the chemistry, manufacturing, and controls section of the NDA
5. Summary of the nonclinical pharmacology and toxicology section of the NDA
6. Summary of the human pharmacokinetics and bioavailability section of the NDA
7. Summary of the microbiology section of the NDA (for anti-infective drugs)
8. Summary of the clinical data section of the NDA, including the results of statistical analyses of the clinical trials
9. Discussion that summarizes benefit and risk considerations related to the drug, including general plans for any proposed additional studies or surveillance the sponsor plans to conduct post-approval

2.6.2 Technical Sections

The NDA is required to contain **technical sections** that include data and information sufficient to enable the FDA to make a knowledgeable judgment as to whether the NDA should be approved. The following technical sections [8] are required.

1. Chemistry, manufacturing, and controls section—describes the composition, manufacture, and specification of the drug substance and the drug product, including
   (i) Drug substance: physical and chemical characteristics and stability; name and address of its manufacturer; method of synthesis

(or isolation) and purification of the drug substance; process controls used during manufacture and packaging; and specifications and analytical methods necessary to assure the identity, strength, quality, and purity of the drug substance and the bioavailability of the substance, including, e.g., specifications relating to stability, sterility, particle size, and crystalline form.

(ii) Drug product: list of components used in manufacturing; composition, specifications, and analytical methods for each component; name and address of each manufacturer of the drug product; description of the manufacturing and packaging procedures and in-process controls for the drug product; such specifications and analytical methods necessary to assure the identity, strength, quality, purity, and bioavailability of the drug product, including, e.g., specifications relating to sterility, dissolution rate, containers, and closure systems; and stability data with proposed expiration dating; batch production records, specifications, and test procedures, including the proposed master production record to be used for manufacturing commercial lots.

(iii) Environmental impact: either a claim for categorical exclusion or an environmental assessment.

2. Nonclinical pharmacology and toxicology section—describes, with the aid of graphs and tables, animals and *in vitro* studies of the drug, including

(i) Pharmacological activity studies: of the drug in relation to its proposed therapeutic indication; studies that otherwise define pharmacological properties of the drug or are pertinent to its possible adverse effects.

(ii) Toxicological effects studies: of the drug as they relate to the drug's intended clinical uses, including studies assessing the drug's acute, subacute, and chronic toxicity; carcinogenicity; and studies of toxicities related to the drug's particular mode of administration or conditions of use.

(iii) Reproductive toxicity studies: of the effects of the drug on reproduction and on the developing fetus.

(iv) Metabolism studies: of the absorption, distribution, metabolism, and excretion of the drug in animals.

(v) For each nonclinical laboratory study subject to the good laboratory practice regulations (GLPs) [63] a statement that it was conducted in compliance with the GLPs, or, if not, a brief statement of the reason for noncompliance.

3. Human pharmacokinetics and bioavailability section—describes the human pharmacokinetic data and human bioavailability data.

4. Microbiology section for an anti-infective drug—describes the microbiology data [64].

   (i) The biochemical basis of the drug's action on microbial physiology.

   (ii) The drug's antimicrobial spectra, including results of *in vitro* preclinical studies demonstrating concentrations of the drug required for effective use.

   (iii) Any known mechanisms of resistance to the drug, including results of any known epidemiologic studies demonstrating prevalence of resistance factors.

   (iv) Clinical microbiology laboratory methods needed to evaluate the effective use of the drug.

5. Clinical data section—describes the clinical trial investigations of the drug, including

   (i) Description and analysis of each clinical pharmacology study of the drug, including a brief comparison of the results of human studies with the animal pharmacology and toxicology data.

   (ii) Description and analysis of each controlled clinical study pertinent to a proposed use of the drug, including the protocol and a description of the statistical analyses.

   (iii) Description of each uncontrolled clinical study, a summary of the results, and a statement explaining why the study is classified as uncontrolled.

   (iv) Description and analysis of any other data or information relevant to an evaluation of the safety and effectiveness of the drug product obtained or otherwise received by the applicant from any source, . . . , including publications or other uses of the drug.

   (v) Integrated summary of efficacy (ISE): An integrated summary of the data demonstrating substantial evidence of effectiveness for the claimed indications. Evidence is also required to support the dosage and administration section of the labeling, including support for the dosage and dose interval recommended, and modifications for specific subgroups (e.g., pediatrics, geriatrics, patients with renal failure).

   (vi) Integrated summary of safety (ISS) and safety updates: An integrated summary of all available safety information about the drug product and updates of safety information.

   (vii) A description and analysis of studies or information related to abuse of the drug.

(viii) Integrated summary of benefits to risks (ISBR): An integrated summary of the benefits and risks of the drug, including a discussion of why the benefits exceed the risks under the conditions stated in the labeling.

(ix–xi) Other documentation regarding IRB and informed consent compliance, use of contract research organizations for study conduct, and auditing of studies.

6. Statistical section—describes the statistical evaluation of clinical data from controlled studies and statistical evaluation of all safety data.

The content and format of the NDA should follow FDA specifications in 21 CRF 314.50 [8] to foster an efficient review process. The NDA including content and format as well as legal requirements may be found at [65]. Guidance for the industry regarding filing electronic NDAs may be found at [66] and at [67].

2.6.3 Integrated Summaries

Preparing the ISE (Section 2.6.2.5.v, vi, viii), ISS, and ISBR represent major efforts on the part of the biostatistician, clinician, and medical writer. The IND/NDA rewrite served notice of the need for including these integrated summaries in the NDA, due primarily to FDA often noting inconsistencies between the clinical and statistical findings in their review of individual trials in the application.

2.6.3.1 Integrated Summary of Efficacy

Efficacy studies begin in Phase II for the purpose of determining whether the drug may be effective in patients, and to determine the dose and frequency of dosing that should be used in the pivotal, confirmatory, proof-of-efficacy trials in Phase III. One must integrate the efficacy findings from Phase II and Phase III trials in order to determine the wording to appear in the labeling regarding effectiveness. Integration has both clinical and statistical interpretations. Meta-analysis methods are helpful statistically in integrating the efficacy findings across trials for the population studied, as well as by the demographics: gender, race or ethnicity, and age.

In addition, one needs to identify the trials that fulfill the statutory requirements for adequate and well-controlled clinical trials. Usually, Phase II trials do not count as adequate. They may be controlled, but are usually inadequate, as they are not designed with sufficient power to provide proof of efficacy. The Phase III pivotal proof-of-efficacy trials carry the weight of substantial evidence of effectiveness and satisfy the statutory requirement for adequate and well-controlled clinical trials. FDA regulation states that there must be two trials (at least for the original NDA). One is generally not sufficient for approval. This goes to the heart of good science, the concept of reproducing a scientific result by confirming it with another study.

One needs to compare and integrate the results of the controlled trials. Clinical dose response or dose comparison trials of effectiveness conducted in Phase II may include placebo, low, middle, and high dose of the drug. In Phase III, the effectiveness of one of these doses (optimal in some sense) is compared to that of the placebo. But there may be other trials that also compare this dose to that of the placebo. So the integration aspect comes in resolving the various estimates of the effectiveness of that dose from several sources. As previously mentioned, meta-analysis can play a central role in the amalgamation or integration of results across several studies for inclusion in the ISE.

2.6.3.2 Integrated Summary of Safety

Safety information is collected in all clinical trials. In developing the ISS, one has to integrate the safety findings from all trials conducted prior to filing the NDA. This includes all trials whether controlled or not. Many Phase III pivotal proof-of-efficacy trials are extended past the double blind, proof-of-efficacy treatment period, to permit the collection of longer term safety data, usually in an uncontrolled manner. Safety data from these extension trials has to be included and integrated in the ISS.

The ISS should include the number of patients exposed to different doses of the drug for different lengths of time; a summary of all AEs and their rates of occurrence; and statistical analysis results of the rates (crude and cumulative time to AE) of occurrence. Koch and Edwards [68] may be seen for crude AE methods. Peace [69] and Peace [70] may be seen for cumulative time-to-event methods. AEs are summarized by body system; e.g., CNS, muscular–skeletal, cardiovascular, gastrointestinal, skin, etc.

Although review of submissions and attendant interaction with pharmaceutical companies require much of their time, FDA employees engage in active research. In the assessment of safety in terms of SAEs, the FDA in conjunction with the International Serious Adverse Events Consortium (SAEC) recently released initial data on the genetic basis of adverse drug events, particularly drug-induced serious skin rashes, such as Stevens–Johnson syndrome and toxic epidermal necrolysis [71].

Any patient who enters a clinical trial but did not complete is considered a dropout. Summary tables of all patients who dropped out prior to study completion, including the reasons for dropout should be presented.

All deaths have to be summarized. Clinical vignettes or descriptions, containing any information about the patient that might be important to a clinician in reviewing mortality information, should be included.

Assay results of clinical laboratory tests (chemistry, hematology, urinalysis, etc.) provide important information about the safety of the drug. These results must be summarized, integrated, and included in the ISS.

This potentially represents a huge effort, as clinical laboratory data are voluminous, with many tests and many times of blood sample collection throughout clinical trials on which assays are performed. There is not very much left to be done in the way of clever analysis, in the presentation of assay test results, and most companies have developed statistical analysis programs that churn out analysis results in rather boilerplate fashion. The book by Gilbert [72] is a good reference.

Meta-analysis methods are helpful statistically in integrating findings from analysis of safety data across trials for the population studied, as well as by demographic characteristics: gender, race or ethnicity, and age. In passing, even though many clinical trials that employ a completely randomized block design (with centers as blocks) are multicenter in nature, analyses of safety data collected from such trials rarely if ever use methods that account for blocking the blocking variables.

The ISS should also include a presentation of the findings from the pre-clinical animal studies of the drug.

2.6.3.3 Integrated Summary of Benefit to Risk

Developing the ISBR of a new drug is challenging. It requires the best thinking of clinicians and statisticians to develop the best and most accurate description of the integrated summary of benefit to risks of drug. Further, this requires clinicians and biostatisticians who thoroughly know the data and the efficacy and safety findings as well as their limitations.

This is still an area that is open for development of novel statistical methodology. One can think of benefit to risk as a ratio of efficacy to risk (the extent to which the drug is unsafe) in some sense. So the question is "How can one take the efficacy measures, the safety measures, particularly AEs and clinical laboratory results, and combine them in some meaningful way to get a numerator and denominator and then study the distribution of the ratios?" Of course this formulation argues for univariate estimates (which could be the quotient of a functional combination of efficacy variables to a functional combination of risk variables) of efficacy and risk.

The lay public, professionals, and legislators often question whether the FDA is doing their job of protecting the nation's health from unsafe drugs getting to the market. This largely is the role of the FDA. They are charged with protecting the public's health in the sense of keeping inefficacious and unsafe drugs, biologics, or medical devices from being marketed. If the efficacy of a pharmaceutical product has been proven, granting marketing approval of the product results largely from the deliberation of its benefits to risk. No product is free of risk. Benefits to risks judgments are important. FDA will allow greater risks for a product if its potential benefit is great—particularly products that are used to treat serious, life-threatening illnesses [73].

2.7 Organizational Structure of the FDA

2.7.1 Overview of FDA Responsibilities

Among the responsibilities of the FDA is the regulation of medical products that must be proven safe and effective before they are allowed to be marketed for use in humans. These products include medicines or drugs used for the treatment and prevention of disease; biologics, including vaccines, blood products, biotechnology products and gene therapy; and medical devices. Although FDA regulates all medical devices for human use, only the most complex medical devices are reviewed by the FDA prior to marketing.

FDA also regulates drugs and devices used for animals, including pets and animals raised for food consumption. Manufacturers of drugs for use in animals (including those used in feeds) must file a regulatory dossier that demonstrates to the FDA that they are safe and effective prior to marketing. Drugs used in animals raised for food consumption are evaluated by the FDA for their safety to the environment and to people who may eat animal products. FDA ensures that drug residues that may remain in these foods are not harmful to those who eat them.

FDA does not have to approve veterinary medical devices prior to marketing. However, they must still be safe, effective, and properly labeled.

FDA's responsibilities have evolved to respond to the challenges of regulating complex and sophisticated industries through a blending of law and science aimed at protecting consumers. To meet their responsibilities, FDA employs about 9000 people who work in various locations around the country. Most of FDA's budget is used to pay its highly skilled and internationally respected work force. FDA employees come from the medical, scientific and public health professions—including biologists, biomedical engineers, chemists, pharmacologists, physicians, toxicologists, veterinarians, and public health education and communication specialists. Products regulated by the FDA reflect about one-quarter of every consumer dollar spent. Dividing FDA's budget by the number of people they protect yields a cost estimate of about one penny per day per person [74].

2.7.2 Centers and Offices of the FDA

The FDA is an agency within the Department of Health and Human Services. Organizationally [75], The FDA consists of six centers and three offices located throughout the country:

Center for Biologics Evaluation and Research (CBER)
Center for Drug Evaluation and Research (CDER)
Center for Devices and Radiological Health (CDRH)

Center for Food Safety and Applied Nutrition (CFSAN)

Center for Veterinary Medicine (CVM)

National Center for Toxicological Research (NCTR)

Office of Chief Counsel

Office of the Commissioner (OC)

Office of Regulatory Affairs (ORA)

Although all the centers require biostatisticians in order to meet their responsibilities, the CBER, CDER, CDRH, CVM, and NCTR are the centers that impact the roles of pharmaceutical industry biostatisticians, in a major way. Three of these CBER, CDER, and CDRH have greater impact on clinical trial biostatisticians than those supporting basic research programs. These offices focus primarily on product review and regulatory policy and are located in the greater Washington, District of Columbia area, particularly in Rockville, Maryland. The organizational structure of these three centers follows. The offices or divisions that have biostatistical responsibility also reflect their organizational structure.

2.7.3 Center for Biologics Evaluation and Research

Office of the Center Director

Office of Management

Office of Compliance and Biologics Quality

Office of Blood Research and Review

Office of Vaccines Research and Review

Office of Communication, Outreach and Development

Office of Biostatistics and Epidemiology (Director)

Deputy Director

Associate Director for Risk Assessment

Associate Director for Research

Director, Division of Biostatistics

Associate Director of Regulatory Policy

Chief, Vaccines Products Branch

Chief, Therapeutics Evaluation Branch

Director, Division of Epidemiology

Office for Information Technology

Office of Cellular, Tissue and Gene Therapies

Additional detail regarding the organization of the Division of Biostatistics in CBER may be found at www.fda.gov/CBER/inside/orglist.htm [76].

2.7.4 Center for Devices and Radiological Health

Office of Management Operations
Office of Device Evaluation
Office of Compliance
Office of Science and Engineering Laboratories
Office of Communication, Education, and Radiation Programs
Office of Surveillance and Biometrics (Director)
  Deputy Director
  Issues Management Staff
  Patient Staff
  Program Management Officer
  Director, Division of Biostatistics
  Deputy Director
  Chief, Cardiovascular and Ophthalmic Devices Branch
  Chief, Diagnostic Devices Branch
  Chief, General Surgical Devices Branch
  Director, Division of Post-Marketing Surveillance
  Director, Division of Surveillance Systems
Office of In Vitro Diagnostic Device Evaluation and Safety

Additional detail regarding the organization of the Division of Biostatistics in CDRH may be found at http://www.fda.gov/cdrh/organiz. html [77].

2.7.5 Center for Drug Evaluation and Research

Office of the Center Director
Office of Regulatory Policy
Office of Management
Office of Training and Communication
Office of Compliance
Office of Information Technology
Office of Medical Policy

Office of Translational Science

Office of Biostatistics (Director)

Director, Division of Biometrics I (supports cardiovascular, renal, neurology, and psychiatric products)

Director, Division of Biometrics II (supports anesthesia, analgesia, rheumatology, metabolic, endocrinology, pulmonary, and allergy products)

Director, Division of Biometrics III (supports gastroenterology, dermatology, dental, reproductive, and urological products)

Director, Division of Biometrics IV (supports anti-infective, ophthalmologic, antiviral, and special pathogens and transplant products)

Director, Division of Biometrics V (supports drug oncology, medical imaging, and hematological and biologic oncology products)

Director, Division of Biometrics VI (supports generic drugs, special safety review activities, and the offices of clinical pharmacology and pharmaceutical sciences)

Office of Clinical Pharmacology (Director)

Office of Executive Programs

Office of Counter-Terrorism and Emergency Coordination

Office of Business Process Support

Office of Surveillance and Epidemiology

Office of New Drugs

Office of Drug Evaluation I

Office of Drug Evaluation II

Office of Drug Evaluation III

Office of Antimicrobial Products

Office of Nonprescription Products

Office of Oncology Drug Products

Office of Pharmaceutical Science

Office of Generic Drugs

Office of New Drug Quality Assessment

Office of Testing and Research

Office of Biotechnology Products

Additional detail regarding the organization of the Office of Biostatistics in CDER may be found at www.fda.gov/cder/Offices/Biostatistics/default. htm [78].

2.8 The FDA Review Process

After receiving an NDA, CDER conducts a technical screening or a completeness review. This review ensures that the NDA contains sufficient data and information to justify "filing" the application. CDER does not want to waste time and resources in reviewing NDAs that are deficient in content and format. NDAs that are incomplete warrant a formal "refuse-to-file" action. The applicant then is sent a letter detailing the decision and deficiencies that form the basis of the action. The letter must be sent within 60 calendar days after the NDA is initially received by CDER [64].

NDAs that are accepted for filing are assigned a team of reviewers. The team consists at a minimum of a lead medical, biopharmaceutical, pharmacology, statistical, chemistry, and microbiology (if an antibiotic) reviewer. The medical reviewer, called the medical officer, is responsible for evaluating the clinical sections and for synthesizing the results of the animal toxicology, human pharmacology, and clinical reviews to formulate the overall basis for a recommended Agency action on the application [64].

The biopharmaceutical review is conducted by the pharmacokineticist, who evaluates the bioavailability of the active ingredient (drug) of the formulation. That is, the pharmacokineticist evaluates the rate and extent to which the active ingredient of the drug is made available to the body (absorption) and the way it is distributed in (distribution), metabolized by (metabolism), and eliminated from the human body (elimination) [64].

The pharmacology and toxicology review is conducted by a team of pharmacologists and toxicologists. They evaluate the results from animal testing and attempt to relate the effects of the drug in animals to its potential effects in humans [64].

The lead statistician (biostatistician or biometrician, depending on the reviewing center) is responsible for evaluating the statistical relevance of the data in the NDA and the methods used to conduct studies as well as the statistical methods used to analyze the data. The statistical review provides the medical officer a better idea of the validity and power of the findings of safety, efficacy, and benefit to risk that will be extrapolated to patients who will use the drug [64]. The office of biostatistics has developed template guidelines regarding the format, organization, and structure of the statistical review of the NDA [79]. The link [80] provides an excellent presentation from a statistical reviewer's perspective of the statistical review of an oncology NDA, including specifications regarding the content and structure of data sets required.

Chemists are responsible for reviewing the chemistry and manufacturing control sections of NDAs. Chemistry reviewers address issues related to drug identity, manufacturing control, and chemical analysis. The reviewing chemist evaluates manufacturing and processing procedures to ensure that the drug is reproducible and stable. If the drug is not stable or not reproducible, the validity of the results from clinical trials would be undermined [64].

Microbiologists evaluate the clinical microbiology section of NDAs for anti-infective or antibiotic drugs. These drugs are used short term to eradicate organisms or microbes that cause infections, and are not expected to affect human physiology. Clinical signs and symptoms of the infection are expected to abate following eradication of the infecting pathogen. The reviewing microbiologist evaluates the drug's *in vivo* and *in vitro* effects on the target microorganisms to establishing effectiveness of the drug.

Prior to NDA approval, CDER uses advisory committees to obtain outside advice and opinions from expert advisors as to the safety, efficacy, and benefit to risk of drugs. Use of advisory committees provides the CDER wider expert input prior to the final decision as to approvability. The CDER may convene an advisory committee meeting for advice on issues other than safety, efficacy, and benefit to risk of a new drug. For example, they may want a committee's opinion about a major indication for an already approved drug, or a special regulatory requirement being considered, such as a boxed warning in a drug's labeling. Advisory committees may also advise CDER on the content of the package insert, or assistance with guidelines for developing particular kinds of drugs, or whether a proposed study for an experimental drug should be conducted. Recommendations by advisory committees are not binding on the CDER, but are considered carefully when deciding drug issues [64].

Additional information regarding FDA NDA review is contained in "Outline for performing NDA review" [81], "Steps and issues in the NDA review process" [82], and "Outline for performing medical review of NDA links to resources" [83]. Figure 2.2 [64] provides a great overview of the NDA review process and contains embedded links for accessing more detailed information.

Prior to 1996, any manufacturer of biologics had to submit both a PLA and an ELA to the CBER for review before engaging in interstate commerce. In 1996, the PLA and the ELA were replaced by a BLA. The BLA is a request to market a new biologic product. Although a BLA simplifies the earlier requirement, it is a large document that requires at least 6 months for FDA CBER review [84]. For additional information regarding BLAs, the links in the references section [85–88] may be accessed.

All centers within the FDA encourage manufacturers to initiate interactions early in the clinical development process (e.g., near the time of filing the IND, end of Phase II, and pre-NDA meetings). A well-managed review process for a BLA begins with interactions between the applicant and the CBER [89].

The link [90] may be used to access information regarding the PMA review process for medical devices.

Although review of submissions (INDs, NDAs, BLAs, PLAs, protocols, emerging risk profiles) and attendant interaction with pharmaceutical companies regarding submissions requires much of their time, FDA employees engage in active research. FDA biostatisticians have contributed heavily to the statistical methodology literature, often take the lead on issues in the larger professional arena, and have contributed in a major way to advancing biostatistics as a scientific discipline.

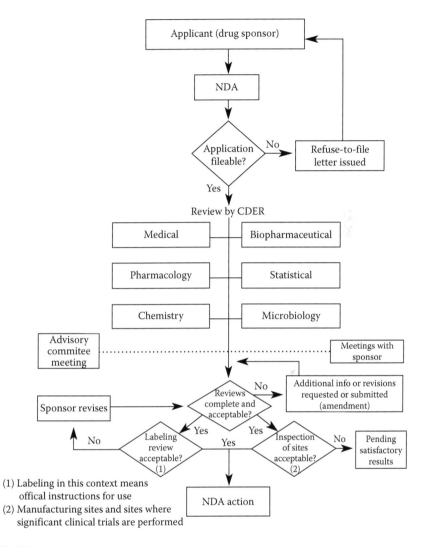

FIGURE 2.2
The NDA review process.

2.9 Labeling and the Package Insert

If an NDA is approved, both the labeling and the package insert must be developed and approved by the FDA prior to marketing. Both attempt to capture and convey what is known about the drug from the NDA (both may be updated as additional information becomes available from SNDA programs for additional indications and from spontaneous adverse event reported after marketing). The FDA-approved label is the official description of the drug product. It includes what the drug is used for; who should take it; AEs or side effects; instructions for use in pregnant women, children, and other populations; and safety information [91]. The labeling is intended primarily for physician use [92].

The package insert is primarily for patient use [93]. It must be distributed when the drug is dispensed. It is written in nontechnical language that is easy to comprehend and is non-promotional. It is scientifically accurate and consistent with the physician labeling. The patient package insert contains information for patients on how to safely use the drug product, and is part of the FDA-approved labeling [91].

If the drug should not be used in certain patients, then the labeling will contain a Boxed Warning. For example, when Cytotec was approved for the prevention of NSAID-induced gastric ulceration in the late 1980s, the labeling contained a black box warning of its potential for inducing abortions (it was in fact used in Europe as an abortifacient agent at the time of its U.S. approval). In addition information about the following must be included:

1. Indications and usage
2. Dosage and administration
3. Dosage forms and strengths
4. Contraindications
5. Warnings and precautions
6. Adverse reactions
7. Drug interactions
8. Use in specific populations
9. Drug abuse and dependence
10. Overdosage
11. Description
12. Clinical pharmacology
13. Nonclinical toxicology
14. Clinical studies
15. References
16. How supplied/storage and handling
17. Patient counseling information

Consumers rely on the product label and the package insert for information on how the drug product should be used. FDA regulates the content (and format) of the labels for biologics, drugs, and medical devices, to ensure that they are accurate and that they provide information that aids consumers to make safe decisions when using the product.

The next time you have a prescription filled at a pharmacy, pull out the package insert and review it. It is very instructive. The product label may be found in Physician Desk References (PDRs), a commercially published compilation of manufacturers' prescribing information, owned by Thompson Corporation of Toronto. They are updated each year. Several years ago, before advances in technology, every physician's office would have a hard copy of the PDR. PDRs are now available electronically, making it easier for the physician to review the labeling and package insert prior to writing a prescription. The package insert is informative to consumers. When a pharmaceutical company begins formulating the clinical development plan for a drug, they should articulate what they want the labeling or package insert to say. This guides the types of studies to be included in the clinical development plan.

The FDA regulates promotional activities. Pharmaceutical companies cannot direct-to-patient advertise, although some advertisements seen on television makes one wonder whether they are in compliance with federal regulation. The advertisements of pharmaceutical products in whatever media cannot overstate claims of efficacy or understate claims of safety; they must be compliant with the product labeling and package insert.

Additional information regarding the product label and the package insert for drugs and biologics may be found at the FDA regulatory Web site [94–96]. The last reference contains information on both content and format (structured product labeling). Information regarding labeling of medical device products may be found at the FDA labeling Web site [97].

2.10 Pharmaceutical Company Organization and Role of the Biostatistician

2.10.1 Pharmaceutical Company Organization Overview

Although most pharmaceutical companies are functionally integrated, they have hierarchical organizational structures. From top down, there is the research and development (R&D) side and the corporate side. Major divisions within R&D are basic research and clinical development. Major divisions within the corporate sector are: sales, marketing, manufacturing, regulatory affairs, medical affairs, and legal affairs.

Areas within the basic research division are (1) pharmaceutical screening and discovery—having responsibility for the discovery, optimization, and development of lead compounds; (2) biological research, which may consist of departments (or labs) of pharmacology, immunology, flow cytometry, genetics/molecular biology, and drug metabolism; (3) chemical research, which may have several "chemistry" departments (e.g., biochemistry, chemical kinetics, etc.), a lab exploring quantitative structure activity relationships (QSAR) of compounds, a department responsible for pharmaceutical formulation optimization, and a scale-up plant—with environmental assessment responsibilities; and (4) preclinical drug safety, which may have several departments or labs with responsibility of characterizing the safety profile of compounds in animals: single dose or acute studies, multiple dose of limited duration studies, range finding studies, subacute or sub-chronic studies, repeat dose studies of 30–90 days, chronic toxicity or carcinogenicity studies, and reproductive toxicology studies.

Areas within the clinical development division are (1) clinical pharmacology (Phase I clinical trials, metabolism, kinetics); (2) clinical operations; and (3) medical departments organized along disease or therapeutic drug development areas: cardiovascular, CNS, anti-inflammatory, antibiotic or anti-infective, antiviral, analgesic, oncology, Alzheimer's, and other disease areas as warranted by the focus of company. Clinical operations may consist of (1) protocol development and monitoring; (2) clinical data management; (3) biostatistics; (4) medical writing; and (5) safety assessment.

The sales, marketing, regulatory affairs, and medical affairs divisions in the corporate side are usually organized along disease or therapeutic lines, depending on the size of the company. Medical affairs area may also have clinical trial operations (protocol development, monitoring, data management, biostatistics, and medical writing), medical communications, and post-marketing or risk management groups. As previously indicated, the primary aim of medical affairs is to extend the product line after the first NDA approval and to manage approved drugs for all indications in terms of risk.

2.10.2 Role of the Biostatistician

Biostatistical thinking and methods have application in virtually every division of a pharmaceutical company. Any area where an experiment or clinical trial needs to be conducted to answer a biological, medical, or other scientific question will benefit by having the input of a biostatistician. Thus pharmaceutical screening and discovery, biological research, chemical research, preclinical drug safety, clinical development, medical affairs, and manufacturing and quality control are areas where the biostatistician should and does contribute.

What can the biostatistician contribute? Many years ago, the role of a biostatistician was seen to be only that of a statistical analyst [1]. He or she most often was not consulted on the design of an experiment, rather the experimenter would conduct the experiment, gather the data, bring the data to the biostatistician, and expect the biostatistician to produce analysis results that were interpretable. Clyde Kramer (lecture at Virginia Polytechnic Institute and State University, 1974) coined the acronym PARC (plan after research completed) for this type of experiment. He went on to say that commuting the letters of the acronym often implied the worth of the experiment.

The role of the biostatistician has progressed over the years. Now biostatisticians are members of discovery, research, and clinical development teams, and are expected to contribute to all logistical aspects of experiments or clinical trials determined to be needed by such teams. Logistical aspects include specifying the research question; choosing the most appropriate experimental design, study planning, study execution—including monitoring, database creation and management, statistical analyses, statistical interpretation, and report generation. In our own experience, greater contributions have been at the front end rather than at the back end. In supporting research and clinical development of pharmaceuticals, the first author has performed analyses of many, many basic research experiments and clinical trials. In many cases, the first author developed innovative analysis methods. While valid data analyses are both necessary and important, it is our belief—based on experience *and* observation—that advances in science, advances in medicines, and advances in the treatment of patients result from well-planned and quality-conducted investigations more so than from any esoteric analysis of data.

Not only are biostatisticians integral members of basic research and clinical development teams, biostatisticians have taken the lead in incorporating principles of decision theory to better guide the entire research and clinical development process at some companies. Others, including myself, have had the responsibility for the clinical development program that led to FDA approval of new drugs as well as approval of new indications for drugs already marketed. Yet others, after functioning as a biostatistician supporting clinical development programs and managing the biostatistics department, have become directors or vice presidents of regulatory affairs and vice presidents of clinical/technical operations. Throughout the broad areas of pharmaceutical research, clinical development, and manufacturing, biostatistical thinking contributes to the attendant processes having better quality and efficiency.

2.11 Concluding Remarks

The path of pharmaceutical clinical development is littered with failed clinical trials—outcomes that are only realized after expending hundreds of millions in investment dollars. It is a rare event when the process confirms that a compound shown to have promise in basic research and preclinical programs is safe and effective in humans. Although there are some exceptions, various estimates of the time required to take a new drug from initial laboratory studies through the clinical development program and FDA approval range from 8 to 15 years. With an average cost per drug of $897 million, including the investment in post-approval studies, companies must focus their efforts on the most promising while identifying probable failures earlier in the process. The sobering reality is that just five out of 5000 compounds introduced to preclinical study continue to human testing, and of the five only one makes it through the long and costly clinical development, NDA submission, and FDA review and approval process.

If the opportunities for failure are not daunting enough, there is the intimidating awareness that a successful drug candidate's revenue producing life cycle of exclusivity will be short lived. The federal Hatch–Waxman Act virtually assures that every new drug brought to market finds a generic competitor waiting to enter the market at the end of its protected patent period.

Although risks plague the route from the time of a drug's discovery until it reaches the consumer, and certain competition awaits the company that successfully navigates the course, research and development is the essence of the pharmaceutical industry. Whether a company is a startup trying to bring a single compound to market or an industry giant, the company must keep a stream of new products in its pipeline. Companies that produce drug candidates that survive the approval process define economic survival in the industry.

There are numerous chances for failure and only a slim likelihood of success in this process. Potential medical benefits for mankind and the monetary rewards for sponsors are driving forces within the industry. The promise of finding new cures and treatment options that improve lives and alleviate suffering is a benevolent yet noble appeal of pharmaceutical research and development. And bringing to market a new drug that achieves blockbuster status and reaps large profits is the ultimate lure that occasionally justifies the financial investment. It is only through the often elusive promise of profit that companies keep coming back to the front lines of research taking risks to create new treatments for disease. Without the promise of financial gain it is unlikely that many of the great advances in the diagnosis and treatment of diseases would have become a reality.

In the pharmaceutical industry, the clinical development division is organized across drug class or therapeutic lines (see Section 2.10). The head (director, senior director, or in some cases vice president) of each development department—such as cardiovascular, antibiotic, or CNS compounds—has staff responsible for one or more compounds. They function as project directors for the drugs in clinical development. The department head may elect to be the project director for some compounds, instead of assigning that responsibility to staff.

A clinical development plan (see Chapter 4) is formulated for each drug candidate. It identifies what Phase I, Phase II, and Phase III protocols or studies need to be developed and conducted in order to gather sufficient evidence to warrant NDA compilation and submission. This plan is the responsibility of the clinical development team. At a minimum, the team includes the project director, a physician if the project director is not a physician, a biostatistician, and representatives from the clinical monitoring, medical writing, clinical data management, regulatory affairs, and project planning departments.

One of the responsibilities of the biostatistician is to make the decision on the number of patients needed for studies. For Phase III, definitive proof-of-efficacy protocols, the first author routinely required enough patients to have a 95% power (the probability of concluding that a drug is efficacious when in fact it is) at a time when the industry norm was 80% power. The reason for doing this was to have a greater opportunity of claiming effectiveness even if the observed margin of efficacy was less than what was thought at the time of designing the protocols. This meant, of course, that a larger number of patients would have to be enrolled, which meant higher costs for conducting the trials. The additional expense is justified, certainly for drugs of blockbuster potential; failure to detect a truly efficacious drug for use in a debilitating disease due to inadequate numbers of patients would be tragic, if not irresponsible or unethical.

Often the relationship between the FDA and pharmaceutical industry personnel is considered adversarial, due in part to the extremely high stakes that are involved. But a component is due to their roles and responsibilities being at opposite ends of the spectrum reflecting the strength of evidence to support claims contained in the regulatory dossier (NDA, SNDA, BLA, and PMA). The pharmaceutical company making the submission to the FDA obviously believes that the strength of evidence is sufficient for approval—else the submission would not be made, and is therefore a proponent of the drug. Becoming a proponent is achieved only after company personnel and expert consultants thoroughly review and analyze the safety and efficacy information collected in the clinical development program and concludes that the compound is efficacious and its potential benefits substantially outweigh its potential risks. The FDA is charged with protecting the public's health in the sense of not allowing inefficacious or unsafe drugs to be marketed and therefore has to take an opposing view—operating during the review process as an opponent of approvability. Only if the submission passes the most comprehensive and stringent review does the FDA feel justified in approving the submission.

Regardless of the due diligence exhibited by the pharmaceutical company in conducting the clinical development program, gathering, reviewing, and analyzing the data generated on the safety and efficacy of a compound, and by the FDA in its review of the submission, recent history makes it clear that neither the FDA nor the U.S. pharmaceutical industry is entirely successful in attaining its goals. This is not unexpected, regardless of how well the pharmaceutical industry and the FDA meet their legal and ethical responsibilities.

First, no drug is approved on the basis of "zero" risk. Drugs are approved on the basis of the benefit in the patient population studied, substantially outweighing the risk in that population. It is impossible to prove definitively that a drug has no risk. The history of FDA regulation recognizes this. Whereas the 1962 Kefauver–Harris Amendment to the Pure Food, Drug and Cosmetics Act requires that efficacy claims be proven, there is no statutory requirement for proof of safety. Second, there are nonzero decision risks associated with claims of efficacy and safety and with the approval process. The FDA following its efficacy review will decide that the drug is efficacious or not.

If the FDA concludes that the drug is not efficacious, then it will not be marketed. This is the correct decision if the drug is truly not efficacious. It is the incorrect decision if the drug is truly efficacious, and not being able to market the drug means a huge loss of research and development dollars to the pharmaceutical company. If the FDA concludes that the drug is efficacious, then it may be marketed if the FDA also concludes that the benefits of the drug outweigh its risks. This is the correct decision, if the drug is in fact efficacious and its benefits outweigh its risks. It is the incorrect decision if the drug is truly not efficacious or if its benefits do not outweigh its risks.

Both the pharmaceutical industry and the FDA control the magnitude of this type of decision error, by requiring that it be no more than 5%, and in almost all cases that it be much less than 5%. It is a fact that the smaller the regulatory or consumer's risk, the larger the population studied prior to approval has to be. To require that it be closer to zero than it already is would lead to a situation where no company could afford the investment dollars or time to bring new drugs to the market.

The clinical development of drugs is a serious business. To achieve success all persons with some responsibility in the design, conduct, monitoring, database creation, biostatistical analyses, report development, and regulatory dossier development must practice and mandate that others practice the highest quality and ethics in all that they do. To do otherwise is not only unprofessional, it is unethical. Quality productivity throughout the research and development process must become the way of doing business.

One should think NDA from the beginning of a clinical drug development project, particularly the content of the labeling or package insert. Pharmaceutical companies should interact with the FDA wisely; too much or too little can cause problems. There are mandated times that pharmaceutical companies should convene meetings with the FDA. There should always be an end of Phase II meeting so at that time the pharmaceutical company can review their Phase III program, particularly the pivotal proof-of-efficacy trials.

Biostatisticians should not only work closely with the clinical project physician, the database management personnel, the medical writers, but also with the clinical monitors to ensure that the protocol is being followed and data are being collected as they should be. Biostatisticians should also interact with in-house regulatory affairs personnel assigned to the clinical development project team, as their job is to know the federal regulations, and provide the link for FDA interaction. There is a need for proactivity to ensure that a quality assured database is available for biostatistical analyses and that analyses are performed soon after all the data have been collected. Proactivity, ethical and quality conduct in meeting responsibilities is required in order for a drug development program to be successful.

References

1. Segreti AC, Leung HM, Koch GG, Davis RL, Mohberg NR, Peace KE (2001): Biopharmaceutical statistics in a pharmaceutical regulated environment: Past, present and future. *Journal of Biopharmaceutical Statistics*; **11**(4): 347–372.
2. U.S. Food and Drug Administration: Section 505(a) of FD&C Act. Federal Food, Drug, and Cosmetic Act: Chapter V—Drugs and devices. Retrieved from http://www.fda.gov/opacom/laws/fdcact/fdcact5a.htm
3. U.S. Food and Drug Administration: Clinical holds and requests for modification: 21 CFR 312.42. Food and drug. Chapter 1: Subchapter D: Drugs for human use. Part 312—Investigational new drug application. Code of Federal Regulations, Title 21. Retrieved from https://www.accessdata.fda.gov/scripts/cdrh/cfdocs/cfCFR/CFRSearch.cfm?fr = 312.42
4. U.S. Food and Drug Administration: Clinical. Part 312—Investigation new drug application: 21 CFR 312. Food and drug. Chapter 1: Subchapter D: Drugs for human use. Code of Federal Regulations, Title 21. Retrieved from https://www.accessdata.fda.gov/scripts/cdrh/cfdocs/cfCFR/CFRSearch.cfm? CFRPart = 312
5. U.S. Food and Drug Administration: Guidance for industry: E6 good. Clinical practice: Consolidated guidance. Retrieved from www.fda.gov/cder/guidance/959fnl.pdf
6. U.S. Food and Drug Administration: The new drug development process: Steps from test tube to new drug application review. In *The CDER Handbook*, Silver Springs, MD. Retrieved from http://www.fda.gov/cder/handbook/
7. Frick H, Elo O, Haapa K, Heinonen OP, Heinsalmi P, Helo P, Huttunen JK, Kaitaniemi P, Koskinen P, Manninen V, Maenpaa H, Malkonen M, Manttari M, Norola S, Pasternack A, Pikkarainen J, Romo M, Sjöblom T, Nikkilä EA (November 12, 1987): Helsinki Heart Study: Primary-prevention trial with gemfibrozil in middle-aged men with dyslipidemia. Safety of treatment, changes in risk factors, and incidence of coronary heart disease. *New England Journal of Medicine*; **317**(20): 1237–1245.
8. U.S. Food and Drug Administration: Content and format of an application: 21 CFR 314.50. Food and drugs. Chapter 1: Subchapter D: Drugs for human use. Part 314—Applications for FDA approval to market a new drug. Code of Federal Regulations, Title 21. Retrieved from http://www.accessdata.fda.gov/scripts/cdrh/cfdocs/cfcfr/CFRSearch.cfm?CFRPart = 314

9. U.S. Food and Drug Administration: Availability for public disclosure of data and information in an application or abbreviated application: 21 CFR 314.430(e) (2)(ii). Food and drugs. Chapter 1: Subchapter D: Drugs for human use. Part 314—Applications for FDA approval to market a new drug. Code of Federal Regulations, Title 21. Retrieved from http://www.accessdata.fda.gov/scripts/cdrh/cfdocs/cfcfr/CFRSearch.cfm?fr = 314.430

10. U.S. Food and Drug Administration: New policies and procedures regarding transparency and public disclosure for FDA Advisory Committees. Retrieved from www.fda.gov/oc/advisory/newacguidance0808.html

11. Griffith E. Risk management for the pharmaceutical industry. Retrieved from www.fujitsu.com/downloads/SVC/fc/article/pharma-risk-mgmt.pdf

12. U.S. Food and Drug Administration (2003): Slide 5 of FDA risk management workshop day 2. Retrieved from www.fda.gov/CDER/meeting/RM/ nelsonday2/sld005.htm

13. U.S. Food and Drug Administration: Supplement type (supplemental new drug application). Retrieved from http://www.fda.gov/Cder/drugsatfda/glossary.htm#S

14. U.S. Food and Drug Administration (1981): The long struggle for the 1906 law. FDA consumer. Retrieved from www.cfsan.fda.gov/~lrd/history2.html

15. U.S. Food and Drug Administration: The Sherley Amendment. Center for Drug Evaluation and Research. Retrieved from www.fda.gov/Cder/about/history/Page7.htm

16. The National Archives: Records of the Food and Drug Administration. Retrieved from http://www.archives.gov/research/guide-fed-records/groups/088.html

17. Meadows M (2006): Promoting safe and effective drugs for 100 years; *FDA Consumer Magazine*. The Centennial Edition: January–February. Retrieved from http://www.fda.gov/fdac/features/2006/106_cder.html

18. U.S. Food and Drug Administration: This week in FDA history. Retrieved from www.fda.gov/centennial/this_week/43_oct_22_oct_28.html

19. Bren L (2007): The advancement of controlled clinical trials. *FDA Consumer Magazine*; 41(2). U.S. Food and Drug Administration, Washington, DC, March–April, 2007. Retrieved from http://www.fda.gov/fdac/features/2007/207_trials.html

20. Peace KE, Parillo AV, Hardy CJ (2008): Assessing the validity of statistical inferences in public health. *Journal of the Georgia Public Health Association*; **1**(1): 10–23.

21. U.S. Food and Drug Administration (2008): Chapter 2: Subchapter 3: Other laws. Regulatory procedures manual 2008. Retrieved from www.fda.gov/ora/compliance_ref/rpm/chapter2/ch2-3.html

22. Arachnoiditis Web Page. FDA's Drug Efficacy Study Implementation (DESI) and Pantopaque. Retrieved from www.arachnoiditis.co.uk/parisian-8.htm

23. Hecht A (1984): A long reach back to assure drug quality—Drug Efficacy Study Implementation program. *FDA Consumer*; Vol. 18, December 1984.

24. U.S. Food and Drug Administration: Center for Drug Evaluation and Research. Retrieved from http://www.fda.gov/cder/about/history/Page37.htm

25. U.S. Food and Drug Administration (2005): Milestones in U.S. food and drug law history. *FDA Backgrounder*. Retrieved from www.fda.gov/opacom/backgrounders/miles.html

26. U.S. Food and Drug Administration: 450.300 OTC drugs—General provisions and administrative procedures for marketing combination products CPG 7132b.16. Compliance policy guides manual. Chapter 4: Human drugs. Retrieved from www.fda.gov/ora/compliance_ref/cpg/cpgdrg/cpg450-300.html

27. Department of Health, Education, and Welfare (1974): Protection of human subjects. *Federal Register*. Retrieved from http://www.hhs.gov/ohrp/documents/19740823.pdf

28. National Institute of Health: National Research Act Pub. L. 93–348. Retrieved from http://history.nih.gov/01docs/historical/documents/PL93-348.pdf

29. Department of Health, Education, and Welfare (1978): Protection of human subjects. *Federal Register*. Retrieved at www.hhs.gov/ohrp/documents/19781130.pdf

30. U.S. Food and Drug Administration: Medical devices: Immunology and microbiology devices; Classification of enterovirus nucleic acid assay. 21 CFR—Part 866. Retrieved from www.fda.gov/OHRMS/DOCKETS/98fr/E8-31213.htm

31. U.S. Food and Drug Administration (2008): Scope food and drugs. Chapter 1: Subchapter A part 58: Good laboratory practice for nonclinical laboratory studies. Code of Federal Regulations, Title 21. Retrieved from http://www.accessdata.fda.gov/scripts/cdrh/cfdocs/cfcfr/CFRSearch.cfm?CFRPart = 58&showFR = 1&subpartNode = 21:1.0.1.1.22.1

32. U.S. Food and Drug Administration: Good laboratory practice: Sections 406, 408, 409, 502, 503, 505, 506, 510, 512–516, 518–520, 721, and 801. Federal Food, Drug, and Cosmetic Act. Retrieved from www.access.gpo.gov/nara/cfr/waisidx_01/21cfr58_01.html

33. U.S. Food and Drug Administration: Good laboratory practice: Sections 351, 354–360F. Public Health Service Act 21, CFR 58: Code of Federal Regulations, Title 21. Retrieved from www.access.gpo.gov/nara/cfr/waisidx_01/21cfr58_01.html

34. Journal of Oncology Practice (2008): ASCO outlines minimum standards and exemplary attributes for research sites: Previews tools to be provided. *Journal of Oncology Practice*; 4(4): 185–187.

35. Avery S (2007): Regulations, ICH Guidelines and good clinical practice (GCP): How do they fit together? Available from Duke Translational Medicine Institute (DTMI), www.dtmi.duke.edu/core-teams/regulatory/ RegulationsICHGuidelinesGCP_2007November.pdf/ preview_popup/file

36. Journal of Oncology Practice (2008): Good clinical practice research guidelines review: Emphasis given to responsibilities of investigators: Second article in a series. *Journal of Oncology Practice*; 4(5): 233–235.

37. U.S. Food and Drug Administration (1998): Protection of human subjects: Categories of research that may be reviewed by the Institutional Review Board (IRB) through an expedited review procedure. *Federal Register*. Retrieved from www.fda.gov/oc/ohrt/irbs/expeditedreview.html

38. U.S. Food and Drug Administration: The Orphan Drug Act. Retrieved at www.fda.gov/orphan/oda.htm

39. Consumer Project on Technology: The Hatch-Waxman Act and new legislation to close its loopholes. Retrieved at www.cptech.org/ip/health/generic/hw.html

40. U.S. Food and Drug Administration: Proposed new drug, antibiotic, and biologic drug product regulations. Code of Federal Regulations, Title 21. Retrieved from http://www.fda.gov/oc/gcp/preambles/48fr/48fr.html

41. U.S. Food and Drug Administration (1987): Part 312, 314, 511, and 514. New drug, antibiotic, and biologic drug product regulations. (Docket No. 82N-0394) 52 FR 8798. Retrieved at http://www.accessdata.fda.gov/scripts/cdrh/cfdocs/cfcfr/CFRSearch.cfm

42. U.S. Food and Drug Administration: Submissions for treatment use. Retrieved at http://edocket.access.gpo.gov/cfr_2001/aprqtr/pdf/21cfr312.35.pdf

43. U.S. Food and Drug Administration (1993): Guideline for the study and evaluation of gender differences in the clinical evaluation of drugs. *Federal Register*. Retrieved at www.fda.gov/cder/Guidance/old036fn.pdf

44. U.S. Food and Drug Administration: Investigational new drug applications and new drug applications. Retrieved from www.fda.gov/OHRMS/DOCKETS/98fr/95n-0010-npr0001.htm

45. U.S. Food and Drug Administration: Fast track, accelerated approval and priority review. Retrieved from www.fda.gov/oashi/fast.html

46. U.S. Food and Drug Administration: Frequently asked questions on prescription drug user fees (PDUFA). Retrieved at http://www.fda.gov/Cder/about/smallbiz/pdufa.htm

47. Peace KE (1989): Some thoughts on the biopharmaceutical section and statistics, ASA Joint Sesquicentennial Meetings, Washington, DC.

48. U.S. Food and Drug Administration: One hundred fifth congress of the United States of America. Retrieved at http://www.fda.gov/cdrh/modact97.pdf

49. The international conference on harmonization of technical requirements for registration of pharmaceuticals for human use: Safety guidelines. Retrieved from www.ich.org/cache/compo/502-272-1.html

50. Peace KE (1995): Considerations concerning subpopulations in the clinical development of new drugs, Annual DIA Meeting on Statistical Issues in Clinical Development, Hilton Head, SC.

51. U.S. Food and Drug Administration: Guidance for industry: Collection of race and ethnicity data in clinical trials. Retrieved at www.fda.gov/CBER/gdlns/racethclin.htm

52. U.S. Food and Drug Administration: One hundred eighth congress of the United States of America. Retrieved at www.fda.gov/cder/Pediatric/S-650-PREA.pdf

53. Federal Register: Notices. Retrieved at www.fda.gov/OHRMS/DOCKETS/98fr/05-21036.pdf

54. Carpenter D (2004): Gatekeeping and the FDA's role in human subjects protection. *Virtual Mentor*; **6**(11). Available at http://virtualmentor.ama-assn.org/2004/11/msoc1-0411.html

55. U.S. Food and Drug Administration: Center for Drug Evaluation and Research Website. Retrieved at www.fda.gov/cder/

56. U.S. Food and Drug Administration: FDA regulations relating to good clinical practice and clinical trials. Retrieved at www.fda.gov/oc/gcp/ regulations.html

57. Johnson J (1988): Past and present regulatory aspects of drug development. In: *Biopharmaceutical Statistics for Drug Development*, Peace KE (ed.), Marcel Dekker, Inc., New York.

58. Thomas L (1977): Biostatistics in medicine. *Science*; **198**: 675

59. Bren L. (November 19, 2008). The advancement of controlled clinical trials. *Quality Digest*, U.S. Food and Drug Administration. Available at: www. qualitydigest. com/inside/fda-compliance-article/advancement-controlled-clinical-trials.html

60. U.S. Food and Drug Administration: Form FDA 1572. Information sheet guidance for sponsors, clinical investigators, and IRBs. Retrieved at www.fda.gov/OHRMS/DOCKETS/98fr/FDA-2008-D-0406-gdl.pdf

61. U.S. Food and Drug Administration: Information for sponsor-investigators submitting investigational new drug applications (INDs). Retrieved at www.fda.gov/CDER/forms/1571-1572-help.html

62. U.S. Food and Drug Administration: Content and format section 312.23. Investigational new drug application. Code of Federal Regulations, Title 21. Retrieved at https://www.accessdata.fda.gov/scripts/cdrh/cfdocs/cfCFR/CFRSearch.cfm?fr = 312.23

63. U.S. Food and Drug Administration: Good laboratory practice for nonclinical laboratory studies: 21 CFR 58. Food and drugs. Chapter 1: Subchapter A. Code of Federal Regulations Title 21. Retrieved from http://www.accessdata.fda.gov/scripts/cdrh/cfdocs/cfcfr/CFRSearch.cfm?CFRPart = 58

64. U.S. Food and Drug Administration: *CDER Handbook*, Silver Springs, MD. Retrieved at http://www.fda.gov/CDER/HANDBOOK/nda.htm

65. U.S. Food and Drug Administration: New drug application process. CDER drug applications. Retrieved at www.fda.gov/cder/regulatory/applications/NDA.htm

66. Levin R: Guidance for preparing electronic NDAs. Retrieved at www.fda.gov/cder/present/dia198/vib.pdf

67. U.S. Food and Drug Administration: Providing regulatory submissions in electronic format—NDA. Retrieved at www.fda.gov/cder/present/dia-498/presrl.pdf

68. Peace KE (ed.) (1990): *Statistical Issues in Drug Research and Development*, Marcel Dekker, Inc., New York.

69. Peace KE (ed.) (1988): *Biopharmaceutical Statistics for Drug Development*, Marcel Dekker, Inc., New York.

70. Peace KE (2009): *Design and Analysis of Clinical Trials with Time-to-Event Endpoints*, Chapman Hall/CRC, Boca Raton, FL.

71. Tilley EE (2009): Certain skin-related adverse drug events may have genetic basis. *Medscape Medical News*; February 17. Retrieved at www.medscape.com/viewarticle/588376

72. Gilbert GS (1993): *Drug Safety Assessment in Clinical Trials*, Marcel Dekker, Inc., New York.

73. U.S. Food and Drug Administration: Opacom. Retrieved at www.fda.gov/opacom/fda101/sld003.html

74. U.S. Food and Drug Administration: FDA organization. Retrieved at www.fda.gov/opacom/7org.html

75. U.S. Food and Drug Administration: FDA organization charts. Retrieved at http://www.fda.gov/oc/orgcharts/orgchart.html

76. U.S. Food and Drug Administration: CBER organizational list. Retrieved at www.fda.gov/CBER/inside/orglist.htm

77. U.S. Food and Drug Administration: CDRH management directory by organization. Retrieved at http://www.fda.gov/cdrh/organiz.html

78. U.S. Food and Drug Administration: CDER office of biostatistics. Retrieved from www.fda.gov/cder/Offices/Biostatistics/default.htm

79. U.S. Food and Drug Administration: Manual of policies and procedures. Center for Drug Evaluation and Research Office of Biostatistics. Retrieved at www.fda.gov/cder/mapp/4000.8NDA.pdf

80. Wilson SE, Zhou F (2006): A statistical reviewer's perspective (PPS presentation). Retrieved from www.fda.gov/cder/present/DIA2006/Zhou.pps
81. Honig S: Outline for performing NDA review. Retrieved at www.fda.gov/cder/reviewer/honig.pdf
82. Moledina N: Steps and issues in the NDA review process. Retrieved at www.fda.gov/cder/reviewer/moledina.pdf
83. Williams G: Outline for performing medical review of NDA links to resources. Retrieved at www.fda.gov/cder/reviewer/dodp2w.pdf
84. Anonymous: The BLA. Biopharm. Retrieved from http://www.highbeam.com/doc/1P3-110472545.html
85. U.S. Food and Drug Administration: Regulatory—License applications refusal to file procedures for biologics license applications. Manual of standard operating procedures and policies. Retrieved at www.fda.gov/cber/regsopp/8404.htm
86. U.S. Food and Drug Administration (2006): Requirements on content and format of labeling for human prescription drug and biological products. *Federal Register*. Retrieved at www.fda.gov/cber/rules/labelcf.htm
87. U.S. Food and Drug Administration (2008): Regulatory—License applications review of product labeling. Manual of standard operating procedures and policies. Retrieved at www.fda.gov/cber/regsopp/8412.htm
88. Food and Drug Administration (2007): Regulatory—The responsibilities of the division of epidemiology (DE/OBE) in the BLA review process. Manual of standard operating procedures and policies. Retrieved at www.bcg-usa.com/regulatory/docs/SOPP/84016.pdf
89. Roland E (2003): FDA review principles. Retrieved at www.ateliersdegiens.org/upload/conferencesG19/Roland.pdf
90. U.S. Food and Drug Administration: Review process. Retrieved at http://www.fda.gov/CDRH/DEVADVICE/pma/review_process.html
91. U.S. Food and Drug Administration: Drugs@FDA instructions: Health information. Retrieved at www.fda.gov/cder/drugsatfda/instructionsHealth.htm
92. U.S. Food and Drug Administration: 21 CFR 201.57—Specific requirements on content and format of labeling for human prescription drug and biological products described in 201.56(b)(1). Food and drug. Chapter 1: Subchapter C: Part 201—Labeling. Code of Federal Regulations. Retrieved at http://www.accessdata.fda.gov/scripts/cdrh/cfdocs/cfCFR/CFRSearch.cfm?fr = 201.57
93. U.S. Food and Drug Administration: 21 CFR 208—Medication guides for prescription drug products. Food and drug. Chapter 1: Subchapter C. Code of Federal Regulations. Retrieved at http://www.accessdata.fda.gov/scripts/cdrh/cfdocs/cfCFR/CFRSearch.cfm?CFRPart = 208
94. U.S. Food and Drug Administration (2006): FDA announces final rule on the requirements for prescribing information for drug and biological products. Retrieved at www.fda.gov/cder/regulatory/physLabel/summary.pdf
95. U.S. Food and Drug Administration: Office of generic drugs. Retrieved at www.fda.gov/cder/ogd/rld/labeling_review_branch.html
96. Gitterman S, Burke L, Levin R (2005): Introduction to SPL changes with the physician labelling rule (ppt presentation). Retrieved at www.fda.gov/cder/Regulatory/ERSR/2006_03_14_SPLv2.ppt
97. U.S. Food and Drug Administration: Labeling. Retrieved at www.fda.gov/cdrh/ode/labeling.html

3

Ethical Considerations in the Design and Conduct of Clinical Trials

3.1 Introduction

Ethics may be thought of as a discipline for dealing with what is good or bad, a set or system of moral values, or a guiding philosophy [1]. Ethics as a philosophy to guide the conduct of clinical trials is a must: from protocol development, to the recruitment of investigators and investigational sites, to the recruitment and treatment of volunteers who participate in the trials, to the monitoring of the trials, to the collection, computerization, and quality assurance of data collected in the trials, to the statistical analysis of the data collected, to the writing and compiling the regulatory dossier, and to the conduct of all who have any responsibility for the design, conduct, and reporting of clinical trials. In the absence of a commitment to ethics, there may be no barriers to prevent inefficient and useless trials from being conducted or to safeguard the health of participants. Having a philosophy of ethics and being bound by a code of ethics ensures that the rights, common decency, and health of clinical trial participants will be paramount, and that the results from clinical trials are presented and reported factually.

The purpose of this chapter is to provide an overview of the evolution of ethical considerations in clinical trials and to impress upon the reader the need for ethical conduct by all individuals with any responsibility in their design, conduct, analysis, and reporting. Toward this end, key milestones in the history and evolution of ethics in clinical research are identified and briefly discussed in Section 3.2. The role of independent review boards is discussed in Section 3.3. Who should practice clinical trial ethics within the context of protocol development, protocol conduct, biostatistical analysis, interpretation, and dissemination of results are presented in Section 3.4. Informed consent is also revisited in Section 3.5 by linking it to sample size determination and power, and arguing that power and sample size should also be included in the informed consent document. Common ethical principles across various codes and regulations are summarized in Section 3.6. Concluding remarks appear in Section 3.7.

3.2 History and Evolution of Ethical Considerations in Clinical Trials: Key Milestones

Fundamental to the evolution of ethical considerations in clinical trials are six key milestones: the Nuremberg Code; the Declaration of Helsinki; the Belmont Report; Section 21, Parts 50 and 56 of the Code of Federal Regulation (21 CFR Parts 50 and 56); Section 45, Part 46 of the Code of Federal Regulation (45 CFR Part 46); and the International Conference on Harmonization (ICH) of Good Clinical Practices (GCP). They form the foundation for the ethical conduct of clinical research today [2] and have been translated into guidelines and requirements in current regulations.

3.2.1 The Nuremberg Code

The modern history of protection of human participants in clinical research began with the discovery of atrocities committed by Nazi physicians—for example, twin experiments. One twin was exposed to a pathogen and then autopsied to determine the natural progression of the disease. The other twin (control) was uninfected and was later sacrificed for comparison with the infected twin [3]. Obviously such an experiment was wholly unethical and inhumane. The judges at the Nuremberg trial had no basis in law to judge the Nazi physicians. They developed 10 principles for this purpose. These principles formed the basis of what came to be known as the Nuremberg Code for research involving human subjects [2]. Appearing below are the 10 basic principles excerpted from the Nuremberg Code [4]:

1. The voluntary consent of the human subject is absolutely essential. This means that the person involved should have legal capacity to give consent; should be so situated as to be able to exercise free power of choice, without the intervention of any element of force, fraud, deceit, duress, overreaching, or other ulterior form of constraint or coercion; and should have sufficient knowledge and comprehension of the elements of the subject matter involved so as to enable him to make an understanding and enlightened decision. This latter element requires that before the acceptance of an affirmative decision by the experimental subject, there should be made known to him the nature, duration, and purpose of the experiment; the method and means by which it is to be conducted; all inconveniences and hazards reasonably to be expected; and the effects upon his health or person which may possibly come from his participation in the experiment. The duty and responsibility for ascertaining the quality of the consent rests upon each individual who initiates, directs, or

engages in the experiment. It is a personal duty and responsibility which may not be delegated to another with impunity.

2. The experiment should be such as to yield fruitful results for the good of society, unprocurable by other methods or means of study, and not random and unnecessary in nature.

3. The experiment should be so designed and based on the results of animal experimentation and a knowledge of the natural history of the disease or other problem under study that the anticipated results will justify the performance of the experiment.

4. The experiment should be so conducted as to avoid all unnecessary physical and mental suffering and injury.

5. No experiment should be conducted where there is an a priori reason to believe that death or disabling injury will occur; except, perhaps, in those experiments where the experimental physicians also serve as subjects.

6. The degree of risk to be taken should never exceed that determined by the humanitarian importance of the problem to be solved by the experiment.

7. Proper preparations should be made and adequate facilities provided to protect the experimental subject against even remote possibilities of injury, disability, or death.

8. The experiment should be conducted only by scientifically qualified persons. The highest degree of skill and care should be required through all stages of the experiment of those who conduct or engage in the experiment.

9. During the course of the experiment, the human subject should be at liberty to bring the experiment to an end if he has reached the physical or mental state where continuation of the experiment seems to him to be impossible.

10. During the course of the experiment, the scientist in charge must be prepared to terminate the experiment at any stage, if he has probable cause to believe, in the exercise of the good faith, superior skill, and careful judgment required of him, that a continuation of the experiment is likely to result in injury, disability, or death to the experimental subject.

The Nuremberg Code is regarded by many as the gold standard for the conduct of clinical trials. However, there are gaps in some areas. For example, it appears to prohibit research involving children or those unable to provide consent on their own. The code makes no provision for consent by parents or legal guardians [5]. Further, the code did not carry the force of law [6].

3.2.2 The Declaration of Helsinki

The Declaration of Helsinki was originally adopted by the World Medical Assembly in June 1964 in Helsinki, Finland. Since then, it has undergone six revisions in 1975, 1983, 1989, 1996, 2000 [7], and 2008 [8]. The original declaration represents a landmark event in the evolution of clinical research ethics as it represents the first major effort of the world medical community to regulate itself with respect to medical research activities. It forms the basis of many documents that followed.

The overriding principle of the original declaration and its revisions is respect for the individual participant, his or her right of self-determination, and the right to make informed decisions regarding participation in research, both initially and during the conduct of the research. The investigator's sole duty is to the participant. While there is always a need for research, the participant's welfare must always take precedence over the interests of science and society, and ethical considerations should always trump laws and regulations. Highlights of the Declaration of Helsinki include [2]

1. The well-being of subjects taking part in research should take precedence over the interests of science and society.

2. Ethical standards regarding respect for persons and protection of subjects' health and rights are articulated.

3. Recognition that some populations are vulnerable (e.g., the physically or mentally handicapped) and require special protection.

4. Stipulation that experimental procedures must be detailed in a protocol for the research, which should be submitted to an ethical review committee. This statement represents one of the first articulations that a protocol is required for a research study and that the protocol should include the scientific reasons and identify what questions the researchers hope to answer by conducting the study.

5. Investigators must submit information obtained (especially monitoring information such as serious adverse events) in the conduct of the research to the ethical review committee.

6. Assessment of risks and benefits to participants or others is required before conducting the research.

7. Subjects must be informed volunteers. If they are unable to give consent themselves, legally authorized representatives must provide consent on their behalf.

8. Subjects have the right to safeguard their own integrity (another application of the principle of respect for persons).

9. Informed consent must be well documented. The context of obtaining informed consent is as important as the information presented in the informed consent document. If the researcher is also the subject's physician, a physician not connected with the research or the subject's medical care should obtain informed consent to minimize undue influence.

The declaration provides requirements for the conduct of biomedical research involving human subjects. Since the original declaration, the number of sections increased from 11 to 34 [9]. For the biostatistician, it is interesting to note that the declaration includes sections on Controlled Clinical Trials, Data Management, and Publication of Results.

A subsection of the latter is entitled Validity of Research Reports and Conflicts of Interest. Here, investigators are obligated to report the methods, results, conclusions, and interpretation of their research fully and accurately.

3.2.3 The Belmont Report

In 1966, Harvard anesthesiologist, Henry Beecher, authored an exposé of numerous unethical experiments that had been published in prominent medical journals [10]. Beecher did not identify the references or investigators of the research. His goal was to increase awareness of broader ethical problems in human experimentation rather than encourage prosecution. He wanted to heighten awareness that unethical research activities in humans were being conducted in the United States that were similar to those of Nazi Germany. His article had a major impact on the development of clinical research regulations. He concluded that consent has to be a goal in clinical research. It may never be fully achievable, but researchers should strive to achieve. It is not merely sufficient to state that consent was obtained. Subjects must be informed and understand the research risks. He also recommended a second safeguard: *an intelligent, informed, conscientious, compassionate, responsible investigator* [2].

The saddest example in the United States of research abuse was the 40 year (1932–1972) Tuskegee Syphilis Study conducted by the Public Health Service [11–13]. Poor and largely uneducated African-American men in rural Tuskegee, Alabama, were injected with the syphilis bacterium without their knowledge in order to study the natural progression of syphilis. *The New York Times* published articles exposing the ethical atrocities of the study in 1972. The study was supposed to last only 6 months. However, since the researchers were getting *good data*, they decided to let the study run; even withholding treatment with penicillin that became widely available in the 1940s.

These revelations spurred Congressional hearings resulting in the National Research Act in 1974, which authorized the formation of the

National Commission for the Protection of Human Subjects of Biomedical and Behavioral Research. The Commission's charge was to consider (1) *the boundaries between biomedical and behavioral research and the accepted and routine practice of medicine*, (2) *the role of assessment of risk–benefit criteria in the determination of the appropriateness of research involving human subjects*, (3) *appropriate guidelines for the selection of human subjects for participation in such research, and* (4) *the nature and definition of informed consent in various research settings* [14].

The Belmont Report is a statement of basic ethical principles and guidelines that should assist in resolving ethical problems arising in the conduct of research with human subjects. The basic ethical principles appearing in the report are Respect for Persons, Beneficence, and Justice. Beneficence means the investigator should act in the best interest of the participant, and in doing so should first do no harm (non-maleficence). Justice pertains to the decision of who has the opportunity to participate in clinical research. Applications of these principles pertain to informed consent, assessment of risk and benefit, and to selection of subjects. Unlike other reports of the commission, the Belmont Report does not make specific recommendations for administrative action by the secretary of the Department of Health, Education, and Welfare (DHEW); rather, the Commission recommended that the Belmont Report be adopted in its entirety, as a statement of the department's policy.

The two-volume appendix (DHEW Publication No. (OS) 78-0013 and No. (OS) 78-0014), containing the reports of experts and specialists who assisted the commission in fulfilling its charge, is available for sale by the superintendent of documents, U.S. Government Printing Office, Washington, District of Columbia 20402.

3.2.4 21 CFR Parts 50 and 56

The FDA is charged by statute with ensuring that the rights, safety, and welfare of human subjects who participate in clinical investigations that support applications for research or marketing permits for products regulated by FDA are protected. Products include food and color additives, drugs for human use, medical devices for human use, biological products for human use, and electronic products. Pertinent sections from the Code of Federal Regulations are 21 CFR Part 50—Protection of Human Subjects, Informed Consent, and 21 CFR Part 56—Standards for Institutional Review Boards [15,16].

3.2.5 45 CFR Part 46

Another regulation enacted for the protection of human subjects under the Department of Health and Human Services (HHS) is 45 CFR 46 [17]. Subpart A provides HHS policy for protection of human research subjects; Subpart B provides additional protections for pregnant women, human fetuses, and neonates involved in research; Subpart C provides additional protections pertaining to biomedical and behavioral research involving prisoners as subjects; and Subpart D provides additional protections for children involved as subjects in research.

3.2.6 International Conference on Harmonization on Good Clinical Practices

Another guideline for the protection of human subjects in clinical trials is the ICH of GCP guideline [18]. The guideline represents an international ethical and scientific quality standard for designing, conducting, recording, and reporting trials that involve the participation of human subjects. This standard ensures that the rights and safety of the trial subjects are protected and that the trial results are credible [19].

The ICH came into existence in April 1990 at a meeting in Brussels [20] among regulatory authorities from Europe, the United States, and Japan, and experts from the pharmaceutical industry. This led to an international, uniform standard for regulatory agencies to accept the results of clinical trials conducted according to the ICH-GCP guidelines on safety, quality, efficacy, and multidisciplinary [19,20].

3.3 Independent Review Boards

Additional ethical and safety nets for the protection of human subjects in clinical trial research protocols are the Investigational Review Board (IRB) and the Data Safety Monitoring Board (DSMB). Both are committees that function independent of the protocol sponsor.

3.3.1 Investigational Review Board

An IRB is a group of at least five independent members whose responsibility is to review, approve, and monitor clinical research protocols (if approved) involving human subjects to ensure that their rights and welfare are protected. An IRB may require changes to the protocol prior to approval or post approval—should such changes be in the best interest of protocol participants. The membership of an IRB must include at least one member of each sex, at least one member whose primary concern is about the scientific activities of the protocol, at least one member whose primary concern is nonscientific, and no member that has a conflict of interest in any aspect of the research being conducted under the protocol. Membership information and functions and responsibilities of IRBs may be found in 21 CFR Parts 50 and 56 [15,16], and 45 CFR Part 46 [17].

3.3.2 Data Safety Monitoring Board

A DSMB is an independent group of experts whose primary responsibility is to monitor safety of clinical trial participants while the trial is ongoing. Usually a DSMB consists of three to seven members. At least one member must be a statistician. At least one member must be a physician who is knowledgeable in the disease being studied in the trial protocol. At least one member must be a physician knowledgeable in areas of major suspected adverse effects. Some protocols, depending on their size and length of time to conduct and the disease area, may require an ethicist as well as a representative of patient advocacy groups. The DSMB has the power to recommend termination of the study based on the review and evaluation of trial data as it accumulates [21].

3.4 Clinical Trial Ethics: Who Should Practice?

Who should practice clinical trial ethics within the context of protocol development, protocol conduct, database creation and quality assurance, biostatistical analysis, clinical study report and interpretation, and dissemination of results is discussed in this section. Raising the question "Who should practice clinical trial ethics?" seems absurd on the face of it. The answer is, everyone with any responsibility in the design and execution of the trial, management and analysis of the data collected, and interpretation or dissemination of clinical trial results. The question is raised to alert readers that clinical trial ethics go beyond that pertaining to the relationship between investigational site personnel and trial participants. All with any responsibility for clinical trial functions should exercise due diligence to ensure that all attendant activities are ethical.

Clinical trial functions include protocol development, all aspects of clinical trial operations, clinical trial data management, biostatistical analysis, writing the clinical trial study report, and disseminating the results.

3.4.1 Protocol Development

Successful development of a quality and ethical protocol requires input from several professionals or experts. These include at the minimum a physician, a biostatistician, and a regulatory affairs expert. Other possible contributors include a data management expert, a field monitoring professional, a medical writer, a clinical safety expert, a preclinical safety scientist, a pharmacologist, a pharmacokineticist, a pharmaceutical formulation chemist, an ethicist, and possibly legal and marketing representatives.

3.4.1.1 The Physician

The physician should have expertise in the disease being studied. This is not always the case in the pharmaceutical industry where the role of the project physician is more toward the overall clinical management of the project. In such cases, the project physician uses consultants who are experts in the disease area and experts in dealing with adverse effects that may arise from the treatment of patients with the drug. The project physician is responsible for ensuring that protocol procedures involving the diagnosis, treatment, or other clinical management of participants not only reflect good medical science, but are also ethical.

3.4.1.2 The Biostatistician

The biostatistician has the responsibility for ensuring that the objective of the protocol is clear and unambiguous and for recommending the most appropriate experimental design for the protocol (see Chapters 6 and 7). It is unethical for the biostatistician to recommend a design based solely upon efficiency at the expense of ethics. For example, requiring all patients in a study of epilepsy to cross over to an alternative treatment even though their seizures are being controlled on the original treatment to which they were randomized, may be unethical (see last two paragraphs of Section 10.7.2.4.2.2 for further discussion). Further, in placebo-controlled clinical trials of a new drug, particularly for diseases with great morbidity, to require as many patients to be assigned to the placebo group as to the drug group may be unethical, particularly since the statistical power is not diminished much by assigning twice as many patients to the drug group as to the placebo group. As sample size determination has both an ethical and an efficacy imperative, it may be unethical to permit a trial (particularly Phase III) to start that is knowingly underpowered [22–25].

The biostatistician also provides the statistical analysis section of the protocol. It is unethical (and unprofessional) for the statistical analysis section to include inappropriate methods for the data to be collected or to include appropriate methods whose validity require the data to satisfy certain assumptions without including plans for checking those assumptions (see Chapter 9). Failure to include statistical monitoring plans that allow early stopping of the trial or early termination of certain treatment arms for safety or efficacy (particularly in placebo-controlled trials) may be unethical, particularly for trials where the natural progression of the disease under study carries great morbidity.

3.4.1.3 Regulatory Affairs Expert

The regulatory affairs expert is responsible for ensuring that the protocol addresses all pertinent federal regulations and guidelines and for filing the protocol and all subsequent amendments with the regulatory agency. It is transparent that the regulatory affairs expert must exercise ethical conduct in carrying out his or her responsibilities. To behave otherwise is to place the sponsor in jeopardy of violating federal regulations.

3.4.2 Clinical Trial Operations

Some pharmaceutical companies include biostatistics, clinical data management, field monitoring, and medical writing under the umbrella of clinical trial operations. Clinical trial operations as defined in this chapter include selection of investigators and investigational sites, recruitment, entry, and treatment of volunteers, and site monitoring for adherence to protocol and state or federal regulations and quality of data collection.

3.4.2.1 Investigator and Site Personnel

Investigators are selected by the protocol sponsor as being qualified to conduct the protocol and having an investigational site (e.g., clinic) that can adequately perform the procedures defined in the protocol. The investigator should be a physician, board certified in treatment of the disease for which the intervention (drug, biologic, or medical device) is being developed, and have extensive experience in the field of clinical trials [26]. Anything that changes in the protocol regarding research activity should be reported by the investigator to the independent IRB that is reviewing and monitoring the clinical trial [26].

Site personnel is the term for any person working at an investigational site with any responsibility for the conduct of a clinical trial. This may include nurses, doctors, pharmacists, technicians, as well as others. They assist in preparing a patient for a procedure, performing a procedure, dispensing trial medication, data collection and recording, and taking care of the patient post-procedure (whether it may be a surgery or observing a patient after taking the treatment).

Investigators and site personnel are the primary targets of the Nuremberg Code, the Declaration of Helsinki, and the Belmont Report with respect to ensuring that rights and welfare of clinical trial participants are protected. Although the investigator and site personnel have contractual responsibilities to the sponsor, these should never trump their responsibility of ensuring the rights and welfare of patients. To behave otherwise is unethical.

3.4.2.2 Field Monitoring

The field monitoring department has responsibility for monitoring clinical trials for adherence to protocols and federal regulations—including those pertaining to ethical conduct of the investigator and site personnel and how human subjects are being treated—as they are being conducted at investigational sites. In addition, field monitors are responsible for ensuring the accuracy of the data collected against the source documents (patient charts) and facilitating the transfer of such data to the sponsor.

Field monitors are called clinical research associates (CRA) at many pharmaceutical companies. Common communications such as telephone conversations, site visits, and written correspondence are the lifelines between the CRA and the clinical trial sites [26]. All aspects of the trial should be documented to permit an audit of "what was to be done," "what was done," and how differences might affect conclusions or inferences. The CRA also functions as a teacher as they instruct site personnel on all aspects of the protocol and their responsibilities under the protocol and contract with the sponsor.

The bulk of the Nuremberg Code, the Declaration of Helsinki, the Belmont Report, 21 CFR Parts 50 and 56, and 45 CFR Part 46 is directed toward ethical treatment of human subjects who participate in clinical trials. Therefore, they are directed more toward what goes on at investigational sites regarding patient care than within the protocol sponsor's facilities. The ICH guidelines, as well as other federal regulations under the auspices of the FDA and Department of HHS (see Chapter 2 for a broad list of Regulations), expand the focus from the clinical trial participant to virtually all activities relating to clinical development of drugs, biologics, and medical devices. Ethical conduct on the part of all persons with responsibility for clinical trial activities is not only a legal requirement, but also goes to the heart of responsible, professional conduct.

3.4.3 Clinical Data Management

The clinical data management department has responsibility for designing the clinical trial database and for ensuring the integrity of data entry and retrieval. It is unethical for any of the clinical data management personnel to knowingly allow data to be entered that is not identical to the data collected. Further, it is unethical and unprofessional to fail to quality assure the data entry or data retrieval processes. See Section 9.2.5 for a fuller discussion.

3.4.4 Biostatistical Analysis

Once the data collected are computerized and quality assured, the biostatistician begins statistical analyses. The aim of statistical analyses is to assess the strength of evidence in support of the trial objective and to produce a valid inference regarding the objective. Assumptions underlying the validity of the analysis methods used should be checked to see if they hold for the data being analyzed (see Section 9.4). If the assumptions do not hold, alternative methods may be used, but require justification.

There are many opportunities for subtle and covert unethical conduct to enter during the analysis process. Some such opportunities are stating that analysis assumptions were checked when they were not, allowing knowledge of the treatment groups to influence values provided for missing or questionable data, or overstating conclusions. In many pharmaceutical companies, the biostatistical department is organizationally located within the clinical development division. The biostatistician's work must not be influenced by the reporting relationship; to do so, would be unethical.

Ideally, the performance of the biostatistician as well as others supporting clinical trial activity in meeting their responsibility should earn an answer of yes to each of the following questions:

1. Was there an a priori commitment to the research objective?
2. Was the endpoint appropriate for the objective?
3. Was the experimental design appropriate for the disease being studied?
4. Was the investigation conducted in a quality manner to eliminate bias and to ensure accuracy of the data?
5. Were steps taken to preserve the integrity of the Type I error?
6. Were the statistical methods for analyses valid (assumptions checked, dropouts appropriately handled, correct variance term used, etc.)?
7. Were the results of statistical analyses properly interpreted (the correct inferred population, impact of multiple endpoints or analyses, etc.)?
8. Was the professional conduct of the biostatistician and others in meeting their responsibilities ethical?

3.4.5 Clinical Trial Study Report

A study report for every clinical trial conducted should be developed, regardless of outcome, whether negative or positive. The medical writer has responsibility for developing and writing the clinical trial study report. The clinical trial biostatistician has responsibility for providing the description of statistical analysis methods and descriptive and inferential results; that is, for ensuring the statistical integrity of the clinical study report. The project clinician has the responsibility of ensuring the integrity of the clinical interpretation of findings. Both the biostatistician and the clinician have the responsibility for ensuring the validity of integrated statistical and clinical findings.

The medical writer should take an objective stance in writing the clinical trial study report, and in general the report should describe what was to be done, what was done, and address how differences affect the findings. Deviations from this stance may be seen as being too strong a proponent of the drug under study and regarded as unethical.

3.4.6 Dissemination of Results

Results of clinical trials are disseminated to regulatory agencies by filing the clinical trial study reports either as components of the new drug application (NDA), or supplemental new drug application (SNDA), or as amendments to the Investigational New Drug Exemption (IND); see Chapter 2 for further discussion. Manuscripts may be developed and submitted to appropriate journals for publication as a way of disseminating clinical trial results. Results from clinical trials may also be disseminated through advertisements. Whatever the route of dissemination, the disseminator is ethically (and legally) bound to ensure that the findings and interpretations of findings are accurately based on the results.

3.5 Informed Consent, Sample Size and Power

The informed consent document should be included in the protocol as an appendix. Instructions on how the document should be reviewed with potential clinical trial participants should also be included. The instructions are to ensure that potential participants are fully informed about all aspects of the trial necessary for them to give consent. Aspects of the trial include the objective, diagnostic, and other medical procedures to be conducted, identification of the drug and control, how participants will be assigned to treatment groups, the benefits to risks of participation, any costs to the patient for participation, identity of site personnel to call if problems related to participation arise, compensation for injuries, and apprising the participant that he or she may voluntarily withdraw at any time without prejudice and schedule of clinic visits.

Although not routinely included in the informed consent document, a case may be made that the power of the trial should also be reviewed with potential participants [22–25].

Many are aware, particularly in Phase III confirmatory proof-of-efficacy trials, that the determination of sample size is an efficacy imperative. That is, in order to confirm a question regarding efficacy of a compound, it is imperative that the sample size of the trial be large enough to provide a priori, a high probability (large power) that the question will be answered.

Sample size determination carries with it *an ethical imperative* as well. Before the authors agree to participate in a clinical trial, we would want to know first that the trial was needed to answer a medically important question (and what that question was), and second, what the likelihood was for the number of planned participants that the question would be answered. Including this second issue in the informed consent document in the protocol would make the informed consent process more ethical.

It is easy to argue that for small trials, we know with relatively large confidence before such trials are conducted, that all we'll be able to say after trial completion is that "we failed to confirm or refute the question." This may be deduced from Table 3.1, which summarizes 90% confidence intervals (CIs) on the difference between—and the ratio of—two treatments (test-T, standard-S), and the length of the CIs for various sample sizes (N) ranging from 10 to 200 per treatment group.

All CIs on the difference between treatments cover 0. Therefore, we cannot conclude that the treatments are different (at the one-sided 5% level of significance). However, all with the possible exception of the interval corresponding to 200 patients per group, are too wide to claim that the treatments are similar. So if at the outset of a trial, we know that it is highly likely that the outcome will be summarized as we can't say that the new treatment is different from the standard, neither can we say that it is similar, why conduct the trial? Unless of course, the primary reason for conducting the trial is pilot in nature: to gain experience with the attendant methods, to gather data for sample size determination of a follow-up confirmatory trial, etc. In which case, patients should be fully informed prior to their decision regarding trial participation.

Having argued that it is ethically imperative to include a statement in the informed consent document regarding the likelihood that the trial will answer the question or objective, we acknowledge that writing such a statement, geared to at most an 8th grade reading level, is challenging. Many, highly educated people find the concept of power difficult to comprehend. Something like the following: *If the drug is δ% more effective than the control,*

TABLE 3.1

90% CIs on Difference (T − S) and Ratio (T/S)

N	CI on (T − S)	CI Length	CI on T/S
10	−36.8%; 36.8%	73.6%	26.4%; 173.6%
25	−23.3%; 23.3%	46.5%	53.4%; 146.6%
50	−16.5%; 16.5%	32.9%	67.0%; 133.0%
100	−11.7%; 11.7%	23.3%	76.6%; 123.4%
200	−08.2%; 08.2%	16.4%	83.6%; 116.4%

there's a $(1 - \beta)$% chance of concluding that the drug is effective, with N patients per treatment group, is a good starting point. Of course, the writer would need to provide the values of δ, β, and N and decide how best to include the Type I error.

3.6 Common Ethical Principles of Various Codes and Regulations

Core ethical principles common to various codes and regulations pertinent to clinical trial research are protection of human subjects, objectivity, honesty, integrity, competence, carefulness, confidentiality, responsible publication, and legality [27].

Protection of human subjects: When conducting research involving human subjects, minimize harm and risk, and maximize benefit. Subjects should be treated with respect and dignity, and their privacy and autonomy should not be compromised. Special precautions should be taken with vulnerable populations. Efforts should be made to distribute benefits and burdens of clinical research evenly.

Objectivity: Strive to avoid bias of any kind (subtle or overt) in experimental design, data analysis, data interpretation, peer review, personnel decisions, report writing, expert testimony, and any other aspect of clinical trial research where objectivity is expected or required. Disclose any personal or financial interests that may affect research design, conduct, or outcome.

Honesty: Strive for honesty in all research activities. Honestly report data, methods and procedures, results, interpretation, and conclusions in all reports and publications. Do not fabricate, falsify, or misrepresent data. Do not deceive colleagues, IRBs, safety or monitoring committees, FDA or other regulatory agencies, or the public. Do not use unpublished data, methods, or results without appropriate permission. Properly acknowledge and give credit for all contributions to research. Never plagiarize.

Integrity: Keep your promises and agreements, act with sincerity, and strive for consistency in objective thought and action. Ensure integrity of data collected in terms of the measurement process, entry, and quality assurance.

Competence: Maintain and improve professional competence and expertise through lifelong educational, learning pursuits, and take steps to promote competence in science, medicine, and research as a whole.

Carefulness: Avoid careless errors and negligence; carefully and critically examine your own work and the work of peers. Keep good records of all activities related to clinical research including design, monitoring, data collection, and correspondence with agencies or journals.

Confidentiality: Protect confidential information including communications.

Responsible publication: Publish in order to advance research and scholarship rather than publishing for the sake of publishing. Avoid wasteful and duplicative publication.

Legality: Know and obey relevant laws and institutional and governmental policies.
　To these we add

Excellence: Strive for excellence in all research activities.

3.7　Concluding Remarks

Clinical trial ethics is not just the act of respecting human rights. It is also the act of all persons with any clinical trial responsibility adhering to the highest standards of medical, scientific, ethical, and professional conduct, thereby ensuring the quality and integrity of a clinical trial. To paraphrase Williams Jennings Bryan, Ethics *"is not a matter of chance, it is a matter of choice; it is not a thing to be waited for, it is a thing to be achieved."*

References

1. Merriam Webster Online Dictionary. Definition of ethics. Retrieved at http://www.merriam-webster.com/dictionary/ethics
2. Perlman DJ (2004): Ethics in clinical research: A history of human subject protections and practical implementation of ethical standards. *SoCRA SOURCE*; 37–41, May.
3. Lifton RJ (1986): *The Nazi Doctors: Medical Killing and the Psychology of Genocide*, Basic Books, New York.
4. U.S. General Printing Office (1949): Trials of war criminals before the Nuremberg military tribunals under Control Council Law No. 10; 2. http://www.ushmm.org/research/doctors/Nuremberg_Code.htm
5. Jonsen AR (1995): The weight and weighing of ethical principles. In: *The Ethics of Research Involving Human Subjects: Facing the 21st Century*, Vanderpool, HY (ed.), University Publishing Group, Frederick, MD, pp. 59–82.
6. Rothman DJ (1995): Research, human: Historical aspects. *Encyclopedia of Bioethics*; 4: 2251–2256.
7. Christie B (2000): Doctors revise declaration of Helsinki. *British Medical Journal*; 321(1266): 913.

8. Williams J (2008): The declaration of Helsinki and public health. *Bulletin of the World Health Organisation*; **86**(8): 650–651. http://www.who.int/bulletin/volumes/86/8/08-050955/en/index.html

9. World Medical Association (1999): Proposed revision of the World Medical Association Declaration of Helsinki. http://www.hks.harvard.edu/case/azt/ethics/hels_rev.html

10. Beecher HK (1966): Ethics and clinical research. *New England Journal of Medicine*; **274**: 1354–1360.

11. Jones JH (1993): *Bad Blood: The Tuskegee Syphilis Experiment*, Free Press, New York.

12. Brunner B (2003): *The Tuskegee Syphilis Experiment*, Tuskegee University, Tuskegee, AL. http://www.tuskegee.edu/Global/Story.asp?s = 1207586

13. US Public Health Service Syphilis Study at Tuskegee (2009): http://www.cdc.gov/tuskegee/timeline.htm

14. The Belmont Report: Ethical principles and guidelines for the protection of human subjects of research: Regulations and ethical guidelines. NIH http://ohsr.od.nih.gov/guidelines/belmont.html

15. FDA Policy for the Protection of Human Subjects (1991): 21 CFR Parts 50 and 56: Informed consent; Standards for Institutional Review Boards for Clinical Investigations [Docket No. 87N-0032] 56 FR 28025 June 18. http://www.fda.gov/ScienceResearch/SpecialTopics/RunningClinicalTrials/ucm118893.htm

16. FDA Policy for the Protection of Human Subjects (2009): 21 CFR Part 50—Protection of human subjects (informed consent); 21 CFR Part 56—Institutional Review Boards; Revised April 1. http://www.fda.gov/AboutFDA/CentersOffices/CDER/ucm090314.htm

17. Public Welfare Department of HHS (2005): CFR 45 PART 46—Protection of human subjects. http://www.hhs.gov/ohrp/documents/OHRPRegulations.pdf

18. European Medicines Agency (2002): ICH topic E 6 (R1): Guideline for good-clinical practice. http://www.emea.europa.eu/pdfs/human/ich/013595en.pdf

19. BBC Home (2006): Good clinical practice, January 16, 2000. http://www.bbc.co.uk/dna/h2g2/A7385682

20. The Official Web Site for ICH: http://www.ich.org/cache/compo/276-254-1.html

21. *Guidance for Clinical Trial Sponsors: Establishment and Operation of Clinical Trial Data Monitoring Committees*, U.S. Dept. of HHS, Food and Drug Administration, March 2006. http://www.fda.gov/downloads/RegulatoryInformation/Guidances/ucm127073.pdf

22. Peace KE (1989): *Some Thoughts on the Biopharmaceutical Section and Statistics*, ASA Joint Sesquicentennial Meetings, Publication of the American Statistical Association, August, Arlington, VA, pp. 98–105.

23. Peace KE (1992): An ethical issue concerning informed consent in clinical trials. *Biopharmaceutical Report*; **1**(2): 3.

24. Peace KE (2005): Making informed consent more ethical. *Drug Information Forum*; **5**(4): 26–27.

25. Peace KE (2008): Commentary: Is informed consent as ethical as it could be? *Bio-IT World*, March 17.

26. Rosenbaum D (1998): *Clinical Research Monitor Handbook: GCP Tools and Techniques*, 2nd edn., CRC Press, Boca Raton, FL.

27. Shamoo A, Resnik D (2003): *Responsible Conduct of Research*, Oxford University Press, New York.

4

Sample Size Considerations in Clinical Trials Pre-Market Approval

4.1 Introduction

Quality clinical research must be well planned, closely and carefully monitored and conducted, and appropriately analyzed and reported. Greater attentiveness to detail at the design stage argues for greater efficiency at the analysis and reporting stages.

An aspect of good design of protocols for new drugs is determining the number of patients required by the clinical investigation to adequately address the objective. Not only is this important on a per-protocol basis, adequate numbers of patients must also be studied within and across the phases of clinical development to support regulatory filing.

Although this chapter could go directly to a presentation on computation of sample sizes, similar to what one would present in a statistics class, a quick review of the phases of clinical trials and their objectives is presented first. Then the clinical development plan and its connection to labeling are discussed. Thereafter the statistical requirements for sample size determination are presented. Proceeding in this manner sets the stage for the recommendations that are made relative to the size of trials in each phase of clinical development pre-market approval. Some philosophical if not controversial issues then follow as well as concluding remarks.

4.2 Phases of Clinical Trials and Objectives

Anyone who has had any involvement with the clinical development program for a new drug knows that the clinical trials comprising the program are categorized as Phase I, Phase II, or Phase III. Although these categories may not be mutually exclusive (nor in some cases mutually exhaustive), there is general agreement as to what types of clinical studies comprise the bulk of the trials within each phase.

4.2.1 Phase I Trials

Phase I trials may consist of "early Phase I" trials, early dose-ranging trials, bioavailability or pharmacokinetic (PK) trials, or mechanism of action studies. Early Phase I trials represent the initial introduction of the drug in humans, in order to characterize the acute pharmacological effect. For most classes of drugs, healthy subjects are enrolled in an attempt to reduce the risk of serious toxicity and to avoid confounding pharmacological and disease effects. The idea is to introduce the drug to humans without inducing acute toxicity.

Early dose-ranging trials, often called dose-tolerance or dose-titration trials, are also most often conducted in healthy subjects. Both the effects of single dosing and multiple dosing schemes are studied. The objective of these trials is to determine a "tolerable" dose range, such that as long as future dosing remains in this range, no intolerable side effects of toxicities would be expected to be seen.

Early Phase I trials and early dose-ranging trials neither establish nor quantitate efficacy characteristics of a drug. These studies have to be conducted first, so that acute pharmacological effects may be described, and a range of tolerable doses determined that guide clinical use of the drug for later studies.

The primary objectives of Phase I bioavailability and PK trials are to characterize what happens to the drug once it is injected into the human body. That is, properties such as absorption, distribution, metabolism, elimination, clearance, and half-life need to be described. These trials also usually enroll healthy subjects and are often called "blood level trials."

Mechanism of action trials attempt to identify how the drug induces its effects. An example is the class of H_2-receptor antagonists, such as cimetidine, ranitidine, famotidine and nizatidine, which by blocking the H_2-receptor reduce the secretion of gastrin, which in turn leads to a reduction of gastric acid production. Another example is the H_1-receptor antagonist, terfenadine (seldane), which by blocking the H_1-receptor reduces histamine release.

Bioavailability or PK studies and mechanism of action studies provide additional information so that the drug may be clinically used more effectively and safer in future studies.

4.2.2 Phase II Trials

Phase II trials represent the earliest trials of a drug in patients. Patients should have the disease under investigation. Patients who enter such trials represent a relatively restricted yet homogeneous population. In some areas of drug development such as oncology, Phase II trials are categorized as Phase IIA and Phase IIB.

Phase IIA trials may include clinical pharmacology studies in patients, and more extensive or detailed PK and pharmacodynamic studies in patients. Phase IIB trials are controlled and represent the initial demonstration of efficacy and safety of a drug at the doses from the clinical pharmacology studies. Also of interest is estimating the effective dose range, characterizing the dose–response curve, and estimating the minimally effective dose. Often it is difficult to distinguish between Phase IIB trials and Phase III trials, particularly in terms of objectives. The primary differences are the inclusion/exclusion criteria and the sample size.

4.2.3 Phase III Trials

Phase III trials may be viewed as extensions of Phase IIB trials. They are larger and the inclusion/exclusion criteria may be less restrictive than those of Phase IIB trials. For a drug to proceed to the Phase III portion of the development program, it must be deemed effective from the Phase IIB program. At this stage, effectiveness has been indicated, but not confirmed.

The primary objectives of the Phase III program are to confirm the effectiveness of the drug in a more heterogeneous population, and to collect more and longer term safety data. Information from Phase IIB provides pilot data for the purpose of sample size determination in Phase III.

For the purpose of obtaining more safety data under conditions that better approximate the anticipated clinical use of the drug, relatively large, uncontrolled, non-comparative trials may also be conducted in Phase III. Since if the drug is given approval to be marketed, it may be used in the elderly, in the renally impaired, etc., and since such patients are usually excluded from other trials, studies in special populations may also be conducted in Phase III.

4.3 The Clinical Development Plan: Pre-Market Approval

As indicated in Section 4.2, the clinical development plan for a new drug includes Phase I, Phase II, and Phase III trials. In viewing the types of trials within each phase of clinical development, it is obvious that the objectives of the trials describe characteristics of a drug that should be known before proceeding sequentially with subsequent clinical use. Further, upon the successful completion of the trials through Phase III, sufficient information should exist for the drug to be approved, to be marketed.

The drug sponsor may wish to include other trials in the clinical development plan particularly to provide a marketing "hook" for launch. Prior to finalizing the clinical development plan, the drug sponsor should formulate draft labeling. The draft labeling should accommodate what is required to be said and what is desired to be said about the compound in the package insert of the marketed product. The clinical development plan then serves as a blueprint for labeling.

Basically, the labeling should communicate characteristics of the drug and give instructions for its use. Usually, the objectives of the trials described in Phase I, Phase II, and Phase III, if met in carrying out the attendant investigations, provide sufficient information to communicate the characteristics of the drug. However, since the population studied pre-market approval is likely to be more homogeneous than the user population post-market approval, and since inferences are based upon group averages, there may be insufficient information from the usual Phase I, Phase II, and Phase III program as to optimal clinical use of the drug, particularly in individual patients.

Therefore, drug sponsors may consider implementing a "Phase III ½" program directed more toward clinical use than toward establishing efficacy as a characteristic of the drug, which in our mind is what the typical pivotal proof-of-efficacy trials in Phase III do. Such a targeted program may be unnecessary if more efficient and more optimal designs and methods, such as response surface methodology, and evolutionary operations procedures are incorporated into the clinical development program as early as Phase II. In addition, being proactive in developing an integrated database consisting of all data collected on a compound, so that meta-analysis and other techniques may be used, should enable the drug sponsor to do a better job at labeling.

4.4 Sample Size Requirements

In presenting the statistical features of sample size determination, it is assumed that a protocol is being developed, and that the project statistician is expected to advice as to the appropriate statistical design, sample size requirements, and provide the data analysis section of the protocol, including appropriate statistical methods. We consider the basis for sample size determination to be a part of design considerations and should be a subsection of the data analysis section of the protocol. There are other subsections of the data analysis section that need to be considered prior to the basis for sample size determination.

4.4.1 Protocol Objectives as Specific Statistical Questions

The data analyses section of the protocol should begin by translating the objectives into specific statistical questions. These should be organized according to whether they address primary efficacy, secondary efficacy, safety, or other (such as quality of life) questions.

If inferential decisions regarding the questions are to be made on the basis of hypothesis testing, the questions should be translated into statistical hypotheses. It is desirable from a statistical viewpoint for the alternative hypothesis (H_a) to embody the research question both in substance and direction [1]. For placebo-controlled studies or for studies in which superior efficacy is the objective, this is routinely the case. For studies in which clinical equivalence is the objective, the usual framing of the objective translates it as the null hypothesis (H_0). In this framework, failure to reject H_0 does not permit a conclusion of equivalence. This will depend on a specification of how much the treatment regimens may truly differ in terms of therapeutic endpoints, yet still be considered clinically equivalent, and the power of the test to detect such a difference. Some authors [2] have suggested reversing the null and alternative hypotheses for equivalence studies, so that a conclusion of equivalence is reached by rejecting the null hypothesis. An attraction of this specification is that the Type I error is synonymous with the regulatory approval or consumer's risk for both efficacy and equivalence studies.

Separate univariate, null, and alternative hypotheses should be specified for each question. The reasons for separate specifications are primarily clarity and insight: clarity because the questions have been clearly elucidated and framed as statistical hypotheses. This sets the stage for appropriate statistical analyses when the data become available. When analyses directed toward the questions occur, it should be clear whether the statistical evidence is sufficient to answer them. Insight is gained from the univariate specifications, as to the significance level at which the tests should be performed. This is true even though the study objective may represent a composite hypothesis.

As an example, suppose that there are three randomized groups in a duodenal ulcer study of a H_2-receptor antagonist (X): placebo group (A), 150 mg group (B), and 300 mg group (C). Further, suppose that the objective of the study is to prove that 300 mg is effective and that it is more effective than 150 mg. There are two separate efficacy questions comprising the study objective: (1) Is 300 mg effective? (2) Is 300 mg more effective than 150 mg? These two questions translate into the two univariate hypotheses:

$$H_{01}: P_c = P_a \quad \text{versus} \quad H_{a1}: P_c > P_a$$

and

$$H_{02}: P_c = P_b \quad \text{versus} \quad H_{a2}: P_c > P_b$$

where P_a, P_b, and P_c represent the true proportions of patients treated with placebo, 150 mg of X, and 300 mg of X, respectively, whose ulcers would heal by the end of 4 weeks of treatment. The study objective is the composite hypothesis for which the null is the logical union of H_{01} and H_{02}, and the alternative is the logical intersection of H_{a1} and H_{a2}. It is therefore clear that if a Type I error of 0.05 were required on the experimental objective, then it would have to be partitioned across the two, separate, univariate hypotheses (questions) using Bonferonni or other appropriate techniques.

Therefore, each question could not be tested at the 0.05 level of significance. The other possible pair-wise comparison: 150 mg of X versus placebo is not a part of the study objective as stated. It may be investigated (preferably using a confidence interval), but it should not invoke a further penalty on the Type I error of the experiment. Further, the global test of the simultaneous comparison of the three regimens is not of direct interest.

Secondary efficacy objectives should not invoke a penalty on the Type I error associated with the primary efficacy objectives. It may be argued that each secondary objective can be addressed using a Type I error of 5%, provided inference via significance testing is preferred. Ninety-five percent confidence intervals represent a more informative alternative. Since the use of confidence intervals implies interest in estimates of true treatment differences, rather than interest in being able to decide whether true treatment differences are some prespecified values, confidence intervals are more consistent with a classification of secondary differences.

Safety objectives, unless they are the primary objectives, should not invoke a penalty on the Type I error associated with the primary efficacy objectives. It is uncommon that a study conducted prior to market approval of a new drug would have safety objectives that are primary. This does not mean that safety is not important. The safety of a drug, in the individual patient, and in groups of patients, is of utmost importance. Questions about safety are very difficult to answer in a definitive way in clinical development programs of a new drug. There are many reasons for this [3]. There may be insufficient information to identify safety endpoints and/or the target population, and inadequate budgets or numbers of patients. Clinical development programs of new drugs should be aggressively monitored for safety within and across trials, but designed to provide definitive evidence of effectiveness. This position is entirely consistent with the statutory requirements [4] for new drug approval in the United States.

4.4.2 Endpoints

After translating the study objectives into statistical questions, the data analyses section should contain a paragraph that identifies and discusses the choice of endpoints reflecting the objectives. It should be clearly stated as to which endpoints reflect primary efficacy, which reflect secondary efficacy, and which reflect safety. An endpoint may be the actual data collected or a function of the data collected. Endpoints are the analysis units on each individual patient that will be statistically analyzed to address study objectives. In an antihypertensive study, actual data reflecting potential efficacy are supine diastolic blood pressure measurements. Whereas it is informative to describe these data at baseline and at follow-up visits during the treatment period, inferential statistical analyses would be based upon the endpoint: change from baseline in supine diastolic blood pressure. Another endpoint of clinical interest is whether patients experienced a clinically significant reduction in supine diastolic blood pressure from baseline to the end of the treatment period. *Clinically significant* is usually defined as a decrease from baseline of at least 10 mmHg or becoming normotensive. Baseline blood pressure should be clearly identified and defined.

4.4.3 Statistical Methods

After specifying the endpoints, the statistical methods that will be used to analyze them should be indicated. The methods chosen should be appropriate for the type of endpoint; for example, parametric procedures such as analysis of variance techniques for continuous endpoints, and nonparametric procedures such as categorical data methods for discrete endpoints. Analysis methods should also be appropriate for the study design. For example, if the design has blocking factors, then statistical procedures should account for these factors. It is prudent to indicate that the methods stipulated will be used to analyze study endpoints, subject to actual data verification that any assumptions underlying the methods reasonably hold. Otherwise, alternative methods will be considered. The use of significance tests should be restricted to the primary efficacy questions (and then only if the study was designed from a sample size point of view to provide definitive answers). Otherwise, confidence intervals should be used. The method for constructing confidence intervals, particularly how the variance estimate will be determined, should be indicated.

Unless there are specific safety questions as part of the study objectives for which sample sizes with reasonable power to address them have been determined, it is usually sufficient to use descriptive procedures for summarizing safety data. Again this position is consistent with statutory requirements [4,5]. If inferential methods are to be used, Edwards et al. [6] provide a large variety, including examples.

The last portion of the statistical methods section should address what methods will be used to address generalizability of results across design blocking factors or across demographic or prognostic subgroups. Most clinical trials require several investigational sites or centers in order to recruit enough patients. Randomization of patients to treatment groups within centers is the standard practice. Therefore, centers represent a design blocking factor. Age, gender, and race, for example, if not stratification factors, would not be design factors. However, it is usually meaningful to explore the extent to which response to treatment is generalizable across such subgroups. Methods for generalizability include descriptive presentations of treatment effects across blocks or subgroups, a graphical presentation of confidence intervals on treatment differences across blocks or subgroups, and analysis of variance models that include terms for interaction between treatment and blocks or subgroups. The assessment of generalizability should follow the assessment of average drug effects across design blocks. If the results don't appear to be generalizable with respect to factors such as age, gender, race, etc., this should be reported, and the assessment of average drug effects redone with such factors appearing as covariates. The interactive effects of treatment group and such factors would not appear in this analysis model.

4.4.4 Statistical Design Considerations

As mentioned previously, sample size determination is considered a part of the overall statistical design of a protocol. Since the statistical analysis methods to be used to analyze the data collected for the protocol should be appropriate for the experimental design, justification for the choice of experimental design should be given. For example, if a crossover design was chosen, why is it appropriate for the disease under study? Then a thorough presentation of the basis for determining sample sizes should ensue. Statistical inferences (i.e., decisions with regards to whether the study objectives have been demonstrated) may be provided via hypothesis tests or via confidence intervals. These may require different sample size determination methods. Appropriate methods should be used.

The well-known per-group sample size (n) formula for parallel designs is

$$n \geq 2\left(\frac{s^2}{\delta^2}\right)[Z_\alpha + Z_\beta]^2 \qquad (4.1)$$

where
  s is an estimate of the standard deviation
  δ is the clinically important difference between groups that is to be detected
  Z_α and Z_β are the appropriate critical points of the standard normal
    distribution corresponding to the magnitudes of the Type I and II errors,
    respectively, or the tables of Fleiss [7] are usually sufficient for hypothesis testing methods based upon non-failure time data

Makuch and Simon [8], Westlake [9], or Bristol [10] provide confidence interval methods.

Hypothesis testing methods and confidence interval methods require estimates of endpoint means and variances of the control group. These estimates may be obtained from the literature or from previous studies. It is a good practice for the biometrics or biostatistics department to develop a file of such information from all studies of company compounds. In obtaining such information, care should be taken to make sure that the information is on a population similar to the target population of the study protocol. If no such information exists, it may still be possible, particularly for dichotomous endpoints, to determine sample sizes by using the worst case of the Bernoulli variance.

As is obvious from the previous sample size formula, sample size procedures also require a clinical specification of the difference (δ) between two comparative groups of interest that is clinically important to detect. For confidence interval procedures, the δ may be thought of as the bound on the allowable clinical difference. Hypothesis testing procedures require the Type I error and the Type II error or the power of the test to detect δ to be specified. Confidence interval methods require the confidence level (the complement of the Type I error) to be specified. They also require specification of either the maximum allowable length of the interval or the degree of certainty of the coverage of the allowable clinical difference.

Sample size determinations yield the estimated numbers of patients required for analyses of efficacy. As such, they represent the number of patients expected to complete or to be efficacy evaluatable. The number of patients, who should be enrolled into the clinical trials, are obtained by dividing the number required for the complete or efficacy evaluatable analyses by the expected proportions of those who enroll, who will complete, or will be evaluatable for efficacy.

In many clinical trials, the primary objective represents more than one question. Consequently, there will be more than one primary endpoint. To ensure that adequate numbers of patients will be enrolled, it is a good practice to compute the sample size required for each question, or endpoint, and then select the largest as the number to be enrolled, provided that all questions are of equal interest. Otherwise, use the number estimated to be adequate for the primary question, but assess the statistical power for this sample size relative to the other questions.

Most pre-market approval studies of new drugs are designed to provide answers to questions of efficacy. Therefore monitoring for efficacy while the study is in progress, particularly in an unplanned, ad hoc manner will almost always be seen to compromise the answers. If it is anticipated that the efficacy data will be looked at prior to study termination, for whatever reason, it is wise to include in the protocol an appropriate plan for doing this. The plan should address Type I error penalty considerations, what steps will be taken to minimize bias, and permit early termination.

The early termination procedure of O'Brien and Fleming [11] is usually reasonable. It allows periodic interim analyses of the data while the study is in progress, while preserving most of nominal Type I error for the final analysis upon scheduled study completion—provided there was insufficient evidence to terminate the study after an interim analysis. Other procedures such as Pocock's [12], or Lan and Demets' [13] may also be used. The paper [14] by the Pharmaceutical Manufacturer's Association (PMA) working group addressing the topic of interim analyses provides a good summary of the concerns about, and procedures for, interim analyses. The sample sizes for early termination, group sequential procedures, such as O'Brien and Fleming's, are determined as per fixed sample size procedures, and then this sample size is spread across sequential groups.

To summarize, the formal statistical basis for sample size determination requires (1) the question or objective of the clinical investigation to be defined; (2) the most relevant endpoints reflecting the objective to be identified; (3) the specification of the difference, δ, between groups in terms of the endpoint that is clinically important to be detected; (4) specification of the magnitudes of the Type I and Type II errors to be specified; and (5) the mean and variability of the endpoint to be estimated from the literature or from previous studies.

Parenthetically, sometimes instead of estimates of the mean and variance of the endpoint being available, an estimate of the coefficient of variation (CV) is. This may be particularly true in bioavailability or bioequivalence studies. The CV may be used instead of the mean and variance by expressing δ as a percent (of the mean). Once one has these ingredients, sample sizes may be determined rather easily.

4.4.5 Numbers in Phase I Program

For clinical trials in the Phase I program, there is no statistical basis for sample size determination. During this phase, only gross estimates of some of the characteristics of the drug are obtained. The number of patients in each Phase I trial is based largely on clinical and/or scientific judgment or comfort. Each trial will usually have from 4 to 24 subjects. The entire program is not likely to have more than 100 subjects. Statistically, it is desirable to have some replication within different dosing levels or under different experimental conditions.

4.4.6 Numbers in Phase II Program

For some trials in the Phase II program, there may be a statistical basis for sample size determination. For example, the data from the Phase I bioavailability or PK studies and from the acute pharmacology studies may provide pilot estimates for sample size determination for more detailed studies of these characteristics. Also, for some drugs, such as anticancer agents, some Phase IIA studies may be viewed as efficacy screens, in which case the single-arm plans of Burdette and Gehan [15], Schultz et al. [16], or Fleming [17] may be used. Further, if pilot estimates exist, it may be possible to statistically determine sample sizes for comparative Phase IIB studies, but it is doubtful that one would want to design such trials to have large power.

In Phase II, much is still not known about a new drug, and there is still the need to proceed cautiously. In Phase II, one is still trying to estimate characteristics of the drug. For single-arm Phase II trials, our practice has been to encourage use of the group sequential plans referenced earlier and/or group sequential estimation plans. The sequential use of groups of patients with relatively small numbers in each group is consistent with proceeding cautiously. For comparative Phase II trials, our practice has been to recommend a sample size based upon 50% power, if sufficient pilot information exists. Parenthetically, for dose–response or dose-comparison studies, the δ corresponds to the difference between the target dose (usually the middle dose) and placebo, and the one-sided Type I error critical point is determined similar to Williams' [18,19] approach. Otherwise, it is recommended that approximately 50 patients per treatment group arm (parallel design) be recruited, and assess a priori the statistical characteristics for this number of patients.

The typical Phase II program will recruit only a few hundred patients in the entire phase.

4.4.7 Numbers in Phase III Program

There is a statistical basis for sample size determination in the Phase III program. The Phase II program should provide estimates of dose and frequency of dosing for the Phase III definitive proof-of-efficacy trials, as well as provide estimates of means and variability for the primary endpoints associated with the dosing regimens.

For the pivotal proof-of-efficacy trials, our practice has been to determine sample size per treatment group sufficient to provide 95% power to detect the clinically important δ with a one-sided Type I error rate of 5%. For other Phase III studies, such as studies in special populations, a power of 50% is recommended.

In determining the sample size for a protocol with multiple questions, one must be able to decide whether the Type I error is an experiment-wise one that is to cover all questions and whether each question should be tested at some level less than 0.05, or whether each question may be tested at the 0.05 level. If for example there were three separate questions comprising the protocol objective and it was decided that the results of the study would be positive only if all questions were answered positively, then using a (Bonferonni) Type I error level of 0.0167 instead of 0.05 would provide a conservative basis for sample size estimation. To be even more conservative, if the endpoint is dichotomous, the worst case of the binomial variance may be used. One would probably want to err in this direction if the estimate of variability from previous studies was not very precise.

The typical Phase III program will recruit several hundred or a few thousand patients in the entire phase.

4.4.8 Other Sample Size Considerations

4.4.8.1 Relative Size of Trials and Detectable Differences

In the previous sections on numbers of patients in Phase II and Phase III trials, a 95% power was recommended for the definitive proof-of-efficacy trials and a 50% power for other trials. Many have responded when suggesting using 50% power, "but that is a coin toss, so why does it matter how many patients we have?" For symmetric null distributions, a power of 50% gives a value of 0 to the quantity Z_β in the sample size formula (Equation 4.1). Therefore, the sample size is basically being determined by the size of the Type I error, the estimate of variability, and the size of the difference δ between groups, which is clinically important to detect. By rewriting the formula, it is easy to see that it becomes the pooled-t statistic being greater than or equal to Z_α, that is, the decision rule for declaring δ to be statistically significant.

It is instructive to reflect the relative size of trials with power lesser than 95% to a trial with 95% power. Relative sizes corresponding to 50%, 75%, and 80% power are summarized in Table 4.1 for a two-sided and one-sided Type I error rate of 5%.

A trial with 50% power would be one-fourth the size of a trial with 95% power if a one-sided alternative hypothesis were used, and would be about 30% as large if a two-sided alternative were used. A trial with 75% power is about one-half the size of a trial with 95% power.

Many use a power of 80% with a two-sided alternative in determining sample size. Sizes of trials corresponding to 80%, 88%, and 95% power and a one-sided alternative relative to a trial with an 80% power and a two-sided alternative are summarized in Table 4.2 for a Type I error rate of 5%.

TABLE 4.1

Size of Trials with Power Less Than 95%
Relative to a Trial with 95%

Power Ratio	Relative Size (Two-Sided) (%)	Relative Size (One-Sided) (%)
50/95	29.6	25.0
75/95	53.5	49.7
80/95	60.0	57.1

TABLE 4.2

Size of Trials with One-Sided H_a
and Various Power Relative to a Trial
with 80% Power and a Two-Sided H_a

Sidedness Ratio	Relative Size (%)
1s80/2s80	79
1s88/2s80	100
1s95/2s80	139

For 80% power, if a one-sided alternative were used rather than a two-sided one, 21% fewer patients would be required. Trials of the same size would have a power of 88% rather than 80%., if a one-sided alternative were used instead of a two-sided one. A trial with 95% power and a one-sided alternative would require approximately 39% more patients than a trial with 80% power and a two-sided alternative.

A primary use of statistical power is in planning the necessary size of a study to be conducted, to detect a difference between groups that is of clinical importance. Often clinicians are overly optimistic in specifying the clinically important difference at the planning stage. It is instructive to reflect what kind of observed differences between groups, relative to the specified design clinically important difference δ, will be detectable as statistically significant once the trial has been completed and the data for analysis has been obtained. Sizes of the observed difference between groups as a percent of the design difference δ, which would be detected as statistically significant appear in Table 4.3 for various levels of power and for both two-sided and one-sided Type I error rates of 5%.

So a trial designed with 50% power to detect a difference δ will be able to detect as statistically significant ($P \leq 0.05$) an observed difference of δ (or larger), assuming that the number of patients who provide data for analysis is the same as that from the sample size determination. On the other hand, if the trial was designed with 95% power, an observed difference as small as 0.5δ would be detected as statistically significant. Strictly speaking, these results hold only if the variance in the observed data is the same as the estimate used in the sample size computation. If the variance in the observed data were smaller (greater) than that used for sample size estimation, then smaller (larger) δs than those in Table 4.3 would be detected as statistically significant.

Since in our experience, the design difference δ is usually larger than the observed difference, it is good practice to design definitive trials with power much larger than 50%. As has been indicated previously, our choice of power for such trials is 95%.

TABLE 4.3

Size of Observed δ between Groups, as a Percent of the Design δ That Can Be Detected as Statistically Significant ($P \leq 0.05$)

Power	Relative Size (Two-Sided) (%)	Relative Size (One-Sided) (%)
50	100	100
75	74	70
80	70	66
95	54	50

An exception to this recommendation occurs in the area of clinical trials conducted to support a Supplemental New Drug Application (SNDA). Here, two identical trials, each with 75% power may be conducted. Each of these trials is about one-half the size of a single trial with 95% power. Each would be expected to detect as statistically significant, a difference between groups as small as 70% δ. So there is a good chance that statistical significance will be reached in each trial, thereby rigidly satisfying the requirement of substantial evidence from two adequate and well-controlled trials. However, it should be indicated in the data analysis section of the protocol for each trial that both trials will be analyzed as a single multi-center trial. Even if not both individual trials reached statistical significance, but the combined trials did and the individual trials demonstrated reproducibility, this should be sufficient evidence of efficacy for approval of a SNDA. A demonstration of reproducibility in two trials, even though not both trials reach statistical significance, in our mind, is consistent with the scientific basis for requiring two trials. Obviously, the analysis of the combined trials would have to show statistical significance in order for one to claim that a drug effect had been established.

4.4.8.2 Three-Arm Efficacy Trial: Dose of New Drug, Placebo, and Dose of Marketed Drug

Often a Phase III trial is conducted comparing a new drug to placebo and to an active drug that is already on the market. One or several doses of the new drug may be studied. The trial discussed here will have only one fixed-dose group of the new drug. In a placebo-controlled, Phase III trial of a new drug, the question is about the (pure) efficacy of the new drug. In an active-controlled, Phase III trial of a new drug, the question is about the relative efficacy, or clinical equivalence on non-inferiority, of the new drug as compared to the active. Since the difference between the new drug and placebo ordinarily would be expected to be larger than the difference between the new drug and the active agent, thereby requiring fewer patients, the question arises as to what is a reasonable strategy with regard to sample size for the three-arm trial.

4.4.8.2.1 Strategy 1

It may be that the presence of the active control is to gain direct comparison information that can be used later for planning other studies, or for marketing purposes, and/or for an internal consistency check. The main objective is to prove that the new drug is effective, as compared to placebo. Thus, the sample size per group should be based upon the new drug versus placebo comparison. After the trial is completed, the inference concerning this comparison should be facilitated with the *P*-value whereas the inference concerning the comparison of the new drug to the active should be facilitated with a confidence interval.

4.4.8.2.2 Strategy 2

If equal or greater interest is in the comparison of the new drug to the active, then the number per group based upon comparing the new drug to the active, N_a, and the number per group for comparing the new drug to placebo, N_p, should be determined. The comparison of the new drug to placebo will be clearly over powered if N_a patients are enrolled in each of the three arms. On the other hand, enrolling N_p patients per each arm, while adequate for the new drug to placebo comparison, will clearly be underpowered for the new drug to active comparison. An alternative is to enroll N_a patients into the new drug and active arms, and N_p patients into the placebo. Since some power is lost in unbalanced allocation of patients to treatment groups, the power of the new drug to placebo comparison may be about what it would be in the balanced case. Of course exact computations can be made, and depending upon the size of N_a and N_p, it may be possible to enroll fewer than N_p patients into the placebo arm and still maintain the same power as N_p patients per arm would provide.

4.4.8.3 Interim Analyses

For more than 25 years, the first author has routinely recommended using group sequential, interim analysis procedures, such as those of O'Brien and Fleming [11] and Pocock [12], providing that recruitment relative to treatment, and resource allocation indicate that interim analyses are logistically feasible. Both procedures allow periodic interim analyses of the data while the study is in progress, and permit study termination at an interim analysis providing there is sufficient evidence of effect. The O'Brien and Fleming procedure preserves most of the Type I error for the final analysis upon scheduled study completion—providing there was insufficient evidence to terminate the study after an interim analysis. This means that very little of the Type I error is allocated at earlier interim analyses and consequently that treatment effects much larger than expected would have to be observed for study termination to occur early. Pocock's procedure allocates the Type I error equally across the planned number of interim analyses.

One advantage of group sequential procedures is that on average they will require fewer patients than fixed sample size procedures. This is consistent with use of the procedures in the hope of being able to terminate a trial early. Terminating a trial of a new drug compared to placebo early, when efficacy is established, rather than going to the planned completion is ethically appealing.

Other reasons why we have recommended rather routine use of group sequential procedures are as follows: (1) studies have to be monitored more closely; (2) data management, including data entry and quality assurance has to occur on an ongoing basis, and data queries have to be resolved quickly; (3) the efficacy evaluatability assessment criteria have to be determined prior to the case report forms coming in-house, and applied in an ongoing manner;

(4) report specifications have to be made prior to the study completion; and (5) statistical analysis programs have to be written and debugged prior to the first scheduled interim analysis. In other words, the technical aspects of good clinical research that one should be doing without incorporating interim analysis procedures have to be done when interim analysis procedures are incorporated. The difference is that we have to be more attentive and pro-active with respect to all operational aspects of the conduct of the trial, or else the main purpose for incorporating interim analysis will be defeated.

There are some disadvantages, which we believe are outweighed by the advantages. First, greater resources may be required. A trial incorporating three interim analyses and one final analysis, if not terminated early, will require more analysis and reporting resources than the same trial if interim analyses were not incorporated. Usually interim analyses are conducted on one or a few variables at each interim analysis, and analysis of the full study data is performed only if the decision is to terminate the trial early. Second, no inferential, interim analysis procedure would allow the full Type I error of 0.05 to be targeted to the final analysis if interim analyses were performed. Therefore for drugs with marginal effects, it may be that statistical significance could not be declared in a trial incorporating interim analyses, when significance could be found in the same trial with no interim analyses. It is good practice for trials in which interim analyses are to be incorporated to be designed with relatively large power. Third, if interim analysis plans are neither well developed nor executed, they may compromise study objectives.

Ideally, the group sequential, interim analysis plan would be included in the protocol. The sample size is determined as a fixed sample size and then spread across the number of analyses. For example, a two group trial with a dichotomous endpoint having 95% power to detect a 20% difference between groups will require approximately 150 patients per group for a total of 300 patients. If two interim analyses plus the possibility of a final analysis were planned, then the first analysis would occur after 100 patients had completed, the second (if necessary) after 200 patients had completed, and the third and last (if necessary) after 300 patients had completed.

Two issues other than sample size need to be addressed in the interim analysis plan: (1) preservation of the Type I error and (2) steps or procedures to minimize bias. The procedures of O'Brien and Fleming, and Pocock, among others if followed preserve the Type I error rate. Minimization of bias can also be achieved. In two separate programs, a NDA and a SNDA, interim analysis procedures were incorporated into the pivotal proof-of-efficacy trials and both applications are approved.

Potential bias was minimized by using an outside vendor. Identity of investigators and patients was concealed from in-house personnel by codes generated by the vendor. Although, of necessity, the data were split into the randomized groups, the groups were identified in random order using labels of A, B, C, and D, whose identity was known only by the vendor. The trials in both programs were dose comparison in nature. Therefore, the vendor, by using a procedure similar to Williams' [18,19], could assess whether significance was achieved and report this back to the sponsor without revealing the identity of each dose group. More about one of these programs will be said in the next section.

One other type of interim analysis, sample size re-estimation, deserves comment. When one is not very sure of the estimate of variability of the primary endpoint that was used to determine the sample size, accumulating data from the trial after it has started may be used to assess the sample size variability estimate, and adjustments to sample size made based upon whether it was an underestimate or an overestimate. Computer programs can be written to perform this exercise so that neither the sponsor nor the analyst has to know the identity of the treatment groups. In fact the data should not be separated into treatment groups for the purpose of looking at group averages. As long as this is done, no Type I error penalty needs to be paid. One reason for this is that from normal theory, the sample mean and sample variance are independent. Two papers on this topic, by Shih [20] and Pedersen and Starbuck [21] may be seen.

4.5 Examples

Four examples of clinical trials illustrating aspects of sample size determination are now considered. The first three trials involve the same formulation of a H_2-receptor antagonist. One trial was a dose-comparison trial, one was a bioequivalence trial, and the other was a trial in the elderly. The fourth example represents two identical dose-comparison trials of a synthetic PGE2 analogue.

The dose-comparison trial (see Chapter 12 for details) and the bioequivalence trial formed the basis of approval for a SNDA of a new formulation of the H_2-receptor antagonist as a single nighttime dose in the treatment of acute duodenal ulcer. The two identical dose-comparison trials formed the basis of approval of a NDA for the synthetic PGE2 analogue in the prevention of NSAID-induced gastric ulcers (see Chapter 13 for details) in osteoarthritic patients. All dose-comparison trials incorporated interim analysis procedures.

4.5.1 H_2-Receptor Antagonist Duodenal Ulcer SNDA Program

To illustrate the importance of numbers on the length of the clinical drug development process, consider three studies that comprised the major part of a program leading to the approval of a change in dosage (and form) of an already approved antiulcer drug. For the first of these studies [22], the original plan at the time of consultation with the biostatistician, called for two separate studies of 300 patients each. One study was to compare dose X to placebo, and the other was to compare dose 1.5 X to placebo. Together, the two studies were to recruit 600 patients at costs for investigators and patients of just over $4.5 million.

The biostatistician recommended (1) amalgamation of the two studies into one, with placebo, dose X, and dose 1.5 X groups, each with 164 patients; and (2) performing an interim analysis at mid-study. The interim analysis would have looked at the two effectiveness comparisons to placebo. If each was effective, then the entire study could be stopped—if effectiveness were the only question. However, if additionally, dose discrimination was of interest, then the placebo arm could be stopped, and the two dose groups run to completion. A conservative estimate of savings would be approximately $1.5 million in investigator and patient costs plus time required to conduct the study.

To make a long story shorter, the final study consisted of four groups: placebo, dose 1/2 X, dose X and dose 1.5 X, each with 164 patients per group. The doses used in the trial were multiples of the 1/2 X formulation, which was already marketed. The objectives were: (1) prove that dose X is effective; (2) prove that dose X is more effective than dose 1/2 X; and (3) establish that dose 1.5 X is no more effective than dose X. Effectiveness was measured as the proportion of patients whose ulcers had healed by the end of 4 weeks of treatment. The sample size of 164 patients per treatment group corresponded to a power of 95% to detect a difference in healing rates of 20% between dose X and placebo (which had an expected in-trial spontaneous healing rate of 50%) with a Type I error rate of 1.67%. Since the objective of the study consisted of three pair-wise comparisons, a Bonferonni approach was taken to split the 0.05 Type I error level across the comparisons. Although an interim analysis was planned and performed, which showed evidence of efficacy and dose–response, the study continued to recruit, and completed 771 patients from more than 50 investigational sites. The final analysis provided little beyond the interim analysis in terms of strength of evidence of effectiveness and dose–response findings. However, twice the amount of safety data was collected, which would not have been the case had the trial stopped early, and other results such as the relationship between healing and smoking habits and healing and ulcer size were better quantitated.

Two interesting aspects of the analyses of this trial should be pointed out. The first is that the interim analysis stopping rule was based upon comparing the target dose (X) to placebo (the primary objective), using William's [18,19] methodology. This approach preserves the Type I error and also permits concluding the existence of dose–response. The second is that analyses were also performed using a model that blocked on 12 cross-classifications of baseline ulcer size and smoking habits (instead of blocking on investigational site). In studies with large numbers of investigators, where one has measurements on strongly prognostic factors, it may be better to give up information on investigational site rather than on the prognostic factors.

The second of these studies was a blood level trial comparing the bioequivalence of a new formulation (Y), at dose X, to that of two doses of 1/2 X, in the marketed formulation. The study was conducted as a two-by-two crossover with 24 normal volunteers. This number corresponded to an 80% power to detect a 20% difference between the mean AUC of the new formulation and the marketed formulation with a Type I error rate of 5% and a coefficient of variation of 34%.

One volunteer dropped out of the study and was not replaced due to the concern that this would extend the date by which the submission could be made. Based upon the 23 subjects who completed the study, the relative bioavailability of the new formulation to the marketed formulation was ±19%; just within the acceptable bioequivalence range of ±20% (at that time). Had one less subject failed to complete or had the study been designed smaller, the study would have likely required to be repeated, thereby delaying the submission.

The third and last of these studies was a clinical trial comparing dose X to placebo in 100 elderly patients. During protocol development the biostatistician argued for a sample size of 0 (don't do the study) for this study as there would likely be enough elderly patients from other trials to examine clinical response in the elderly population. Prior to completion of the elderly protocol, a search of the database for the four-arm, dose-comparison trial discussed above found that among 101 elderly patients, 42 were on placebo or dose X. The comparison of these two groups revealed 95% confidence limits of 10.3%–75.6%, in terms of ulcer healing—evidence that dose X was effective in the elderly (It should be noted that since the elderly were a subset, treatment groups were compared at baseline and found comparable). The take-home message from this example is that a clinical trial may not be needed to answer every question of clinical interest, and conducting unnecessary trials may delay submissions.

4.5.2 Two Identical Studies in the Prevention of NSAID-Induced Gastric Ulceration

A few years ago, the first author had the responsibility of running a large-scale clinical research program of a synthetic prostaglandin (PGE2) analogue. Clinical and statistical evidence from the program formed the primary basis for NDA approval in the United States, of the drug in the prevention of NSAID-induced gastric ulcers in osteoarthritic patients requiring NSAIDs in the management of their arthritic symptoms.

The clinical research program consisted of two identical protocols. Osteoarthritic patients who had upper gastrointestinal (UGI) pain and who were without gastric ulcer upon endoscopic evaluation were randomized in balanced, double-blind fashion to either a placebo group, a 100 μg drug group, or a 200 μg drug group, and the placebo or drug administered four times daily. Patients were to return for follow-up endoscopy and other clinical evaluations after 4, 8, and 12 weeks of study medication administration.

The objectives of the protocols were (1) to demonstrate the effectiveness of the drug in the prevention of gastric ulcers and (2) to assess the effectiveness on UGI symptom relief.

The efficacy parameters were (1) prevention of ulcer development, as confirmed by endoscopy at weeks 4, 8, or 12; (2) UGI pain relief as derived from pain ratings recorded by the patient in a daily diary; and (3) relief of other UGI symptoms. Of these, the prevention of ulcer development was primary. Patients rated UGI pain according to the scales:

UGI day-pain rating scale:

0 = None = I had no abdominal pain

1 = Mild = I had some abdominal pain but it did not interrupt my normal activities

2 = Moderate = I had some abdominal pain sufficient to interrupt my normal activities

3 = Severe = I had severe disabling abdominal pain

UGI night-pain rating scale:

0 = None = I had no abdominal pain

1 = Mild = I had some abdominal pain but I went back to sleep

2 = Moderate = I had abdominal pain sufficient to keep me awake for long periods

3 = Severe = I had severe abdominal pain that kept me awake most of the night

The ratings were recorded on a diary that was provided by the sponsor as part of the case report forms. The diaries were collected at each follow-up visit.

Per-protocol sample size determinations revealed 450 evaluatable patients would be needed to address the primary objective. The numbers were determined on the basis of a 5% one-sided, Type I error rate and a 95% power to detect a 15% difference in ulcer development rates, given an expected ulcer rate of 25% in the placebo group.

The primary efficacy endpoint was the proportion of patients with ulcers by 12 weeks. The secondary endpoint was the proportion of patients without daytime or nighttime pain. The Mantel–Haenszel [23] or Fisher's exact test was (to be) used for statistical analyses of the endpoints.

No plans were provided in the protocol for any formal, statistical, interim analyses of the efficacy endpoints. We did however monitor the studies closely and aggressively computerized the data. We knew on a weekly basis, the status of the studies as to entry, completion, and ulcer development, without splitting the data into the three treatment groups. Table 4.4 summarizes such data at about the halfway point, during the conduct of the studies.

TABLE 4.4

Enrollment/Completion Status of Patients
at Study Midpoint

Protocol	Patients Entered	Patients Completed
1	275	132
2	253	130
1 and 2	528	262

Ignoring study and treatment group and based upon patient information in the computerized database, we noticed that the incidence of ulcer development may range from a crude rate of 8.4% to a worst-case rate of 27.4% (Table 4.5).

Parenthetically, comparable rates were also observed among patients whose case report form data had not yet been computerized (Table 4.6). However, all the ulcers could have been in one of the treatment groups. If this were the case, the incidence within that group could have been three times as high, or anywhere from 25.2% to 82.2%. We therefore felt compelled, on ethical grounds, to hold a meeting with the Food and Drug Administration (FDA) to discuss plans for performing an interim analysis of the studies, with the possibility of stopping the studies early.

TABLE 4.5

Ulcer Rates of Completed Patients in the Database

Patients	No Ulcer	Ulcer	Unknown	% Ulcer
215	156	18	41	8.4[a]
215	156	18	41	10.3[b]
215	156	18	41	27.4[c]

[a] Crude or best case estimate (an underestimate).
[b] Reduced estimate.
[c] Worst-case estimate (an overestimate).

TABLE 4.6

Ulcer Rates of Completed Patients Not
in the Computerized Database

Patients	No Ulcer	Ulcer	Unknown	% Ulcer
43	34	5	4	11.6[a]
43	34	5	4	12.8[b]
43	34	5	4	20.9[c]

[a] Crude or best case estimate (an underestimate).
[b] Reduced estimate.
[c] Worst-case estimate (an overestimate).

We met with the FDA and discussed the data, our procedures for stopping the trials, collecting any remaining data and statistical analyses. Among the information we presented at the meeting is that contained in Tables 4.4 through 4.8.

Table 4.7 reflects 215 patients with 18 ulcers being split in a reasonably balanced way across three treatment groups, with numbers of ulcers per group reflecting a reasonable, but perhaps conservative dose–response relationship. Table 4.8 reflects comparative analyses of the data in Table 4.7 using confidence intervals and Fisher's exact test (expected to be more conservative than the Mantel–Haenszel test).

It should be stressed that Table 4.7 represents a reasonable distribution of the total number (18) of ulcers under an assumption of dose proportionality. At the time of our meeting with the FDA, the blind had not been broken, nor had we separated the data according to blinded group labels. Since we had not planned to do a formal interim analysis at the protocol development

TABLE 4.7

Crude Ulcer Rates of Completed Patients in Database: Possible Grouping Reflecting Dose Proportionality

Group	Patients	No Ulcer	Ulcer	Unknown	% Ulcer
A	70	58	0	12	0.0[a]
B	71	53	6	12	8.5[b]
C	74	45	12	17	16.2[c]
All	215	156	18	41	8.4[d]

[a] Worst case = 17.1%, reduced estimate = 0%.
[b] Worst case = 25.4%, reduced estimate = 10.2%.
[c] Worst case = 39.2%, reduced estimate = 21.1%.
[d] Worst case = 27.4%, reduced estimate = 10.3%.

TABLE 4.8

Comparison of Ulcer Rates Based on Completed Prophylaxis Patients in Database: Possible Grouping Reflecting Dose Proportionality: *P*-Values and Confidence Intervals

Comparison[a]	% Difference	Std. Er.	90% CI[b]	*P*-Value[c]
B − A (BC)	8.5	0.033	3.1%; 13.9%	0.015/0.028
C − A (BC)	16.2	0.043	9.2%; 23.2%	0.000/0.000
B − A (WC)	8.3	0.069	−2.9%; 19.6%	0.162/0.304
C − A (WC)	22.1	0.073	7.9%; 36.3%	0.003/0.005
B − A (R)	10.2	0.039	3.7%; 16.7%	0.014/0.027
C − A (R)	21.1	0.054	12.2%; 30.0%	0.000/0.000

[a] BC, best case; WC, worst case; R, reduced.
[b] Normal approximation.
[c] Fisher's exact test (one-sided/two-sided).

stage, we wanted to make the case to the FDA that we should perform an interim analysis on ethical grounds, and if dose–response was observed, that we may be able to stop the studies early based upon a demonstration of prophylaxis efficacy. We wanted to be convincing that if an interim analysis was done, then it would be performed in a statistically valid, bona-fide manner.

There were three issues that received considerable discussion at the meeting with the FDA. These were (1) When to terminate the trials? (2) To what extent should blinding be maintained during the interim analysis? (3) At what Type I error level should we conduct the interim analysis?

Three possibilities were considered as to when termination would occur. We could terminate immediately; we could terminate based upon enrollment after 4 additional weeks; or we could continue entry until the interim analysis was completed and then decide on the basis of that analysis. The first two of these possibilities exact no penalty on the Type I error, provided we were prepared to live with the results. The third however, would, and is consistent with the philosophy for performing interim analyses.

Blinding considerations consisted of asking "to what extent should investigators, patients and company personnel be blinded as to the results of the interim analysis?" The primary concern was that if we failed to terminate the studies on the basis of the interim analysis results, the act of having performed the interim analysis would not compromise the study objectives.

As to the size of the Type I error for the interim analysis, we could take the O'Brien and Fleming approach and use 0.005 and if there was insufficient evidence to stop, allow the studies to continue to completion and conduct the final analysis at the 0.048 level. Another possibility was to use a two stage Pocock procedure that would allocate a Type I error of 0.031 to each stage. Yet another possibility was to conduct the interim analysis at the 0.01 level with the final analysis being conducted at a level determined as per Lan and Demets [13] or Peace and Schriver [24], if insufficient evidence existed for termination at the interim analysis.

The agency was receptive to us performing an interim analysis subject to us providing them with written plans. Such plans should address the three issues noted above, as well as any others that would reflect positively on the scientific and statistical validity of the exercise.

We developed and submitted the plan to the agency. We addressed blinding considerations during the interim analysis so as to minimize bias. We selected a Type I error rate of 0.01. Our stopping rule was as follows: terminate the trial if the P-value for the high dose group compared to placebo was less than or equal to 0.01. Parenthetically, it should be noted that the high dose being effective at the 0.01 level infers dose–response via an argument similar to Williams' [18,19]. In addition, the power of the combined interim analysis was about the same as each individual study at the design stage.

To make a long story shorter, we were able to terminate the trials, perform complete analyses, generate study reports, and compile the submission.

Even though the interim analysis was not planned at the protocol development stage, through attentive monitoring and taking a proactive approach to clinical trial/data management, we were able to recognize that an interim analysis was justified on ethical grounds. By working prospectively with the U.S. regulatory agency, a bona fide interim analysis was performed. This led to earlier termination of the program, and consequently, the submission was made and approved earlier than it otherwise may have been.

4.6 Philosophical Issues

In this section, five topics, which may be philosophical if not controversial, are considered. The first is what we've called "axioms of drug development [3]." The second is "sample size: efficacy or ethical imperative?" The third is "whether to have fewer but larger trials or greater but smaller trials [25]?" The fourth is one-sided versus two-sided tests [1,26–30]. The fifth is "amalgamation of Phase IIB and Phase III trials."

4.6.1 Axioms of Drug Development

One of the major goals of clinical research and development of a new drug is to accumulate sufficient evidence of its efficacy and safety. When this has been accomplished, the registrational dossier may be compiled and submitted for a regulatory marketing approval decision. The sequential nature of the phases of clinical development together with the desire to accumulate sufficient evidence of the efficacy (a statutory requirement) and safety of a new drug suggest two axioms [3] of clinical drug development.

> **Axiom 1**: Drugs in clinical development are considered inefficacious until proven otherwise.
>
> **Axiom 2**: Drugs in clinical development are considered safe until proven otherwise.

These axioms may be translated into null and alternative hypotheses as follows:

> **Axiom 1**: H_{0e}: the drug is not efficacious versus H_{ae}: the drug is efficacious
>
> **Axiom 2**: H_{0s}: the drug is safe versus H_{as}: the drug is not safe.

The clinical development of a new drug will proceed until which time the following decisions are reached: (1) it is declared unsafe (rejection of H_{0s}), or

(2) until it is declared inefficacious (acceptance of H_{0e}), or (3) until it is proven to be efficacious (rejection of H_{0e}) and it has not been declared unsafe. From the hypotheses constructs, the risk associated with decision (2) is a Type II error; and the risks associated with decisions (1) and (3) are Type I errors.

Decision (1) is not likely to be reached based upon statistical analyses, and more often than not, it will be made prior to reaching Phase III. Decision (2) could be reached in Phase II or Phase III, but most likely it will be reached in Phase IIB. Decision (3) would be reached in Phase III, and basically represents the goal of Phase III.

So basically, unless the new drug sponsor decides to curtail clinical development on the basis of safety concerns, and/or on the basis of inefficacy in Phase IIB, clinical development programs will proceed into Phase III, and continue until either H_{0e} is accepted or H_{0e} is rejected—decision (3) is reached. As has been discussed previously in this paper, the way decision (3) is currently reached is by having two adequate and well-controlled trials, both demonstrating statistical significance of drug effects.

It is appealing to develop inferential sequential, statistical procedures that would permit efficacy to be determined based upon the cumulative information on efficacy. If the information on safety at that time does not contradict H_{0s}, then let the regulatory dossier be filed, and hopefully reviewed and approved quickly.

At the time of termination of the development program based upon the demonstration of efficacy, it is unlikely that information would exist as to the optimal use of the drug. As a condition to approval, such studies could be conducted, and the labeling expanded. The attraction of this is that the drug would get on the market more quickly, and sales of the drug could begin funding research to learn more about the drug. The notion that adequate information on every possible characteristic of a drug has to be developed pre-market approval is unrealistic. After all, learning doesn't stop with submission of a regulatory dossier. Safety, for example, needs to be continuously monitored. The cumulative safety information that is available on a drug at one point in time is merely a snapshot of future safety information.

4.6.2 Sample Size: Efficacy or Ethical Imperative?

We design the Phase III pivotal proof-of-efficacy-trials with large power. Apart from good science, we do so because it is imperative that we prove efficacy. Therefore, we could think of the determination of sample size as being mandated by an efficacy imperative. However, should there also be an ethical imperative? For example, should anything be said in the informed consent section of the protocol about adequacy of the sample size to address a medically relevant question? How many patients would enter a trial if they knew that there was only a 10% power, say, to detect the minimal, clinically significant difference?

4.6.3 Larger versus Smaller Trials

Clinical development budgets are fixed (or at least finite). For a fixed budget, particularly for Phase III, a larger number of smaller trials could conceivably be conducted for the same costs, as could a fewer number but larger trials. Which is better? Suppose for arguments sake that the trials to be conducted will be of a new drug versus a control. Suppose further that whenever it is concluded based upon the results of a single trial, that the new drug is better than the control, the new drug will be added to the treatment armamentarium. The question "Which is better, fewer but larger trials, or greater but smaller trials?" may then be answered [cf. 26 and its references].

To do so, let (1) P denote the probability that a drug deemed superior from a clinical trial is in fact a superior drug; (2) α denote the probability of concluding a false positive result; (3) $1 - \beta$ denote the probability of concluding a true positive result; (4) and R denote the ratio of the average or expected number of false positive results (FPR) to true positive results (TPR). Now R may be written as

$$R = \frac{\text{Expected \#(FPR)}}{\text{Expected \#(TPR)}} = \left[\frac{1 - P}{P}\right] \times \left[\frac{(\alpha)}{(1 - \beta)}\right] \tag{4.2}$$

Table 4.9 reflects values of R for various values of $(1 - \beta)$ and P, for a Type I error rate (α) of 0.05.

The numbers within the parentheses to the right of the ratio values in Table 4.9, represent the percent of new drugs found superior to the control, which may be false positive results. For example, for new drugs with a value of $P = 0.05$, which have been deemed superior from controlled trials with a power of 40%, 70% may in fact be false positive results, rather than true positive results, This number becomes 20% for new drugs with a value of P of 0.20 and trials with 80% power.

One notes that R is small whenever P is large and/or power is large. We have no control over P (although it may be argued that having high quality drug discovery programs would produce candidate compounds with larger P than otherwise, as would insistence of total quality throughout the drug research and development phases) and it cannot be easily estimated [26].

TABLE 4.9

Values of R for Various Values of $(1 - \beta)$ and P for $\alpha = 0.05$

$1 - \beta$	P: 0.05	0.20	0.50
40%	2.38 (70%)	0.50 (33%)	0.13 (11%)
80%	1.19 (54%)	0.25 (20%)	0.06 (06%)
100%	0.95 (49%)	0.20 (17%)	0.05 (05%)

However, we have control over the power of a study. Therefore, in the setting discussed, it is better to have fewer but larger trials, rather than more but smaller trials.

4.6.4 One-Sided versus Two-Sided Tests

Whether to analyze data using one-sided or two-sided tests has stimulated a lot of debate. Readers may wish to review references [1,27–30]. Briefly, the authors' position is that the alternative hypothesis should embody the research question, both in substance and direction. Whether a one-sided or two-sided analysis or inference is appropriate should follow accordingly.

In clinical efficacy trials of a new drug, the research question is "is the drug efficacious?" Therefore, the alternative hypothesis is directional (one-sided), particularly for placebo-controlled trials. If the trial is a confirmatory pivotal proof-of-efficacy trial, a one-sided alternative is consistent with the trial being confirmatory. For it to be two-sided says at the design stage that you don't know what question you're trying to confirm. To use a two-sided P-value for inference at the analysis stage, theoretically presents a multiple range test type of problem. Therefore, logically the results can't be viewed as confirmatory.

We should also have internal consistency with respect to directionality. For example, suppose we have a dose–response trial with placebo, dose 1, and dose 2 of a new drug. The null and alternative hypotheses are H_{0e}: $P_0 = P_1 = P_2$ versus H_{ae}: $P_0 < P_1 < P_2$, where P_0, P_1, P_2 represent the probability of responding while on placebo, dose 1, or dose 2, respectively. If however, the trial could only be conducted with the highest dose and placebo, then the null and alternative hypotheses should be: H_{0e}: $P_0 = P_2$ versus H_{ae}: $P_0 < P_2$, rather than the alternative being H_{ae}: $P_0 \neq P_2$.

To operate with a two-sided 5% Type I error level in placebo-controlled efficacy trials of a new drug, is really operating with a 2.5% Type I error level.

4.6.5 Amalgamation of Phase IIB and Phase III Trials

In some areas of drug development, for example in the development of drugs to treat some forms of cancer, the primary response measure in the Phase IIB program is different from the primary response measure in the Phase III program. For patients with advanced stages of disease, the usual primary measure of efficacy in Phase IIB is response rate, whereas it is survival rate in Phase III. Typically, the Phase IIB and Phase III programs are conducted in different patients.

An alternative to this may be to design a large trial in which the goals of Phase IIB and Phase III are amalgamated. We might envision a multi-stage group sequential trial, in which the goals of Phase IIB are addressed in early stages and goals of Phase III are addressed in later stages.

It is unclear whether there has to be a Type I error penalty paid on addressing the Phase III goals for having addressed the Phase IIB goals. A reasonable strategy would be to design the trial as a Phase III trial with respect to sample sizes and allocate the 5% Type I error across the stages in which the goals of Phase III are addressed. Such a plan would appear to save at least the number of patients usually included in Phase IIB.

4.7 Concluding Remarks

The statistician, clinician, and upper management should understand that sample size estimation for pre-market approval studies is an important exercise. It should not be taken lightly nor as "game playing." However, one should realize that there is a need to balance numbers with practical considerations, but in so doing, all involved need to understand the risks involved by going with smaller rather than larger studies. For example, a truly efficacious drug may be discontinued from further clinical development due to the results from a small trial, when the problem is low power rather than true inefficacy.

In addition, all research should be conducted with a total commitment to quality, and with imaginative and creative research and development teams, who aren't merely satisfied with adhering to status quo, but who will also incorporate innovative approaches, which will lead to the shortest possibly time for safe and efficacious drugs to be marketed and available to patients.

Finally, we have not presented numerous examples of sample size determination, particularly the technical details. Rather, we have focused on the bases for sample size determination and suggested criteria for choosing sample sizes for clinical trials in the clinical development plan. For assistance with computational aspects, for a variety of trials and endpoints, the excellent book by Chow et al. [31] may be seen.

References

1. Peace KE (1989): The alternative hypothesis: One-sided or two-sided? *Journal of Clinical Epidemiology*; **42**: 473–476.
2. Hauck WW, Anderson S (1983): A new procedure for testing equivalence in comparative bioavailability and other trials. *Communications in Statistical Theory and Methods*; **12**: 2663–2692.
3. Peace KE (1987): Design, monitoring, and analysis issues relative to adverse events. *Drug Information Journal*; **21**: 21–28.

4. Food and Drug Administration (1987): New drug, antibiotic, and biologic, drug product regulations; final rule. 21 CFR Parts 312, 314, 511, and 514; **52**(53): 8798–8857; Thursday, March 19.

5. Food and Drug Administration (1988): *Guidelines for the Format and Content of the Clinical and Statistical Sections of New Drug Applications*, Center for Drugs and Biologics, Office of Drug Research and Review, Rockville, MD.

6. Edwards S, Koch GG, Sollecito WA (1989): Summarization, analysis, and monitoring of adverse events. In: *Statistical Issues in Drug Research and Development*, Peace, KE (ed), Marcel Dekker Inc., New York, pp. 19–170.

7. Fleiss J (1981): *Statistical Methods for Rates and Proportions*, 2nd edn., John Wiley & Sons, New York.

8. Makuch R, Simon R (1978): Sample size requirements for evaluating a conservative therapy. *Cancer Treatment Reports*; **62**: 1037–1040.

9. Westlake WJ (1988): Bioavailability and bioequivalence of pharmaceutical formulations. In: *Biopharmaceutical Statistics for Drug Development*, Peace, KE (ed.), Marcel Dekker Inc., New York, pp. 329–352.

10. Bristol DR (1989): Sample sizes for constructing confidence intervals and testing hypotheses. *Statistics in Medicine*; **8**: 803–811.

11. O'Brien PC, Fleming TR (1979): A multiple testing procedure for clinical trials. *Biometrics*; **35**: 549–556.

12. Pocock S (1977): Group sequential methods in the design and analysis of clinical trials. *Biometrika*; **64**: 191–199.

13. Lan KKG, Demets DL (1983): Discrete sequential boundaries for clinical trials. *Biometrika*; **70**: 659–670.

14. Pharmaceutical Manufacturers Association Biostatistics and Medical Ad Hoc Committee on Interim Analysis (1991): Interim analysis in the pharmaceutical industry. *Controlled Clinical Trials*; **14**: 160–173.

15. Burdette WJ, Gehan EA (1970): *Planning and Analysis of Clinical Studies*, Charles C. Thomas, Publisher, Spingfield, IL.

16. Schultz JR, Nichol FR, Elfring GL, Weed SD (1973): Multiple stage procedures for drug screening. *Biometrics*; **29**: 293–300.

17. Fleming TR (1982): One-sample multiple testing procedure for phase II clinical trials. *Biometrics*; **38**: 143–151.

18. Williams DA (1971): A test for differences between treatment means when several dose levels are compared with a zero dose control. *Biometrics*; **27**: 103–117.

19. Williams DA (1972): The comparison of several dose levels with a zero dose control. *Biometrics*; **28**: 519–531.

20. Shih WJ (1992): Sample size re-estimation in clinical trials. In: *Biopharmaceutical Sequential Statistical Applications*, Peace, KE (ed.), Marcel Dekker Inc., New York.

21. Pedersen R, Starbuck R (1992): Interim analysis in the development of and antiinflammatory agent: Sample size re-estimation and conditional power analysis. In: *Biopharmaceutical Sequential Statistical Applications*, Peace, KE (ed.), Marcel Dekker Inc., New York.

22. Valenzuela J, Dickson B, Dixon W, Peace KE, Putterman K, Young MD (1985): Efficacy of a single nocturnal dose of cimetidine in active duodenal ulcer. *Post Graduate Medicine*; **78**(8): 34–41.

23. Mantel N, Haenszel W (1959): Statistical aspects of the analysis of data from retrospective studies of disease. *Journal of the National Cancer Institute*; **22**: 719–748.

24. Peace KE, Schriver RS (1987): *P*-values and power computations in multiple-look trials. *Journal of Chronic Diseases*; **40**: 23–30.
25. Peace KE (1990): Regulatory or consumers risk (letter to the ed.). *Journal of Clinical Epidemiology*; **43**(9): 1013–1014.
26. Peace KE (1991): One-sided or two-sided *p*-values: Which most appropriately address the question of efficacy? *Journal of Biopharmaceutical Statistics*; **1**(1): 133–138.
27. Dubey S (1991): Some thoughts on the one-sided and two-sided tests. *Journal of Biopharmaceutical Statistics*; **1**(1): 139–150.
28. Fisher L (1991): The use of one-sided tests in drug trials: An FDA advisory committee member's perspective. *Journal of Biopharmaceutical Statistics*; **1**(1): 151–156.
29. Overall J (1991): A comment concerning one-sided tests of significance in new drug applications. *Journal of Biopharmaceutical Statistics*; **1**(1): 157–160.
30. Koch GG (1991): One-sided and two-sided tests and *P*-values. *Journal of Biopharmaceutical Statistics*; **1**(1): 161–169.
31. Chow S-C, Shao J, Wang H (2003): *Sample Size Calculations in Clinical Research*, 2nd edn., CRC Press, Taylor & Francis Publishing Group, Boca Raton, FL.

5

Sequential, Group Sequential, Stochastic Curtailment, and Adaptive Design Procedures in Clinical Trials

5.1 Introduction

Increasing use of statistical procedures that permit analyses of data collected in clinical trials prior to a trial reaching its preplanned conclusion has occurred over the last 30 years. Ideally, details of such procedures are incorporated into the protocol at the design stage. In doing so, the procedures from a statistical methodological point of view can be clearly presented. In addition, steps to be taken to ensure that by conducting such procedures the integrity of the trial will not be compromised, should also be clearly and unambiguously specified.

Basically such procedures permit the analyses of specified efficacy or safety endpoints as data accumulate over specified stages of a trial. Some of the more commonly used procedures are reviewed and discussed in this chapter. These include sequential procedures, group sequential procedures, stochastic curtailment procedures, and adaptive design methods.

5.2 Sequential Procedures

Two categories of sequential procedures should be distinguished. The first is applicable when conducting an experiment that produces outcomes (responses of interest) to experimental interventions prior to subjecting additional experimental units to the interventions. For a single intervention, the response of interest on a specific experimental unit would be known prior to enrolling the next experimental unit. For two interventions, responses on pairs of experimental units would be known prior to enrolling the next pair. Statistical theory applicable to this setting that permits sequential probability analyses of accumulating data with a view toward early termination is widely known; see, for example, Wald's sequential probability ratio test [1], Bross [2], Armitage [3,4], Armitage et al. [5], McPherson and Armitage [6], and Armitage [7,8].

In clinical trials, comparing interventions for the treatment of some disease, primarily due to staggered entry and the length of the intervention period, several patients are usually entered before data for analysis become available. Therefore, sequential methods of the above authors have not been widely incorporated into clinical trials. Sequential methods applicable to this clinical trial setting are referred to as group sequential or interim analysis procedures.

5.3 Group Sequential Procedures

Many authors have contributed to the evolution of group sequential or interim analysis procedures, for example, Colton and McPherson [9], Pocock [10], O'Brien and Fleming [11], McPherson [12], and Lan and DeMets [13]. Early termination rules may be formulated a priori using these methods, but a deeper understanding of group sequential procedures is gained by knowing how the associated P-values and power are computed; particularly if the trial is terminated based upon the results at an interim stage.

Detailed design, decision, and computational aspects of P-values and power for clinical trials in which group sequential procedures (i.e., interim analyses of accumulating data) are planned [14] appear in this section. Background theory and an application sufficient to understand and to illustrate the procedures are also presented. In addition, definitions of the term P-value and power, appropriate for a trial in which interim analyses are planned, are proposed.

5.3.1 Definitions

The definitions of P-value and power for a fixed-sample-size, single-stage (with no interim analyses) trial extend to trials with planned multistage, interim analyses. The definition utilizes their interpretation as rejection probabilities in a manner that reflects the sequential stages of the trial. First recall the definitions of the Type I and Type II errors associated with making a decision about a null hypothesis, H_0, versus a specific alternative hypothesis, H_a.

A Type I error occurs when a decision maker rejects H_0 when it is true. The magnitude of this decision error is typically denoted by α. A Type II error occurs when a decision maker fails to reject H_0 when it is false. The magnitude of this decision error is typically denoted by β. The *power* of a test of H_0 versus H_a, based upon the test statistic T, is defined to be the complement of the Type II error and is denoted by $1 - \beta$. So power is the probability of rejecting H_0 when H_0 is false—and should be rejected. (It should be pointed out that one utility of α, β, and T and the manner in which H_0 is false (H_a: $\delta \neq 0$), lies in the computation of the necessary sample size.)

The data collected would be summarized by the value t of the statistic T and H_0 rejected if t falls in the rejection or critical region (C). At the design stage, the critical region is determined from the probability distribution of T under H_0 and α. Alternatively, the P-value may be computed at the end of the trial and compared to α. If $P \leq \alpha$, then H_0 is rejected.

The term P-value abbreviates probability value and is invariably linked to significance testing. It is doubtful that the first use of the abbreviation is known. Fisher certainly used the term [15]. Toddhunter cites examples of significance testing in the eighteenth century [16]. A distinction should be made between significance testing and hypothesis testing. We reserve use of the term hypothesis testing for designed investigations, where the question of interest is embodied in H_a, and significance testing otherwise. It is noted that the statistical methods used to produce a P-value for designed investigations may be the same as those to produce P-values in unplanned or inadequately designed investigations or even in "data reduction"—which often occurs in preclinical investigations.

No doubt the term P-value was originally used in a fixed-sample experiment where the only analysis occurred after all data were collected. The computation of P-value involves finding the appropriate tail area(s) of the distribution of T under H_0. If rejection is desired for large values of T (a one-sided alternative with $\delta > 0$), then the P-value $P = P_r\,[T \geq t \mid H_0]$ (read: P equals the probability that T is greater than or equal to t given that H_0 is true). If the null hypothesis is true, P is the probability of observing the summary value t of the data or a value more extreme. If the test based upon T is a size α test, then P may be thought of as that portion of α that reflects the strength of the data against H_0, providing $P \leq \alpha$. It is clear that P is a rejection probability.

Group sequential trials are generally designed from a sample size viewpoint as a fixed-sample-size trial. Then group sequential methodology is used to specify the *interim analysis plan*; i.e., the decision rules for reacting to analyses of the data at the various stages. Typically, decision rules for a group sequential trial with k-analysis stages may be formulated as follows:

Stage 1: Reject H_0 if t_1 falls in C_1 and stop; else continue to

Stage 2: Reject H_0 if t_2 falls in C_2 and stop; else continue to...

Stage k: Reject H_0 if t_k falls in C_k; else stop and do not reject;

where C_i is the critical region associated with the test procedure and t_i is the value of the test statistic T based on all the data at the ith analysis stage, $i = 1, 2, \ldots, k$. Whether the trial proceeds to a subsequent stage is conditional on the outcome at the current stage. If the trial is terminated at an interim analysis stage, say r, then one knows that t_1 did not fall in C_1, t_2 did not fall in

$C_2, \ldots, t_{r-1}$ did not fall in C_{r-1}, and t_r fell in C_r. In this case, one knows intuitively that the *overall P-value $P_r \leq \alpha$* and that it is a rejection probability. Further P_r reflects the strength of the data as observed and summarized through T against H_0. It is the sum of contributions from each of the r stages and is written as $P_r = P_1 + P_{2.1} + \cdots + P_{r(r-1)\ldots1}$.

It is the probability of observing the components of the vector $(t_1, t_2, \ldots, t_r)$ *sequentially*. Under H_0, P_1 is the probability of observing t_1 or a more extreme value $(T \geq t_1)$; $P_{2.1}$ is the probability of observing a value less extreme than t_1 $(T < t_1)$, and observing t_2 or a more extreme value; $\ldots$; $P_{r(r-1)\ldots1}$ is the probability of observing a value less extreme than t_1, and observing a value less extreme than t_2, and, $\ldots$, and observing a value less extreme than t_{r-1}, and observing t_r or a value more extreme.

The functional form of T is the same at each analysis stage. It is a function of all the data at the rth analysis stage and may be expressed as a function of its forms at earlier analysis stages, denoted by $T_1, T_2, \ldots, T_{r-1}, T_r$. The computation of P_1 proceeds as in the single-stage trial. Computations of the remaining contributions to P_r require finding the appropriate content from the joint null distribution of the test statistics T_i. This involves the evaluation of multiple integrals or multiple sums depending on whether the null distribution is continuous or discrete.

In a single-stage, fixed-sample-size trial, the computation of power involves finding the appropriate tail area of the distribution of the test statistic under H_a. For $\delta > 0$, $1 - \beta = P_r[T \geq Z_\alpha \mid \delta]$, where Z_α determines the critical region of size α. If a multistage trial is not terminated prior to the rth analysis stage, the overall power $(1 - \beta)_r$ will consist of contributions from each stage, and is written as

$$(1 - \beta)_r = (1 - \beta)_1 + (1 - \beta)_{2.1} + \ldots + (1 - \beta)_{r(r-1)\ldots1}$$

Under H_a, $(1 - \beta)_r$ is the probability of T_1 falling in C_1, $(1 - \beta)_{2.1}$ is the probability of T_1 falling out of C_1 and T_2 falling in $C_2, \ldots$, and $(1 - \beta)_{r(r-1)\ldots1}$ is the probability of T_1 falling out of C_1 and T_2 falling out of C_2 and $\ldots$ and T_{r-1} falling out of C_{r-1} and T_r falling in C_r.

The computations of the individual contributions to the overall power are similar to those of the corresponding contributions to the overall P-value.

5.3.2 Computational Aspects of the Contributions from Each Planned Interim Analysis to Overall P-Value and Power

The case for $k = 3$ for a one-sided alternative H_a: $\delta > 0$ and for statistics with continuous distributions is presented. Extending the results to two-sided alternatives and $k > 3$ is straightforward. The methodology for statistics with discrete distributions may be obtained by performing summation operations instead of the integration operations. The contributions to the *overall P-value* are

$$P_1 = \int_{t_1}^{\infty} f(t_1)dt_1,$$

$$P_{2.1} = \int_{-\infty}^{t_1} \int_{t_2}^{\infty} f(t_1, t_2)dt_2 dt_1,$$

and

$$P_{3.12} = \int_{-\infty}^{t_1} \int_{-\infty}^{t_2} \int_{t_3}^{\infty} f(t_1, t_2, t_3)dt_3 dt_2 dt_1,$$

where under H_0, $f(t_1)$ is the probability density of T_1, $f(t_1, t_2)$ is the joint (bivariate) probability density of (T_1, T_2), and $f(t_1, t_2, t_3)$ is the joint (trivariate) probability density of (T_1, T_2, T_3). Values of P_1, $P_{2.1}$, and $P_{3.12}$ may be obtained from the cumulative distribution functions of T_1, (T_1, T_2) and (T_1, T_2, T_3) if they exist in closed form, or if they have been sufficiently tabulated, or by using numerical integration techniques.

In clinical trials, particularly those designed to provide definitive evidence of efficacy, sample sizes are usually sufficiently large to draw on central limit theory. This permits the distribution of T to be viewed as normal, and the distribution of (T_1, T_2, T_3) to be viewed as multivariate normal.

Now the *computation of P_1* is straightforward. It is the area in the tail of the normal density (with mean μ and σ_1^2). The density may be standardized by the transformation $z_1 = (t_1 - \mu)/\sigma_1$. Thus $P_1 = \int_{z_1}^{\infty} \phi(w_1)dw_1 = 1 - \varphi(z_1)$, where ϕ and φ are the normal zero-one density and distribution functions, respectively. These are extensively tabulated and are available in elementary statistics texts and computer software programs.

In order to compute $P_{2.1}$, the double integral of the bivariate normal density of (T_1, T_2) over the region $T_1 < t_1$ and $T_2 < t_2$ must be evaluated. If stages 1 and 2 were independent, then T_1 and T_2 would be also, $\rho_{12} = 0$ and $P(t_1, t_2) = P(t_1)p(t_2)$. Consequently, the double integral could be evaluated as the product of two single integrals; i.e., $P_{2.1} = \phi(z_1)(1 - \phi(z_2))$, where $z_2 = (t_2 - \mu)/\sigma_2$. However, stages 1 and 2 are not independent (T_2 is a function of the data used in T_1, plus the data on patients available between the two stages). So the double integral would have to be evaluated or tables of the bivariate normal distribution used. Some tables [17] exist. However, the numerical evaluation can be accomplished by expressing the double integral as a single integral. This latter integral is instructive in that it reflects the nature of the dependence of stages 1 and 2.

To *compute* $P_{2.1}$, write $P(t_1, t_2)$ as $P(t_1)P(t_2 \mid t_1)$, and transform T_1 and $T_2 \mid T_1 = t_1$ by z_1 and

$$z_{2.1} = \frac{(t_2 - \mu_{2.1})}{\sigma_{2.1}} = \left[\frac{t_2 - \{\mu_2 + (\sigma_2\rho_{12})z_1\}}{\sigma_{2.1}} \right] = \frac{\sigma_2(z_2 - \rho_{12}z_1)}{\sigma_{2.1}},$$

where $\sigma_{2.1}$ is the positive square root of $\sigma_{2.1}^2$. With these transformations, $P_{2.1}$ becomes

$$P_{2.1} = \int_{-\infty}^{z_1} \int_{z_{2.1}}^{\infty} \varphi(w_2 \mid w_1)\phi(w_1)dw_2dw_1 \quad p_{2.1} = \int_{-\infty}^{z_1} \{1 - \varphi(z_{2.1})\}\phi(w_1)dw_1,$$

upon iterating the integral. Note that $z_{2.1} = \sigma_2(z_2 - \rho_{12}z_1)/\sigma_{2.1}$. Thus the value of $\{1 - \varphi(z_{2.1})\}$ is dependent not only on the value t_2 of the test statistic T at the second stage, but also on the value t_1 at the first stage.

The *computation of* $P_{3.12}$ is similar to that of $P_{2.1}$. The integral of the trivariate normal density has to be evaluated:

$$P_{3.12} = \int_{-\infty}^{z_1} \int_{-\infty}^{z_{2.1}} \int_{z_{3.12}}^{\infty} \phi(w_3 \mid w_1, w_2)\phi(w_2 \mid w_1)\phi(w_1)dw_3dw_2dw_1.$$

This is accomplished by numerically evaluating a double integral—that reflects the dependence of the analysis at the third stage upon the analyses at the first two stages.

To obtain this latter integral, $P(t_1, t_2, t_3)$ is expressed as $P(t_1)P(t_2 \mid t_1)P(t_3 \mid t_1, t_2)$. Then $T_1, [T_2 \mid T_1 = t_1]$ and $[T_3 \mid T_1 = t_1 \text{ and } T_2 = t_2]$ are standardized using the transformations

$$z_1 = \frac{(t_1 - \mu)}{\sigma_1},$$

$$z_{2.1} = \frac{(t_2 - \mu_{2.1})}{\sigma_{2.1}}$$

$$z_{3.12} = \frac{(t_3 - \mu_{3.12})}{\sigma_{3.12}} = \left[\frac{t_3 - \{\mu + \sigma_3 az_1 + \sigma_3 bz_2\}}{\sigma_{3.12}} \right] = \sigma_3 \frac{(z_3 - az_1 - bz_2)}{\sigma_{3.12}}$$

where $z_3 = (t_3 - \mu)/\sigma_3$, $a = (\rho_{13} - \rho_{12}\rho_{23})/(1 - \rho_{12}^2)$, $b = (\rho_{23} - \rho_{12}\rho_{13})/(1 - \rho_{12}^2)$, $\sigma_{3.12} = \sigma_3(1 - a\rho_{13} - b\rho_{23})^{1/2}$, and where ρ_{ij} is the correlation between T_i and T_j. This yields

$$P_{3.12} = \int_{-\infty}^{z_1} \int_{-\infty}^{z_{2.1}} \int_{z_{3.12}}^{\infty} \phi(w_3 \mid w_1, w_2)\phi(w_2 \mid w_1)\phi(w_1)dw_3dw_2dw_1;$$

which may be written as

$$P_{3.12} = \int\limits_{=\infty}^{z_1} \int\limits_{-\infty}^{z_{2.1}} \{1 - \varphi(z_{3.12})\}\phi(w_2 \mid w_1)\phi(w_1)dw_2 dw_1,$$

upon iterating the integral. The above integral with the transformations $z_1, z_{2.1}$, and $z_{3.12}$ reflects the interdependence of the three analysis stages.

The computation of the **overall power** closely parallels that of the overall *P*-value. Formally, the differences are that the density under the alternative hypothesis replaces the density under the null hypothesis and the critical points of the boundaries of the critical regions replace the t_i. In clinical trials comparing two treatments, H_0 reflects $\mu = \delta = 0$ and H_a reflects $\mu = \delta$. In this setting under normal theory, the alternative distribution of (T_1, T_2, T_3) is multivariate normal with mean vector (δ, δ, δ) and variance–covariance matrix Σ.

The **boundary points of the critical regions** may be found using Pocock [10] or O'Brien and Fleming [11] methodology or that of many others. They may also be found by the method described herein for computing the overall *P*-value. In doing this the experimenter would have to specify the partitioning of α (note that National Bureau of Standards [18] refer to this as the spending function approach) into additive components:

$$\alpha = \alpha_1 + \alpha_{2.1} + \cdots + \alpha_{k(k-1)\ldots 1}.$$

The relative size of the components would reflect whether there was a preference for being able to stop earlier rather than later or vice versa or whether there was indifference.

After the components are specified, the critical point c_1 for the first critical region is obtained as in the single-stage, fixed-sample-size trial. That is, for $\delta > 0, c_1$ satisfies

$$\alpha_1 = 1 - \varphi\left\{\frac{(c_1 - \mu)}{\sigma_1}\right\} = 1 - \varphi\left(\frac{c_1}{\sigma_1}\right).$$

The critical point c_2 for the second critical region satisfies

$$\alpha_{2.1} = \int\limits_{-\infty}^{c_1/\sigma_1} \{1 - \varphi(z_2)\}\phi(w_1)dw_1,$$

where $z_2 = \left\{(c_2/\sigma_2 - \rho_{12}w_1)/(1 - \rho_{12}^2)^{1/2}\right\}$. The integral may be solved numerically with respect to c_2 provided σ_1, σ_2, and ρ_{12} are known, specified or determinable. Similar integrals permit the determination of c_k for $k > 2$.

5.3.3 A Three-Stage, Two-Treatment Trial

To illustrate the determination of the critical regions and P-value and power computations, a clinical trial with three planned analysis stages comparing the effects, τ_A and τ_B, of treatments A and B is considered. The statistic T_i is $\overline{X}_{Ai} - \overline{X}_{Bi}$, where $\overline{X}_{Ai}(\overline{X}_{Bi})$ denotes the mean of the response variable measured on each of the N_i individuals on treatment A (B) available at the ith analysis stage, $i = 1, 2, 3$. The distribution of $X_{Ai}(X_{Bi})$ is assumed normal with mean μ and variance σ^2. Thus the distribution of T_i is normal with mean $\mu_i = \mu = \tau_A - \tau_B = \delta$ and variance $\sigma_i^2 = 2\sigma^2/N_i$. From Section 5.3.2, (T_1, T_2, T_3) is multivariate normal with mean vector (δ, δ, δ) and variance–covariance matrix Σ, which may be expressed as

$$\Sigma = \begin{bmatrix} 1 & (1+r)^{-1} & (1+r+s)^{-1} \\ (1+r)^{-1} & (1+r)^{-1} & (1+r+s)^{-1} \\ (1+r+s)^{-1} & (1+r+s)^{-1} & (1+r+s)^{-1} \end{bmatrix} \cdot \frac{2\sigma^2}{N},$$

where $N = N_1, (1+r)^{-1} = N/N_2$, and $(1+r+s)^{-1} = N/N_3$. For this variance–covariance structure, it may be shown that

$$\rho_{12} = (1+r)^{-1/2} = \left(\frac{N}{N_2}\right)^{-1/2},$$

$$\rho_{13} = (1+r+s)^{-1/2} = \left(\frac{N}{N_3}\right)^{-1/2},$$

$$\rho_{23} = (1+r)^{1/2}(1+r+s)^{-1/2} = \left(\frac{N}{N_2}\right)^{-1/2} \times \left(\frac{N}{N_3}\right)^{-1/2},$$

$$1 - \rho_{12}^2 = r(1+r)^{-1} = \left(1 - \frac{N}{N_2}\right),$$

$$a = 0,$$

and

$$b = (1+r)^{1/2}(1+r+s)^{-1/2} = \rho_{23},$$

where the general form of a and b appear in Section 5.3.2.

The transformation equations of Section 5.3.2 become

$$Z_i = \frac{(t_i - \delta)}{\sigma_i}; \quad i = 1, 2, 3,$$

$$Z_{2.1} = \frac{(Z_2 - \rho_{12}Z_1)}{(1 - \rho_{12}^2)^{1/2}} = r^{-1/2}\left\{(1 + r)^{1/2}Z_2 - Z_1\right\}$$

$$= \left\{\frac{N_1}{(N_2 - N_1)}\right\}^{1/2}\left\{\left(\frac{N_2}{N_1}\right)^{1/2}Z_2 - Z_1\right\},$$

and

$$Z_{3.12} = \frac{(Z_3 - \rho_{23}Z_2)}{(1 - \rho_{23}^2)^{1/2}}$$

$$= s^{-1/2}\left\{(1 + r + s)^{1/2}Z_3 - (1 + r)^{1/2}Z_2\right\}$$

$$= \left\{\frac{N_1}{(N_3 - N_2)}\right\}^{1/2}\left\{\left(\frac{N_3}{N_1}\right)^{1/2}Z_3 - \left(\frac{N_2}{N_1}\right)^{1/2}Z_2\right\}.$$

In the case of equal numbers ($r = s = 1$ or $N_2 = 2N_1$ and $N_3 = 3N_1$) of observations between analysis stages, $Z_{2.1} = \sqrt{2}Z_2 - Z_1$ (note: $\sqrt{2}Z_2 = $ square root of 2 times Z_2), and $Z_{3.12} = \sqrt{3}Z_3 - \sqrt{2}Z_2$.

For this case, the critical point, c_1, for the first planned interim analysis satisfies $1 - \Phi(c_1/\sigma_1) = \alpha_1$; the critical point, c_2, for the second planned interim analysis satisfies

$$\int_{-\infty}^{c_1/\sigma_1}\left[1 - \Phi\left\{\left(\frac{\sqrt{2}c_2}{\sigma_2}\right) - w_1\right\}\Phi(w_1)dw_1\right] = \alpha_{2.1};$$

and the critical point, c_3, for the third or final planned analysis satisfies

$$\int_{-\infty}^{u_1}\int_{-\infty}^{u_{2.1}}\left[1 - \Phi\left\{\left(\frac{\sqrt{2}c_3}{\sigma_3}\right) - \sqrt{2}w_2\right\}\Phi(w_2)\Phi(w_1)dw_2dw\right] = \alpha_{3.12},$$

where $u_1 = c_1/\sigma_1$ and $u_{2.1} = (\sqrt{2}c_2/\sigma_2) - u_1$. The above equations for determining c_i contain σ_i, which is $\sqrt{2}\sigma/\sqrt{N}$, so that knowledge of σ is required. This may be dodged by solving iteratively for $c_i^* = c_i/\sigma_i$ instead of for c_i; then $c_i = c_i^*\sigma_i$.

The above equations for determining c_i may also be used for determining the contributions to the overall P-value. Formally, c_i would be replaced by t_i, α would be replaced by P, and the resulting integrals evaluated. The common population standard deviation would have to be specified in these evaluations.

In addition, the above equations for determining c_i may also be used to determine the contributions to the overall power. Formally, c_i would be replaced by $(c_i - \delta)$, α would be replaced by $(1 - \beta)$, and the resulting integrals evaluated; σ would also have to be specified in these evaluations.

5.3.4 Application

An application of the methods discussed for a clinical trial comparing two treatments with a total of three stages (note that only the first two stages would reflect "interim" analyses) is presented. Three cases are presented. The first uses the conditional partitioning of α [14] referred to as alpha spending by DeMets and Lan [17] method. The second uses the Pocock [10] method. The third uses the O'Brien/Fleming method [11].

The **design of a trial** incorporating group sequential decision rules usually begins with determining the number of patients required to detect a clinically important treatment effect (δ) with specified magnitudes of the Type I and Type II errors using single testing procedures. For the application considered, 135 patients in each treatment group are needed to detect a 20% treatment group difference in terms of proportions of patients responding, with a Type I error of 5% and a power of 95%, and an expected response rate of 40% in the control treatment group. The sample size formula based on the normal approximation of the binomial was used. The approximation is known to be good for response rates in the 40%–60% range. The estimate of sample size is conservative $\{\sigma^2 = 0.50$ instead of $\sigma^2 = p_1(1 - p_1) + p_2(1 - p_2) = (0.4)(0.6) + (0.6)(0.4) = 0.48\}$. Parenthetically, our practice for many years has been to use the worst case of the binomial variance when designing clinical trials with dichotomous primary efficacy endpoints, particularly Phase III pivotal proof of efficacy trials.

The **total possible number of stages** or planned group sequential analyses is then decided ($k = 3$ in the application considered). Then the **number of patients between stages** (to be accrued and available for analysis) or the total to be accrued and available at the time of the analysis at each stage is specified. The number to be accrued between each stage is usually taken as the single testing sample size number divided by the total number of planned stages ($135/3 = 45$ for the application considered). Departures from such balance are possible. Next, the **nominal critical point** (NCP) is specified for each stage. Finally, the **decision rules are formulated in terms of the NCPs**.

5.3.4.1 Conditional Partitioning of α or α Spending Method

The NCPs for the conditional partitioning of α approach are determined by a computational program that solves the integral equations of Section 5.3.3 (involving $\alpha_1, \alpha_{2.1}, \alpha_{3.12}$) for the C_i (or for the C_i/σ_i). This requires the clinical team to choose the appropriate values of the $\alpha_1, \alpha_{2.1}, \alpha_{3.21}$. The values chosen for this application reflect partitioning of the overall Type I risk into equal conditional Type I risks ($\alpha_1 = 0.02, \alpha_{2.1} = 0.02$) at the interim stages that were twice that of the conditional Type I risk ($\alpha_{3.21} = 0.01$) at the final stage.

TABLE 5.1

Design Aspects of a Three-Stage Trial: Conditional Partitioning of α

Analysis Stage	N_i[a]	Variance[b]	α[c]	α[d]	C_i/σ_i[e]	C_i	Power[f]
1	45	0.5/45	0.0200	0.0200	2.054	0.2165	0.4384
2	90	0.5/90	0.0200	0.0278	1.914	0.1427	0.3582
3	135	0.5/135	0.0100	0.0221	2.012	0.1224	0.1231
Group sequential total	135		0.0500	0.0699			0.9197
Fixed total	135	0.5/135	0.0500	0.0500	1.645	0.1000	0.9500

[a] Number (N_i) of treated patients planned in each group at each stage.
[b] Variance $= \sigma^2 = 0.5/N_i$ when the true response rate in the common referenced population is 0.5 (conservative estimate).
[c] Conditional Type I error allocated to each stage; symbolically $\alpha_{r(r-1)(r-2)}$.
[d] Nominal Type I error at each stage.
[e] Standardized normal deviate.
[f] Conditional on not stopping at the earlier stage; symbolically, $(1 - \beta)_{r(r-1)(r-2)}$.

Table 5.1 summarizes all planning aspects of the trial, the results of determining the C_i, the contributions to the overall P-value, and the contributions to the overall power. The contributions to P_r and $(1 - \beta)_r$ in the application were computed using a computer program written by Robert Schriver [19].

The conditional nominal Type I risks at stages 1, 2, and 3 (column 5) are 0.02, 0.0278, and 0.0221, respectively. The conditional power (CP) (last column) at each stage, computed as discussed in Section 5.3.3, is 0.4384, 0.3582, and 0.1231, respectively.

To reflect decision aspects, suppose the trial continues to the second stage and suppose that by the second stage 49 of 90 patients on treatment A responded and 36 of 90 patients on treatment B responded for an observed difference of 14.44% in response rates. Using the decision rules from the conditional partitioning of α approach, statistically there would be a basis for stopping the trial; i.e., 14.44% is greater than 14.27%. Logically the P-value would be <0.04 $(0.02 + 0.02)$. When computed, it is found to be 0.0393.

5.3.4.2 Pocock's Method

To obtain the NCPs for Pocock's procedure [10], enter his Table 1, p. 193, with the total number of planned stages, read off the nominal significance levels (NSLs), and convert the NSLs to the corresponding normal deviates. Table 5.2 summarizes design aspects of the trial if Pocock's method is used. The conditional Type I risks (column 4) are 0.0221, 0.0221, and 0.0221 and the CP (last column) are 0.4550, 0.3190, and 0.1433, respectively, at stages 1, 2, and 3.

5.3.4.3 The O'Brien/Fleming Method

For O'Brien and Fleming's procedure [11], enter their Table 1, p. 551, with the number of planned stages, reading off the value of the quantity $p(N, \alpha)$

TABLE 5.2

Design Aspects of a Three-Stage Trial: Pocock's Method

Analysis Stage	$N_i{}^a$	Variance[b]	α^c	$C_i/\sigma_i{}^d$	C_i	Power[e]
1	45	0.5/45	0.0221	2.012	0.2100	0.4550
2	90	0.5/90	0.0221	2.012	0.1500	0.3190
3	135	0.5/135	0.0221	2.012	0.1224	0.1433
Group sequential total	135		0.0663			0.9173
Fixed total	135	0.5/135	0.0500	1.645	0.1000	0.9500

[a] Number (N_i) of treated patients planned in each group at each stage.
[b] Variance $= \sigma^2 = 0.5/N_i$ when the true response rate in the common referenced population is 0.5 (conservative estimate).
[c] Nominal Type I error at each stage.
[d] Standardized normal deviate.
[e] Conditional on not stopping at the earlier stage; symbolically, $(1 - \beta)_{r(r-1)(r-2)}$.

and substituting it into the formula on p. 552. The formula produces (nominal) decision rules in terms of a 1 *df* chi-square statistic of which the square root is the absolute value of a standard normal deviate. The formula may incorporate unequal numbers of patients between stages. Table 5.3 summarizes design aspects of the trial if the O'Brien/Fleming method was used. The conditional Type I risks (column 4) are 0.0016, 0.0184, and 0.0441 and CP (last column) are 0.1459, 0.5808, and 0.2197, respectively, at stages 1, 2, and 3.

5.3.4.4 Minimum Detectable Difference

The element in the C_i column in the bottom rows of the Tables 5.1 through 5.3 reflects the fact that a fixed-sample-size trial, designed as the one discussed to

TABLE 5.3

Design Aspects of a Three-Stage Trial: O'Brien/Fleming's Method

Analysis Stage	$N_i{}^a$	Variance[b]	α^c	$(C_i{}^2/\sigma_i{}^2)^d$	C_i	Power[e]
1	45	0.5/45	0.0016	8.721	0.3113	0.1459
2	90	0.5/90	0.0184	4.361	0.1556	0.5808
3	135	0.5/135	0.0441	2.907	0.1038	0.2197
Group sequential total	135		0.0641			0.9464
Fixed total	135	0.5/135	0.0500	2.706	0.1000	0.9500

[a] Number (N_i) of treated patients planned in each group at each stage.
[b] Variance $= \sigma^2 = 0.5/N_i$ when the true response rate in the common referenced population is 0.5 (conservative estimate).
[c] Nominal Type I error at each stage.
[d] Square of standardized normal deviate = Chi-square with 1 df.
[e] Conditional on not stopping at the earlier stage; symbolically, $(1 - \beta)_{r(r-1)(r-2)}$.

detect a 20% difference in response rates with 5% Types I and II risks, will furnish statistical evidence ($P \leq 0.05$) of a real difference if the observed difference (δ) is greater than or equal to 10%. The elements from the C_i column in the first two rows of the tables reflect the minimum observed differences in response rates necessary for the trial to satisfy the statistical stopping rule at the first two stages.

At stage 1, a minimum difference of 21.65% would be needed according to the conditional partitioning of α given in Table 5.1. A minimum difference of 21% (Table 5.2) would need to be observed if Pocock's method is used. A minimum difference of 31.13% would need to be observed (Table 5.3) if the O'Brien and Fleming methodology is used.

Whereas group sequential methods preserve the overall Type I risk, interim stages do exact a penalty on the minimum observed difference needed for statistical significance if the trial continues to the last stage. If there is insufficient evidence for the trial to stop at an interim stage, the minimum observed differences necessary to claim statistical significance at the final stage are 12.24%, 12.24%, and 10.38%, for the conditional partitioning of α, Pocock's, and O'Brien/Fleming's methods, respectively. These are to be contrasted with a minimum observed difference of 10% for the trial if no interim analyses were planned and conducted.

5.3.4.5 Power

The CP for each stage appears in the last column of Tables 5.1 through 5.3. At stage 1, the CP for the conditional partitioning of α, Pocock's, and O'Brien/ Fleming's method are 0.4384, 0.4450, and 0.1459, respectively. At stage 2, the CP for the conditional partitioning of α, Pocock's, and O'Brien/Fleming's method are 0.3582, 0.3190, and 0.5808, respectively. At stage 3, the CP for the conditional partitioning of α, Pocock's, and O'Brien/Fleming's method are 0.1231, 0.1433, and 0.2197, respectively.

If there is insufficient evidence for the trial to stop at an interim stage, the overall power for the conditional partitioning of α, Pocock's, and O'Brien/ Fleming's methods are 0.9197, 0.9173, and 0.9464, respectively. These are to be contrasted with a power of 0.9500 for the trial if no interim analyses were planned. Therefore, including interim analysis procedures penalizes power slightly; with the O'Brien/Fleming procedure being penalized the least.

5.3.5 Summary

One objective of Section 5.3 was to provide definitions of P-value and power reflecting the stages of multistage, group sequential, or interim analysis trials, as well as across stages. This was accomplished in Section 5.3.1. The definitions are consistent with those for fixed-sample-size, single-stage trials. They are rejection probabilities and mirror the strength of the data as observed and summarized through the test statistic against the null hypothesis.

Another objective was to present detailed, pedagogical aspects of the computation of *P*-values and power for multistage trials. This was accomplished in Sections 5.3.2 through 5.3.4. The computations require direct evaluation of multiple integrals (providing the distribution of the test statistic is continuous).

The third objective was to illustrate how to design a multistage clinical trial incorporating group sequential methods. This was accomplished primarily in Section 5.3.4.

Most premarket approval clinical trials of new drugs are designed to provide answers about questions of efficacy. Therefore, monitoring for efficacy while the clinical trial is in progress, particularly in an unplanned, ad hoc manner, is almost always seen to compromise the answers. If it is anticipated that efficacy data will be analyzed—even if only descriptively summarized, prior to termination of the trial, for whatever reason, it is wise to include in the data analysis section of the protocol an appropriate plan for doing this. The plan should address Type I error penalty considerations, what steps will be taken to minimize bias, and permit early termination.

The early termination procedure of O'Brien and Fleming [11] is usually reasonable. It allows periodic interim analyses of the data while the trial is in progress, while preserving most of the nominal Type I error for the final analysis upon scheduled trial completion—providing there was insufficient evidence to terminate the trial after an interim analysis. Trials utilizing this methodology would only be stopped at an earlier stage providing differences much larger than anticipated were observed.

Other procedures such as Pocock's [10], or the alpha spending function approach of Lan and DeMets [17], or the conditional partitioning of alpha approach [14] may also be used. The paper [20] by the Pharmaceutical Manufacturers' Association Working Group addressing the topic of interim analyses provides a good summary of the concerns about, and procedures for, interim analyses. The sample sizes for early-termination, group-sequential procedures, such as O'Brien and Fleming's, are determined as per fixed-sample-size procedures, and then this sample size is spread across sequential groups.

5.4 Stochastic Curtailment

5.4.1 Introduction

Curtailment has been used in the quality control area for a long time. For example, if the number of defective items in a sample of size 20 from a batch is greater than 5, then the batch is rejected. This means that when 5 defective items are observed sequentially (at anytime before inspecting 20), there is no need to inspect further. More recently the concept of stochastic curtailment has been adopted in pharmaceutical clinical trials for planned (or unplanned) interim analyses [21–24]. Since then, stochastic curtailment has been used in a variety of areas, and there is hardly a unique specification of the method.

In pharmaceutical clinical trials, stochastic curtailment is widely used for stopping a clinical trial for either a positive or a negative outcome, but most often the latter is targeted. Therefore, stochastic curtailment is actioned when the probability of a positive outcome, conditional on the data available at a given interim analysis, becomes too small. This is the conditional-probability approach to stochastic curtailment. This means that CP is used for early stopping. CP is defined as the probability that the outcome at the end of the trial will be statistically significant given the current interim data. An advantage of this method is that there is no restriction as to when an interim analysis is conducted, and thus has great attraction in monitoring pharmaceutical clinical trials.

There are other stochastic curtailment methods; e.g., a Bayesian predictive-power (PP) approach [25,26]. This approach averages the CP over the posterior distribution of the treatment effect parameter. Other procedures include those based on conditional probability ratios [22,27,28] that utilize likelihood ratio tests to decide whether the test statistic at the end of the trial is consistent with the accumulated data.

5.4.2 Methods

Following the scenario and notation used in Section 5.3.3, we describe stochastic curtailment methods for early stopping of a clinical trial of two treatments with continuous data. These methods may be easily extended to multiple arms studies [28,29].

Without loss of generality, consider the two-sided hypothesis testing problem

$$H_0: \delta = \tau_A - \tau_B = 0 \quad \text{versus} \quad H_a: \delta = \delta_a \neq 0,$$

where δ represents the difference between the two treatment groups (A and B) in a K-stage sequentially conducted (for example, $K=3$ in Section 5.3.3) clinical trial. The null hypothesis (H_0) may be tested using the normalized test statistic:

$$T_i = \frac{\overline{X}_{Ai} - \overline{X}_{Bi}}{\sqrt{\dfrac{S_{Ai}^2}{N_{Ai}} + \dfrac{S_{Bi}^2}{N_{Bi}}}}$$

where
  N_{Ai}, N_{Bi} denote the sample sizes
  $\overline{X}_{Ai}, \overline{X}_{Bi}$ denote the sample means
  S_{Ai}, S_{Bi} denote the sample standard deviations of treatment groups A and B, respectively, at the ith analysis stage

T_i may be regarded as the test statistic with information level $N_i = N_{Ai} + N_{Bi}$ from the ith interim analysis with N_K reflecting the information at the last analysis stage. For illustration, we assume that T_i is normally distributed with unknown mean δ and variance 1—which is reasonable for sufficiently large trials.

The conventional decision is made based on the critical value of C_K for the test statistic T_K to reject hypothesis H_0 if $|T_K| \geq C_K/\sqrt{N_K}$ and accept H_0 otherwise. The value of N_K is determined to ensure a power of $1 - \beta$ in the design of the clinical trial.

In stochastic curtailment, CP is employed to inform the decision as to when to stop the trial. Here CP is defined as the probability that the estimated treatment effect $\hat{\delta} = (\overline{X}_{AK} - \overline{X}_{BK})$ at the end of the trial will be significant given the cumulative data on the parameter (δ) at the ith interim analysis.

Mathematically CP may be expressed as

$$CP(i, \delta) = P\left(\frac{|T_K| \geq C_K}{\sqrt{N_K}} \Big| T_i, \delta\right)$$

Based on this definition, Lan et al. [21] suggested using $CP(i, \delta_a)$, i.e., the CP under H_a as a criterion. If $CP(i, \delta_a)$ is less than a specified threshold γ_0, the trial should be stopped at the ith interim analysis stage in favor of the null hypothesis H_0. In order for the trial to be stopped in favor of H_a, $CP(i, 0)$ should be calculated and H_a accepted if $CP(i, 0)$ is greater than some threshold $1 - \gamma_1$. At the ith interim analysis stage ($i \leq K$), this leads to the following rule:

Accept H_a if

$$|T_i| \geq C_K\sqrt{\frac{N_K}{N_i}} + z_{1-\gamma_1}\sqrt{\frac{N_K - N_i}{N_i}}$$

Accept H_0 if

$$|T_i| \leq C_K\sqrt{\frac{N_K}{N_i}} - \frac{\delta_1(N_K - N_i)}{\sqrt{N_i}} - z_{1-\gamma_0}\sqrt{\frac{N_K - N_i}{N_i}}$$

where $z_{1-\gamma_0}$ and $z_{1-\gamma_1}$ are the $1 - \gamma_0$ and $1 - \gamma_1$ normal deviates. Therefore, for the predetermined sample size N_K, the stopping boundaries may be parameterized by the triplet (C_K, γ_0, γ_1).

Jennison and Turnbull [22] present an alternative procedure. They use $CP(i, \hat{\delta})$, where $\hat{\delta}$ is an estimate of δ based on the data at the ith interim analysis. Pepe and Anderson [30] suggest a small $CP(i, \hat{\delta} + se(\hat{\delta}))$ as an indication that H_0 is favored, where se denotes standard error.

Another alternative to the CP approach in Lan et al. [21] is the so-called Bayesian type of PP approach proposed in Jennison and Turnbull [22]. PP is defined as the CP integrated over the posterior distribution π of the unknown δ, given the data. It may be seen that for a noninformative prior, the PP is independent of any parameters. In the case of normal data with information level N_i at the ith interim analysis stage, the posterior distribution of PP can be shown to be $N(T_i/N_i, 1/N_i)$. Based on this posterior, the following criterion is proposed:

Accept H_a if

$$|T_i| \geq C_K \sqrt{\frac{N_i}{N_K}} + z_{1-\gamma_1} \sqrt{\frac{N_K - N_i}{N_K}}$$

Accept H_0 if

$$|T_i| \leq C_K \sqrt{\frac{N_i}{N_K}} - z_{1-\gamma_0} \sqrt{\frac{N_K - N_i}{N_K}}.$$

A criterion for stopping clinical trials may also be derived using the conditional-probability ratio in [27,31].

Debates on the CP approach have centered on the arbitrariness of its evaluation on the basis of the value of δ_a under the alternative hypothesis H_a. This led Betensky [32] to consider alternative rules for early stopping in favor of H_0. A comprehensive review and other approaches can be found in Jennison and Turnbull [33].

Again, in stochastic curtailment, data are accumulated at each interim analysis stage. At each interim analysis, the behavior of future data is projected and is used to assess the possible outcomes of the trial as to whether the trial should be stopped or continued. It may be more appropriate to consider a version of CP evaluated under H_0 to mitigate concerns about arbitrariness. This version of CP is a stochastic curtailment tool and is defined as

$$CP(i) = P\left(\frac{|T_K| \geq C_K}{\sqrt{N_K} \mid T_i}\right), \quad \delta = 0$$

which measures how far the current observations deviate from the null hypothesis. Note that, at each interim analysis i, $1 \leq i \leq K$, $CP(i)$ is a random variable ranging from 0 to 1 having mean $\alpha = 1 - \Phi(C_K/\sqrt{N_K})$. At the last stage (i.e., the Kth stage), $CP(K)$ follows a Bernoulli distribution with probability $1 - \alpha$ at 0 and α at 1.

This conditional-probability measures the extent to which the current data are inconsistent with H_0. Therefore, if $CP(i)$ falls below some threshold value γ_0, the continuation of the trial is unlikely to favor H_a, and if $CP(i)$ rises above some threshold $1 - \gamma_1$, then the trial should be stopped and H_0 rejected. This corresponds to the curtailment rule as follows:

Stop the trial and conclude H_a if $CP(i) > 1 - \gamma_1$,
Stop the trial and conclude H_0 if $CP(i) < \gamma_0$.

This leads to the following early stopping rules at interim analysis $i \leq K$:

Accept H_a if

$$|T_i| \geq C_K \sqrt{\frac{N_K}{N_i}} + z_{1-\gamma_1} \sqrt{\frac{N_K - N_i}{N_i}}$$

Accept H_0 if

$$|T_i| \leq C_K \sqrt{\frac{N_K}{N_i}} - z_{1-\gamma_0} \sqrt{\frac{N_K - N_i}{N_i}}$$

The Type I error for the sequential test is

$$P\left(\text{stopping at } K, |T_i| \geq C_K \sqrt{\frac{N_K}{N_i}} \,\middle|\, \delta = 0 \right),$$

which is always larger than α (when $K \geq 2$). Also, the upper boundary is identical with that for early stopping using CP [21]. This leads to the stopping boundaries for T_i with the design triplet parameters $(C_K, \gamma_0, \gamma_1)$ for fixed N_K. In practice, we may choose $(C_K, \gamma_0, \gamma_1)$ to control the Type I error and power (or the expected sample size).

The methods presented in this section are for continuous, non-time-to-event data. The methods may be easily extended for categorical and time-to-event data [33,34].

5.4.3 Application

Extending the example in Section 5.3.4, assume that the trial continues to the second stage and that by the second stage, 49 of 90 patients on treatment A responded and 36 of 90 patients on treatment B responded for an observed difference of $\hat{\delta} = \hat{p}_A - \hat{p}_B = 49/90 - 36/90 = 13/90 = 0.1444$ (14.44%) as illustrated in Table 5.1. Using the decision rules from the conditional partitioning of approach, there would be a statistical basis for stopping the trial based on $\hat{\delta} = 0.1444 > C_2 = 0.1427$. Furthermore, the P-value should be <0.04 (0.02 + 0.02) and when computed it is found to be 0.0393.

To illustrate the decision rules from the conditional-probability point of view in stochastic curtailment, we follow the approach of Proschan et al. [34] to cast the group sequential approach into the Brownian motion framework for a unified theory. Following this framework, the trial information fraction at this second stage is $t_{(2)} = N_{(2)}/N_K = 90/135 = 2/3 \approx 0.6667$ with other trial information fractions: $t_{(0)} = 0$ at the beginning of the trial, $t_{(1)} = 45/135 = 1/3 = 0.3333$ at the first stage of the trial, and $t_{(3)} = 1$ at the end of the trial. At the second stage, we calculate the associated Z-statistic $Z(t_{(2)})$

$$Z(t_{(2)}) = \frac{\hat{p}_A - \hat{p}_B}{\sqrt{\frac{\hat{p}_A(1-\hat{p}_A)}{N_K} + \frac{\hat{p}_B(1-\hat{p}_B)}{N_K}}} = 2.402,$$

and the so-called Brownian B-value $B(t_{(2)}) = \sqrt{t_{(2)}} \times Z(t_{(2)}) = 1.962$. Therefore, given the observed data at the second stage of $B(t_{(2)}) = b = 1.962$, and the B-value at the end of trial is $B(1) = B(t_{(3)}) = b + B(1) - B(t_{(2)})$, which is approximately normally distributed with variance $1 - t_{(2)}$ and mean

$$E[B(1)|B(t_{(2)}) = b] = b + \delta(1 - t_{(2)}),$$

where δ is the expected z-score at the end of the trial and is called the drift parameter. Therefore, the conditional probability illustrated in Section 5.4.2 can be explicitly expressed as

$$CP(2, \delta) = 1 - \Phi\left[\frac{z_{\alpha/2} - E[B(1)|B(t_{(2)}) = b)]}{\sqrt{1 - t_{(2)}}}\right] = 1 - \Phi\left[\frac{z_{\alpha/2} - [b + \delta(1 - t_{(2)})]}{\sqrt{1 - t_{(2)}}}\right]$$

And at the second stage, the empirical estimate for $\hat{\delta} = B(t_{(2)})/t_{(2)} = 2.942$. The conditional probability is calculated from the above equation as $CP(2, \hat{\delta}) = 0.956$. This means that conditional on the observed data at second stage, the probability to reject the null hypothesis at the end of the trial will be 0.956, which provides statistical evidence to stop the trial at this stage. This conclusion is consistent with that from the conditional partitioning of alpha approach in Section 5.3.4, and again confirms the statistical decision rule to stop the trial at the second stage.

5.5 Adaptively Designed Clinical Trials

5.5.1 Introduction

In recent years, some pharmaceutical companies have implemented adaptive clinical trials. The theory and research attendant to adaptive designs in clinical trials support the argument that their incorporation will lead to improved efficiency, reduced costs, and conduct time. However, incorporation of adaptive designs in clinical trials has been slow primarily due to their complexity in planning and execution.

In consensus, an adaptively designed clinical trial is a trial that allows adaptations or modifications to aspects of the trial after its initiation without undermining the validity and integrity of the trial. An adaptive design usually consists of multiple stages. At each stage, data analyses are conducted, and adaptations are made based on updated information to maximize the probability of success.

Adaptive design is a data-driven sequential approach that is flexible and allows modification of the trial in order to detect futility early and accrue cost efficiency. In addition, adaptive design is decision oriented and incorporates learning from the trial sequentially so that Bayesian methodology and computer simulation come into play. However, the flexibility of adaptive design must not compromise the validity and integrity of the trial or the development process.

Adaptive design methods represent a revolutionary approach in the biopharmaceutical industry. Under the adaptive design philosophy, the company can substantially improve the chances for success of a trial with potentially reduced costs. Bayesian approaches provide tools for optimizing trial designs and development plans. Clinical trial simulation offers a powerful tool to design and monitor trials. Adaptive design, the Bayesian approach, and clinical trial simulation combine to form a powerful suite of statistical methodology to significantly impact successful drug development programs. Extensive research and publications can be found in the literature; cf. [35–38] and the references within.

There is an array of clinical trials in the literature that utilize adaptive designs. The more notable ones are group-sequential design, sample-size-adjustable design, drop-loser design (DLD), adaptive-randomization design, adaptive dose-finding design, biomarker-adaptive design (BAD), and multiple adaptive design. We summarize and outline the methods and approaches in adaptively designed clinical trials in the following sections.

5.5.2 Group Sequential Design

Group sequential design (GSD) is the most prominent adaptive method used in clinical trials. As illustrated in Sections 5.2 through 5.4, an adaptive design allows for early termination of a trial due to efficacy or futility, based on the results of interim analyses. GSD was originally developed to obtain clinical benefits under economic and ethical constraints. For trials with a positive result, early stopping allows a new drug to reach the market sooner with less development costs and fewer patients exposed. If a negative result is indicated, early stopping avoids wasting resources.

There are fundamentally three different types of GSDs. The first is the early efficacy stopping design, the second is the early futility stopping design, and the third is the design that allows stopping for early efficacy or futility.

5.5.3 Sample-Size Reestimation Design

A sample-size reestimation (SSR) design is commonly referred to as an adaptive design that allows for sample-size adjustment or reestimation based on the results from interim analyses [35]. Sample size determination for a clinical trial is mathematically based on pilot estimates of efficacy endpoints and their variability, and a guesstimate of how effective (δ) the new treatment will be as compared to the control treatment. Misspecification of these parameters is inevitable, which can lead to an underpowered or overpowered design, neither of which is desirable. We know that if a clinical trial is underpowered, clinically meaningful differences may not be detected, and consequently could preclude a potentially effective drug from being delivered to patients. On the other hand, a trial that is overpowered could result in unnecessary exposure of many patients to a potentially harmful compound, particularly if the drug is not effective. Therefore, it is practically desirable to reestimate the sample size based on the effect size or its variability from the ongoing trial.

As illustrated in Chang [35], there are two types of SSR procedures based on blinded data as well as unblinded data. This design is more applicable when there are no good or reliable estimates of the effect size and its variability. Sample size adjustment or reestimation may be done from the criteria for treatment effect size, CP, and reproducibility probability. For example, when a trial continues to an interim analysis stage, one can reestimate sample size from the observed effect size at this interim stage, so that the CP that the test statistic rejects the null hypothesis of no effect at the end of the trial reaches some desired level [39]. Another option is to reestimate the sample size necessary for the power conditional on the new postulated effect size at this interim stage, to achieve a desired level [40]. Intuitively, SSR can be done at any interim analysis stage, but one should be cautious in the early stages when the estimated effect size is usually not stable enough to produce an informative estimate to carry out a reliable SSR. Therefore, we recommend that SSR be performed at the earliest interim stage at which the interim data can produce an informative and reliable estimate of the effect size.

It is well known that if the only interest at an interim analysis stage—for the purpose of SSR—is whether the variance estimate used at the design stage is not an underestimate, then the sample size may be reestimated upward without paying a Type I error penalty (see Section 10.12.1 for an example). This is certainly true for normally distributed data since the mean and variance estimates of samples from a normal distribution are independent, and at an interim analysis stage, only the variance estimate (and not the estimate of the effect size) needs to be examined. Of course all interim analyses should be conducted under a plan that ensures that the integrity of the data and trial are not compromised. Such a plan should provide sufficient logistical detail that is unambiguous, easily followed, and adequately documented so that a reviewer will understand why inferences from the analyses are believable.

5.5.4 Drop-Loser Design

A DLD is an adaptive design with multiple stages [35]. At each stage, interim analyses are conducted to drop the losers based on prespecified criteria which leads to the eventual retention of the best arms. Of course, if there is a control group, it is usually retained for the purpose of comparison. A Phase II clinical trial is often a dose–response trial to assess a treatment effect. If there is treatment effect, the goal becomes finding the appropriate dose and frequency of dosing for the Phase III trials. The traditional design is not efficient with respect to time and resources because the Phase II efficacy data are not pooled with data from Phase III trials, which are the pivotal trials for confirming efficacy. Hence it is desirable to combine Phases II and III to use the data more efficiently as well as to reduce the time required for the drug development. Thus the DLD may be best for Phase II/III seamless trials.

5.5.5 Adaptive-Randomization Design

An adaptive-randomization–allocation design (ARD) is a design that allows modification of randomization schedules while conducting the trial. It is well known that in clinical trials, a goal of randomization is to ensure balance with respect to patient characteristics among treatment groups. However in ARD, especially the response-adaptive randomization (RAR) as discussed in Hu and Rosenberger [37], the allocation probability for patients to be entered is based on responses of previous patients, and ethical considerations dictate having a larger probability of allocating new patients to a superior treatment group. This response randomization can be deemed as a DLD with a seamless allocation probability of shifting from an inferior arm to a superior arm. Well known response-adaptive models include the randomized play-the-winner (RPW), an optimal model that minimizes the number of failures. Other RARs, such as utility adaptive randomization, also have been proposed that are combinations of RAR and treatment-adaptive randomization designs [37].

5.5.6 Biomarker-Adaptive Design

BAD refers to a design that allows for adaptations using information obtained from biomarkers. A biomarker is a characteristic that is objectively measured and evaluated as an indicator of normal biologic or pathogenic processes or pharmacologic response to a therapeutic intervention. A biomarker can be a classification, prognostic, or predictive marker as discussed in Chow and Chang [38]. A BAD can thus be used to select a more appropriate patient population, to identify and profile the course of disease and to help in developing personalized medicine.

5.5.7 Multiple Adaptive Designs

A multiple adaptive design (MAD) is a combination of several adaptive designs described [38] in the previous sections. A commonly considered MAD includes, but is not limited to, the combination of adaptive GSD,

DLD, and adaptive seamless-trial design. This has intuitive appeal, but the statistical inference is practically difficult if not impossible. Therefore, appropriate simulations to evaluate possible outcomes and performance for MAD in clinical trials are required at the planning stage of such trials.

5.6 Concluding Remarks

The first author began incorporating group-sequential methods into prospective clinical trials more than 30 years ago when he was director of clinical biostatistics at A.H. Robins Pharmaceuticals, Richmond, Virginia. At that time, when the data from a completed trial was available for statistical analyses, the biostatistician analyzed the data and generated a stand-alone biostatistical report, replete with methods, results, interpretations, and conclusions. The statistical report was sent to the in-house clinical trial MD, where it was to form the basis for generating the clinical study report (in fact, the statistical report would be included as an appendix).

Invariably, the MD would find data on some patients deemed to be inevaluatable for efficacy, and would request reanalyses excluding data on those patients. This led to additional time to issue the final clinical study report, was a drain on resources, and was of doubtful scientific validity. So group sequential interim analysis procedures were introduced into protocols for prospective Phase III clinical trials. The selling point was that such procedures might lead to being able to stop a trial earlier, thereby representing a potential savings of development dollars, and possible earlier filing of the NDA.

Whereas this is true, perhaps the greater benefit accrued from forcing all aspects of clinical data management to be performed more quickly and with greater quality. This included more frequent site monitoring, getting the data collection forms in-house sooner for database entry and quality assurance—including blinded efficacy evaluatability review, developing and validating biostatistical analysis programs, and developing the mock clinical study report. Once data has been reviewed and considered efficacy evaluatable and an interim analysis performed, the decision as to efficacy evaluatability cannot be changed upon review of data for the next interim analysis. Thus, designing clinical trials to include interim analysis may lead not only to earlier stopping and fewer patients (ethical and cost savings imperatives) exposed to an unapproved drug, but also forces better real-time management of all activities attendant to the conduct, management, and analysis of the trials.

In addition to the publications previously referenced in this chapter, others of relevance to the issues discussed appear as references [41–56]. The last four [53–56] are computer programs for group-sequential methods and adaptive designs. Among these four, [55] is a free R package in reference to [33,34] and is available free from CRAN (http://www.r-project.org). The last one is a free FORTRAN program and is a companion to the book by Jennison and Turnbull [33].

References

1. Wald A (1947): *Sequential Analysis*, John Wiley, New York.
2. Bross I (1952): Sequential medical plans. *Biometrics*; **8**: 188–205.
3. Armitage P (1954): Sequential tests in prophylactic and therapeutic trials. *The Quarterly Journal of Medicine*; **91**: 225–274.
4. Armitage P (1957): Restricted sequential procedures. *Biometrika*; **44**: 9–26.
5. Armitage P, McPherson CK, Rowe BC (1959): Repeated significance tests on accumulating data. *Journal of the Royal Statistical Society (A)*; **132**: 235–244.
6. McPherson CK, Armitage P (1971): Repeated significance tests on accumulating data when the null hypothesis is not true. *Journal of the Royal Statistical Society (A)*; **134**: 15–25.
7. Armitage P (1971): *Sequential Methods in Medical Research*, Blackwell, Oxford, U.K.
8. Armitage P (1975): *Sequential Medical Trials*, 2nd edn., John Wiley & Sons, New York.
9. Colton T, McPherson KL (1976): Two stage plans compared with fixed-sample-size and Wald SPRT plans. *Journal of the American Statistical Association*; **71**: 353: 80–86.
10. Pocock SJ (1977): Group sequential methods in the design and analysis of clinical trials. *Biometrika*; **2**: 191–199.
11. O'Brien PC, Fleming TR (1979): A multiple testing procedure for clinical trials. *Biometrics*; **35**: 549–559.
12. McPherson K (1982): On choosing the number of interim analyses in clinical trials. *Statistics in Medicine*; **1**: 25–36.
13. Lan KKG, DeMets DL (1983): Discrete sequential boundaries for clinical trials. *Biometrika*; **70**(3): 659–663.
14. Peace KE, Shriver R (1987): *P*-value and power computations in multiple look trials. *Journal of Chronic Diseases*; **40**(1): 23–30.
15. Fisher RA (1925): *Statistical Methods for Research Workers*, Oliver and Boyd, Edinburgh, U.K.
16. Toddhunter I (1865): *A History of the Mathematical Theory of Probability from the Time of Pascal to That of Laplace*, Macmillan, London, U.K.
17. DeMets DL, Lan KK (1994): Interim analysis: The alpha spending function approach. *Statistics in Medicine*; **13**(13–14): 1341–1352; Discussion 1353–1356.
18. National Bureau of Standards (1959): *Tables of the Bivariate Normal Distribution and Related Functions*. U.S. Dept of Commerce, Washington, DC, Applied Mathematics Series 50.
19. Schriver R (1980): Three-stage clinical trials, SmithKline and French Labs Internal Memorandum.
20. Pharmaceutical Manufacturers Association Biostatistics and Medical Ad Hoc Committee on Interim Analysis (1993): Interim analysis in the pharmaceutical industry. *Controlled Clinical Trials*; **14**: 160–173.

21. Lan K, Simon R, Halperin M (1982): Stochastically curtailed tests in long-term clinical trials. *Communications in Statistics*; **1**: 207–219.
22. Jennison C, Turnbull B (1990): Statistical approaches to interim monitoring of medical trials: A review and commentary. *Statistical Science*; **5**: 299–317.
23. Betensky R (1997a): Conditional power calculations for early acceptance of H_0 embedded in sequential tests. *Statistics in Medicine*; **16**: 465–477.
24. Betensky R (1997b): Early stopping to accept H_0 based on conditional power: Approximations and comparisons. *Biometrics*; **53**: 794–806.
25. Herson J (1979): Predictive probability early termination plans for phase II clinical trials. *Biometrics*; **35**: 775–783.
26. Spiegelhalter D, Freedman L, Blackburn P (1986): Monitoring clinical trials: Conditional or predictive power? *Controlled Clinical Trials*; **7**: 8–17.
27. Xiong X (1995): A class of sequential conditional probability ratio tests. *Journal of the American Statistical Association*; **90**: 1463–1473.
28. Leung D, Wang TG, Amar D (2003): Early stopping in favor of H_0 in a three-arm sequential trial. *Journal of the Royal Statistical Society* (C); **52**: 139–152.
29. Siegmund D (1993): A sequential clinical trial for comparing three treatments. *Annals of Statistics*; **21**: 464–483.
30. Pepe MS, Anderson GL (1992): Two-stage experimental designs: Early stopping with a negative result. *Applied Statistics*; **41**: 181–190.
31. Jennison C (1992): Bootstrap tests and confidence intervals for a hazard ratio when the number of observed failures is small, with application to group sequential survival studies. In: *Computing Science and Statistics*, Springer, New York, pp. 89–97.
32. Betensky R (2000): Alternative derivations of a rule for early stopping in favor of H_0. *American Statistician*; **54**: 35–39.
33. Jennison C, Turnbull B (2000): *Group Sequential Methods with Applications to Clinical Trials*, Chapman & Hall/CRC, Boca Raton, FL.
34. Proschan MA, Lan G, Wittes JT (2007): *Statistical Monitoring of Clinical Trials: A Unified Approach*, Springer, New York.
35. Chang, M (2008): *Adaptive Design Theory and Implementation Using SAS and R*, Chapman & Hall/CRC, Boca Raton, FL.
36. Chow SC, Shao J, Wang H (2008): *Sample Size Calculations in Clinical Research*. 2nd edn., Chapman & Hall/CRC, Boca Raton, FL.
37. Hu, F, Rosenberger WF (2006): *The Theory of Response-Adaptive Randomization in Clinical Trials*, John Wiley & Sons, New York.
38. Chow SC, Chang M (2008): Adaptive design methods in clinical trials—A review. *Orphanet Journal of Rare Diseases*; **3**: 11 (open access at http://www.ojrd.com/content/3/1/11).
39. Cui L, Hung HMJ, Wang SJ (1999): Modification of sample size in group sequential clinical trials. *Biometrics*; **55**: 321–324.
40. Lawrence J (2002). Design of clinical trials using an adaptive test statistic. *Pharmaceutical Statistics*; **1**: 97–105.
41. Jennison C, Turnbull BW (1984): Repeated confidence intervals for group sequential clinical trials. *Controlled Clinical Trials*; **5**: 33–45.
42. Tsiatis AA, Rosner GL, Mehta CR (1984): Exact confidence intervals following a group sequential test. *Biometrics*; **40**: 797–804.
43. Tsiatis AA, Rosner GL, Tritchler DL (1985): Group sequential tests with censored survival data adjusting for covariates. *Biometrika*; **72**(2): 365–373.

44. Jennison C, Turnbull BW (1985): Repeated confidence intervals for the median survival time. *Biometrika*; **72**(3): 619–625.

45. Jennison C (1987): Efficient group sequential tests with unpredictable group sizes. *Biometrika*; **74**(1): 155–165.

46. Wang SK, Tsiatis AA (1987): Approximately optimal one-parameter boundaries for group sequential trials. *Biometrics*; **43**: 193–199.

47. Ghosh BK, Sen PK (1991): *Handbook of Sequential Analysis*, Marcel Dekker, New York.

48. Peace KE (1992): *Biopharmaceutical Sequential Statistical Applications*, CRC Press, Boca Raton, FL.

49. Reboussin DM, DeMets DL, Kim KM, Lan KK (2000): Computations for group sequential boundaries using the Lan-DeMets spending function method. *Control Clinical Trials*; **21**(3): 190–207.

50. Rosner GL, Tsiatis AA (2006): The impact that group sequential tests would have made on ECOG clinical trials. *Statistics in Medicine*; **8**(4): 505–516.

51. Mehta CR, Bauer P, Posch M, Brannath W (2007): Repeated confidence intervals for adaptive group sequential trials. *Statistics in Medicine*; **26**(30): 5422–5433.

52. van der Laan MJ (2008): The construction and analysis of adaptive group sequential designs. U.C. Berkeley Division of Biostatistics Working Paper Series. Working Paper 232. http://www.bepress.com/ucbbiostat/paper232

53. The ADDPLAN Software: http://www.addplan.com/node/88 (accessed Oct. 10, 2009).

54. PASS Group Sequential Tests: http://www.ncss.com/passsequence.html (accessed Oct. 09, 2009).

55. Anderson KM (2009). *gsDesign: An R Package for Designing Group Sequential Clinical Trials, Version 2.0 Manual* (a free R package from CRAN: http://www.r-project.org).

56. Jennison CJ, Turnbull BW (2000): Group sequential methods with applications to clinical trials; http://people.bath.ac.uk/mascj/book/programs/general (accessed Oct. 09, 2009).

6

Biostatistical Aspects of the Protocol

A protocol has to be developed for each clinical trial. A most important responsibility of the statistician or biostatistician assigned to the protocol is to provide its statistical content. This includes ensuring that the objectives are clear; recommending the most appropriate design (experimental design and determination of sample size) for the condition being studied; assessing the adequacy of endpoints to address study objectives; assigning participants to protocol interventions to minimize bias; and developing the statistical analysis section. In addition, it is imperative that the biostatistician provides a review of the protocol for completeness and consistency.

Sections 6.1 through 6.5 provide a simple outline for a protocol. Biostatistical input to these sections is discussed.

6.1 The Background or Rationale

In the background or rationale section, sufficient information should be given to set the stage for the clinical trial for which the protocol is being developed. This requires integrating the results (with references) of previous studies that have bearing on the current protocol. The section should end with something like this: *Therefore this study is being conducted to . . . (assess the efficacy of drug D in the treatment of patients diagnosed with disease X; as an example).*

6.2 Objective

The objective or research question of the protocol should be defined so that it is unambiguous. For example, in an investigation about the antihypertensive efficacy of drug D in some defined population, the statement "The objective of this investigation is to assess the efficacy of drug D" is ambiguous. It provides only general information as to the question "Is D efficacious?" The statement "The objective of this investigation is to assess whether drug D is superior to placebo P in the treatment of hypertensive patients with diastolic blood pressure (DBP) between 90 and 105 mmHg for six months" is better—as the hypertensive population to be treated and what is meant by efficacious in a comparative sense are specified.

However, the data or endpoint(s) upon which antihypertensive efficacy will be based is (are) not specified. DBP is stated, but how will it be measured?—Using a sphygmomanometer or a digital monitor? Will DBP be measured in the sitting, standing, or supine position? Further, what function of the DBP will be used?—The change from baseline to the end of the treatment period? Or whether the patient achieves a therapeutic goal of normotension (DBP $\leq$ 80 mmHg) by the end of the treatment period?

If there is more than one question or objective, one should identify which is primary versus which is secondary. See Section 6.4.1 for further discussion.

6.3 Plan of Study

The plan of study entails all that is to be done in order to enroll and treat patients, monitor the study, ensure patient safety, and collect valid data. The study population has to be specified. Design aspects of the study, including all procedures to be used in the diagnoses, treatment, or management of patients must be delineated.

6.3.1 Study Population

Characteristics of the population of patients to be entered into the protocol must be specified. This is typically accomplished by specifying inclusion and exclusion criteria appropriate for the disease and drug under study. In specifying these criteria, one has to be cognizant that patients entered must have the disease under study, that the condition of the patient must not compromise patient safety by participating in the protocol, and that the patients entered should enable the efficacy of the drug under study to be determined (absence of masking or confounding factors).

The inclusion criteria specify the demography of the patient population, their disease characteristics, acceptable vital signs ranges, acceptable clinical laboratory tests ranges, etc. Exclusion criteria are generally the complement of the inclusion criteria, with delineation of a subset that specifically excludes patients from entry. For example, non-menopausal females who are pregnant or who do not agree to practice an acceptable form of birth control during the intervention period are excluded; as are patients who do not agree to abstain from using concomitant medications that may mask or interfere with the activity of the drug under study. Inclusion/exclusion criteria essentially define the population to be studied. Therefore, they provide general descriptors of the population to which inferences from analyses of the data collected pertain.

6.3.2 Study Design

The study design subsection should identify the type of study; the treatment or intervention groups, and how patients who qualify for the protocol will be assigned to treatment groups; what measures will be taken to ensure the absence of bias; requirements relative to patients taking medications other than those constituting the assigned intervention; and all procedures that are required by the protocol in order to diagnose, treat, ensure patient safety, and collect data.

6.3.2.1 Type of Study

The type of study should be described. Is the study prospective? What type of control (placebo, positive, historical, etc.) will be used? Is it single or multicenter? Is the study parallel, crossover, stratified, or some other type?

6.3.2.2 Treatment Group Specification and Assignment

The treatment groups and the interventions (drug, dose, etc.) that patients in the groups will receive should be specified. Then how patients will be assigned to the treatment groups to remove assignment bias should be articulated. The gold standard is to randomly assign patients to the groups in balanced fashion. Minor departures from balance are acceptable and may be more ethical. For example, for a placebo control trial of a new drug, our preference is to recommend that twice as many patients be randomly assigned to the drug than to placebo. This reduces the number of patients assigned to placebo by one-sixth, and ensures that twice as many patients are assigned to the drug group as to the placebo group. A two-to-one departure from balance has a relatively small impact on power.

6.3.2.3 Packaging to Achieve Blinding

Intervention group medications should be packaged so that neither the patient nor personnel (physician, research nurse, or assistant) who will either treat, assign medication, draw blood, administer procedures, or collect data knows the identity of the interventions. This requires interaction between the protocol biostatistician (who will generate the randomization schedule) and the formulation or packaging chemists (who will package the medication). Both have to thoroughly know the protocol, particularly the drug, dose, and frequency of dosing of intervention medications, when patients are at the clinic for medication dispensing, and how many days are between visits.

6.3.2.4 Concomitant Medication

The protocol should indicate whether any medications other than those comprising the treatment or intervention groups are permitted while the patient is participating in the protocol. Generally, any medication, prescription, or over the counter (OTC), that would mask, cloud, or otherwise interfere with the effect of the intervention medications should be excluded.

6.3.2.5 Procedures

All procedures required for enrolling, diagnosing, treating, or medically monitoring patients should be clearly identified and described. This applies to all phases: pretreatment, during treatment, or post treatment, of the protocol. Providing a study schema at the end of the protocol that identifies procedures to be administered by day of study is helpful.

Observers (personnel who see patients that result in data collection and recording) should be specified. The assignment of observers to patients should be made to try to eliminate or minimize the introduction of observer variability into the trial. For example, in hypertension studies, different observers for different patients are permitted, but each patient should have the same observer throughout the trial.

Procedures for recording the data to be collected in the trial should be specified. Whether data are to be recorded on paper data collection forms (DCFs) or electronically requires protocol sponsor personnel to interact with site personnel to ensure proper and valid recording of data.

6.3.3 Problem Management

In this section of the protocol, criteria for dealing with problems related to patient safety or that may compromise study objectives if left unattended should be specified. For example, clinically significant changes in clinical laboratory parameters; criteria for discontinuing study drug, including severe adverse events; actions to be taken for protocol deviations or violations, including taking prohibited drugs, missed visits, dropouts, etc. should be specified. Contact information from the investigational sites to the protocol sponsor for problem management should be clearly delineated.

6.4 Statistical Analysis Section

There are many ways that one may organize the content of the statistical analysis section. One organization is to have six sections or paragraphs: study objectives as statistical hypotheses; endpoints; statistical methods;

statistical monitoring procedures; statistical design considerations; and subset analyses [1].

6.4.1 Study Objectives as Statistical Hypotheses

6.4.1.1 Primary, Secondary, Safety, or Other Objectives

It is important to classify study objectives according to those that reflect primary efficacy, those that reflect secondary efficacy, those that reflect safety, and those that reflect other questions of interest (e.g., quality of life). Then the objectives within each classification should be translated into statistical questions.

6.4.1.2 Translating Protocol Objectives into Statistical Hypotheses

If inferential decisions regarding the questions are to be made on the basis of hypothesis or significance testing, the questions should be translated into statistical hypotheses. It is desirable from a statistical viewpoint, for the alternative hypothesis (H_a) to embody the research question, both in substance and direction [2]. For placebo-controlled studies or for studies in which superior efficacy is the objective, this is routinely the case. For studies in which clinical equivalence (or noninferiority) is the objective, the usual framing of the objective translates it as the null hypothesis (H_0). In this framework, failure to reject H_0 does not permit a conclusion of equivalence or noninferiority. This will depend on a specification of how much the treatment regimens may truly differ in terms of therapeutic endpoints, yet still be considered clinically equivalent or noninferior, and the power of the test to detect such a difference. Some authors [3–6] have suggested reversing the null and alternative hypotheses for equivalence studies, so that a conclusion of equivalence is reached by rejecting the null hypothesis. An attraction of this specification is that the Type I error is synonymous with the regulatory approval or consumers risk for both efficacy and equivalence or noninferiority studies.

Separate univariate, null, and alternative hypotheses should be specified for each question. The reasons for separate specifications are primarily clarity and insight: clarity because the questions have been clearly elucidated and framed as statistical hypotheses. This sets the stage for appropriate statistical analyses when the data become available. When analyses directed toward the questions occur, it should be clear whether the statistical evidence is sufficient to answer them. Insight is gained from the univariate specifications, as to the significance level at which the tests should be performed. This is true even though the study objective may represent a composite hypothesis.

Secondary efficacy objectives should not invoke a penalty on the Type I error associated with the primary efficacy objectives. It may be argued that each secondary objective can be addressed using a Type I error of 5%, providing inference via significance testing is preferred. Ninety-five percent confidence intervals represent a more informative alternative. Since the use of confidence intervals implies interest in estimates of true treatment effects, rather than interest in being able to decide whether true treatment effects differ from some prespecified values, confidence intervals are more consistent with a classification of secondary.

Safety objectives, unless they are the primary objectives, should not invoke a penalty on the Type I error associated with the primary efficacy objectives. It is uncommon that a study conducted prior to market approval of a new drug would have safety objectives that are primary. This does not mean that safety is not important. The safety of a drug, in the individual patient, and in groups of patients, is of utmost importance. Questions about safety are very difficult to answer in a definitive way, in clinical development programs of a new drug. There are many reasons for this [7]. There may be insufficient information to identify safety endpoints and/or the target population, and inadequate budgets or numbers of patients. Clinical development programs of new drugs should be aggressively monitored for safety within and across trials, but designed to provide definitive evidence of effectiveness. This position is entirely consistent with the statutory requirements [8] for new drug approval in the United States.

Sections 4.4.1 and 7.5.1 may be seen for more specifics regarding translating protocol objectives into statistical questions.

6.4.2 Endpoints

Data collected in the protocol reflecting primary efficacy, secondary efficacy, safety, or other objectives should be identified. Then endpoints to be statistically analyzed to address protocol objectives should be defined. An endpoint may be the actual data collected or a function of the data collected. Endpoints are the analysis units on each individual patient that will be statistically analyzed to address study objectives. In an antihypertensive study, actual data reflecting potential efficacy are supine DBP measurements. Whereas it is informative to describe these data at baseline and at follow-up visits during the treatment period, inferential statistical analyses are usually based upon the endpoint: change from baseline in supine DBP. The reason for this is that change from baseline within each treatment group is an indicator of the extent to which the drug received in each group is effective.

Another endpoint of clinical interest is whether a patient experienced a clinically significant reduction in supine DBP from baseline to the end of the treatment period. Clinically significant is usually defined as a decrease from baseline of at least 10 mmHg or becoming normotensive (DBP $\leq$ 80 mgHg). This definition of an endpoint essentially dichotomizes DBP at the end of treatment.

Section 4.4.2 may be seen for further discussion of endpoints.

6.4.3 Statistical Methods

Statistical methods that will be used to analyze the data collected and the endpoints should be described. The methods chosen should be appropriate for the type of data or endpoint; e.g., parametric procedures such as analysis of variance techniques for continuous endpoints, and nonparametric procedures such as categorical data methods for discrete endpoints. Analysis methods should also be appropriate for the study design. For example, if the design has blocking factors, then statistical procedures should account for these factors. It is prudent to indicate that the methods stipulated will be used to analyze study data and endpoints, subject to actual data verification that any assumptions underlying the methods reasonably hold. Otherwise, alternative methods will be considered.

The use of significance tests may be restricted to the primary efficacy questions. Otherwise, confidence intervals should be used. The method for constructing confidence intervals, particularly how the variance estimate will be determined, should be indicated.

Unless there are specific safety questions as part of the study objectives, for which sample sizes with reasonable power to address them have been determined, it is usually sufficient to use descriptive procedures for summarizing safety data. Again this position is consistent with statutory requirements. If inferential methods are to be used, Edwards et al. [9] and Sogliero-Gilbert [10] provide a variety of methods.

The last portion of this section should identify methods to be used to address generalizability of results across design-blocking factors or across demographic or prognostic subgroups. Methods for generalizability include descriptive presentations of treatment effects across blocks or subgroups, a graphical presentation of confidence intervals on treatment differences across blocks or subgroups, and analysis of variance models that include terms for interaction between treatment and blocks or subgroups.

Section 4.4.3 may be seen for further detail regarding the statistical methods section.

6.4.4 Statistical Monitoring Procedures

Most clinical trials of new drugs are designed to provide answers to questions of efficacy; this is particularly true for Phase III trials, as they are typically the pivotal proof of efficacy trials. Therefore, monitoring for efficacy while the study is in progress, particularly in an unplanned, ad hoc manner, will almost always be seen to compromise the integrity of such trials. If it is anticipated that the efficacy data will be summarized or statistically analyzed prior to study termination, for whatever reason, it is wise to include an appropriate plan for doing this in the protocol. The plan should address Type I error penalty considerations, what steps will be taken to minimize bias, and permit early termination.

The early termination procedure of O'Brien and Fleming [11] is usually reasonable. It allows periodic interim analyses of the data while the study is in progress, while preserving most of nominal Type I error for the final analysis upon scheduled study completion—providing there was insufficient evidence to terminate the study after an interim analysis. Other procedures such as Pocock's [12], or Lan and Demets [13], may also be used, as well as publications by numerous authors. The paper [14] by the PMA Working Group addressing the topic of interim analyses provides a good summary of the concerns about, and procedures for, interim analyses. The sample sizes for early termination, group sequential procedures, such as O'Brien and Fleming's, are determined as per fixed-sample-size procedures, and then this sample size is spread across sequential groups.

Safety data, particularly serious adverse events should be monitored for all trials as the data accumulate [15–17]. The group sequential procedures referenced above may be used for these purposes. However, unless the trial has been designed to provide statistical evidence regarding some safety objective, it is unclear that a prespecified overall Type I error rate should be preserved [7]. The idea is to be alerted as early as possible about any events that may reflect possible safety concerns so that appropriate intervention may be taken. Often, the repeated confidence interval method of Jennison and Turnbull is helpful [18].

The subsection on statistical monitoring procedures should begin with a paragraph that specifies what data and endpoints will be sequentially monitored (analyzed); when such monitoring will occur (calendar time or cumulative number of patients at each planned analysis); how the data will be quality assured; and specification of procedures to be followed to minimize bias or otherwise jeopardizing the integrity of the study. Section 4.4.8.3 and Chapter 5 may be seen for more detailed discussions about interim analyses monitoring procedures.

6.4.5 Statistical Design Considerations

The statistical, experimental design for the study should be described. Is the experimental design parallel using a completely randomized design (CRD)? Or is the design parallel using a completely randomized block design (CRBD)? Or is the design a two-sequence, two-period, two-treatment crossover design $(2 \times 2 \times 2)$? Or is a balanced incomplete block design (BIBD) used? What are the stratification variables if any? What type of control (placebo, positive, historical, etc.) will be used? Is it single or multicenter? The type of experimental design used in the trial impacts the type of statistical methods that will be used to analyze data collected.

Once the design is known, the number of clinical trial participants necessary to provide valid inferences to protocol objectives may be determined [19]. This requires one to know what the objectives are in terms of statistical questions; i.e., what is the δ in each separate alternative hypothesis? Specifying δ requires collaboration between the biostatistician and the clinician.

The specification of δ is the responsibility of the clinician or medical director, and requires careful thinking and exploration by both the biostatistician and the medical expert. A δ too large may lead to failure to answer the question due to too small a sample. A δ too small would increase costs of conducting the investigation and may not be accepted as clinically meaningful.

Once δ is specified, the magnitude of the Type I error α, and the statistical power $1 - β$ or degree of certainty required to detect δ must be specified. Then an estimate of variability, $σ^2$, of the data or endpoint reflecting the question is needed. When the biostatistician has the inputs δ, α, $1 - β$, and an estimate of $σ^2$, the sample size may be computed using well-known sample-size formulae, sample-size computational software programs, or using simulation techniques.

Sections 4.4 and 4.5 may be seen for more detailed discussions regarding sample size determinations, including examples of sample sizes for several clinical trials.

6.4.6 Subset Analyses

The last subsection of the statistical or data analysis section should identify what subsets or subpopulations among trial participants will be investigated or subjected to statistical analyses. Both the gender rule and the demographic rule (see Section 2.3) identify subpopulations indexed by age, gender and race, or ethnicity. But other subpopulations may be of interest; e.g., levels of disease severity. In addition, methods to be used for investigating subsets or performing analyses of subsets should be specified. How one views the objective of subset investigation will dictate the type of analyses [20].

If the objective is to provide valid inferences of treatment effects within subpopulations, then one could stratify the protocol by subpopulation and design the trial to have sufficient power and numbers of participants to assess the effectiveness of treatment in each subpopulation. This would seldom be required if ever. Few if any drug sponsors could afford to conduct such clinical trials. Alternatively, step-down procedures may be helpful in providing valid inferences with subpopulations. The recent article by Alosh and Huque [21] provides an alternative method.

What is of interest is to assess whether the treatment effects in the total population are generalizable across subpopulations. This can be assessed by introducing subpopulation and treatment-by-subpopulation as fixed effects into the analysis model and noting the size of the *P*-value for the interaction term. Large *P*-values are consistent with an interpretation of treatment effects being generalizable across subpopulations, whereas small *P*-values provide evidence that treatment effects differ across some subpopulations. Since clinical trials are not usually designed to have large power to detect significant interactions, many biostatisticians use a *P*-value of less than or equal to

0.10 to quantify small. Some suggest that the protocol should be stratified by subpopulation to ensure balance across treatment groups in terms of subpopulations.

In addition to interaction tests to address generalizability of treatment effects across subpopulations, descriptive tables of treatment effects and graphical presentations of confidence intervals on treatment effects by subpopulation are helpful. In such graphical presentations, the centers of the confidence intervals representing random variation about a horizontal line are indicative of generalizability of treatment effects. Lack of generalizability requires the biostatistician to identify what subpopulations are discrepant, and then through collaboration with the clinician and/or monitoring or investigational site assess whether there are explanations for the discrepancies.

After the statistical analysis section has been finalized and the protocol approved, the project biostatistician should develop the statistical analysis plan (SAP). The SAP should follow the data analysis section but would contain greater specificity. The SAP serves as a blue print for biostatistical analyses of the data and endpoints. It should be developed so that if the project biostatistician has to be replaced, the new biostatistician would not require much time to become fully engaged with analyses. An example of a statistical analysis plan for a protocol is presented in Chapter 7.

6.5 Administration

The major sections of the administration section of the protocol specify review and informed consent procedures and requirements, record-keeping procedures and investigational-site monitoring plans.

6.5.1 Review and Consent Requirements

The informed consent document should be developed and included in the protocol (usually as an appendix). Instructions on how the document should be reviewed with potential clinical trial participants so that they are fully informed about all aspects of the trial necessary for them to give consent should also be included. Aspects of the trial include the objective, diagnoses, and treatments to be received, how participants will be assigned to treatment groups, the benefits to risks, any costs to the patient for participation, schedule of clinic visits, etc.

Although not routinely included in the informed consent document, a case may be made that the power of the trial should also be reviewed with potential participants [22–24].

6.5.2 Record Keeping

The record-keeping section of the protocol identifies what records and/or documentation are to be kept, by whom and where. Most of this pertains to the investigational sites as they must provide and maintain a central file for documents pertinent to conducting the protocol. Such documents include a copy of the final protocol plus any amendments, a copy of the DCF, a copy of the investigational brochure, identification of all site personnel who have some responsibility for conducting the trial at the site, and specification of what that responsibility is, copies of correspondence from the drug sponsor including results of the drug sponsor monitoring visits, numerous regulatory documents, including the good clinical practice guidelines, etc.

In addition, patient records (source documents) are to be kept to facilitate quality assurance review of the data recorded on the DCF. Also, careful records of dispensing study drugs to participants, and the return of drugs, must be kept to permit assessment of compliance. If the trial is double blinded, the blinded assignment (coding memorandum or randomization schedule) of drugs to participants must be kept in a secure place, and only opened on a per-participant basis, if identity is needed by the principal investigator to provide the best medical care for the participant.

6.5.3 Monitoring

Specifics of how the conduct of the protocol will be monitored at participating investigational sites should be presented in the monitoring section of the protocol. Drug sponsors typically recruit investigational sites based on previous clinical trial experience and/or the reputation of lead investigators at the sites. They will then visit the sites to ensure that their facilities are adequate to conduct the planned protocol.

The monitoring plan includes the frequency of drug sponsor monitoring visits, from the initiation visit, to the final closeout visit, and interim visits in between. Specific dates of such visits are usually not possible to specify. The initiation visit is usually scheduled to coincide with delivery of packaged study drugs. At this visit, the sponsor's monitor will open the package of medication and inventory its contents, and ensure that its contents are securely housed. In addition, the monitor will go over the protocol and mock DCF with the investigator and assistants who will perform assessments on trial participants.

The first (interim) visit after the initiation visit occurs after one to three patients have been entered to assess whether the patients satisfy protocol entry criteria and to ensure that data are being collected and recorded properly. Other interim visits may be scheduled after a specified number of patients have been entered. The final closeout visit is scheduled after all patients have been entered and completed and all queries from the sponsor to the site have been answered.

The drug sponsor should develop a checklist to identify what activities will be conducted at each visit. This list is usually shared with investigational site personnel prior to each visit.

6.6 Protocol References Section

The protocol is a scientific document providing information as to how it will be conducted. Accordingly, it should contain a list of references to permit a reviewer to crosscheck the information provided and referenced.

6.7 Concluding Remarks

Quality clinical research must be well planned, closely and carefully monitored, utilize procedures that ensure quality collection and management of data, use appropriate statistical analysis procedures, and properly interpret the results so that inferences are valid and without bias. The first step in this process is to develop a quality protocol for every clinical trial.

References

1. Peace KE (2005): Statistical section of a clinical trial protocol. *The Philippine Statistician*; **54**(4): 1–8.
2. Peace KE (1989): The alternative hypothesis: One-sided or two-sided? *Journal of Clinical Epidemiology*; **42**: 473–476.
3. Hauck WW, Anderson S (1983): A new procedure for testing equivalence in comparative bioavailability and other trials. *Communications in Statistical Theory and Methods*; **12**: 2663–2692.
4. Petrie A, Sabin C (2005): *Medical Statistics at a Glance*, Wiley Blackwell, New York.
5. Lesaffre E (2008): Superiority, equivalence, and non-inferiority trials. *Bulletin of the NYU Hospital for Joint Diseases*; **66**(2): 150–154.
6. Liu JP, Chow SC (1999): *Design and Analysis of Bioavailability and Bioequivalence Studies*, CRC Press, LLC, Boca Raton, FL.
7. Peace KE (1987): Design, monitoring, and analysis issues relative to adverse events. *Drug Information Journal*; **21**: 21–28.
8. Food and Drug Administration (1987): New drug, antibiotic, and biologic, drug product regulations; Final rule. 21 CFR Parts 312, 314, 511, and 514; **52**(53): 8798–8857; Thursday, March 19.

9. Edwards S, Koch GG, Sollecito WA (1989): Summarization, analysis, and monitoring of adverse events. In: *Statistical Issues in Drug Research and Development*, Peace, KE (Ed.), Marcel Dekker, Inc., New York, pp. 19–170.
10. Sogliero-Gilbert G (ed.) (1993): *Drug Safety Assessment in Clinical Trials*, Marcel Dekker, Inc., New York.
11. O'Brien PC, Fleming TR (1979): A multiple testing procedure for clinical trials. *Biometrics*; **35**: 549–556.
12. Pocock S (1977): Group sequential methods in the design and analysis of clinical trials. *Biometrika*; **64**: 191–199.
13. Lan KKG, Demets DL (1983): Discrete sequential boundaries for clinical trials. *Biometrika*; **70**: 659–70.
14. PMA Biostatistics and Medical Ad Hoc Committee on Interim Analysis (1993): Interim analysis in the pharmaceutical industry. *Control Clinical Trials*; **14**: 160–173.
15. Herson J (2009): *Data and Safety Monitoring Committees in Clinical Trials*, Chapman & Hall/CRC, Arlington, VA.
16. Piantadosi S (2005): *Clinical Trials: A Methodologic Perspective*, Wiley-Interscience, New York.
17. Proschan MA, Lan KKG, Wittes JT (2005): *Statistical Monitoring of Clinical Trials: A Unified Approach*, Springer, New York.
18. Jennison C, Turnbull BW (1984): Repeated confidence intervals for group sequential clinical trials. *Controlled Clinical Trials*; **5**: 33–45.
19. Peace KE (2006): Importance of the research question relative to analysis. *Philippine Statistical Association Newsletter*; **1**(1): 7–9.
20. Peace KE (1995): Considerations concerning subpopulations in the clinical development of new drugs. In *Annual DIA Meeting on Statistical Issues in Clinical Development*, Hilton Head, SC.
21. Alosh M, Huque MF (2009): A flexible strategy for testing subgroups and overall population. *Statistics in Medicine*; **28**(1): 3–23.
22. Peace KE (2008): Commentary: Is informed consent as ethical as it could be? *Bio-IT-World*, March 17.
23. Peace KE (2005): Making informed consent more ethical. *Drug Information Forum*; **5**(4): 26–27.
24. Peace KE (1992): An ethical issue concerning informed consent in clinical trials. *Biopharmaceutical Report*; **1**(2): 1–2.

7

The Statistical Analysis Plan

7.1 Introduction

The purpose of this chapter is to provide details regarding statistical characteristics and plans for conducting statistical analyses of efficacy of a drug T in the prevention of acute kidney injury (AKI). Details of the trial, including the statistical analysis section, appear in the protocol [1].

The objective as stated in the protocol appears in Section 7.2. Efficacy data to be collected in the trial and protocol schema appear in Section 7.3. Primary and secondary efficacy endpoints as functions of these data appear in Section 7.4. The objective, translated as statistical hypotheses, appears in Section 7.5. Protocol design features appear in Section 7.6. Details of planned statistical analyses are presented in Section 7.7, including identification of populations upon whom analyses of efficacy are performed.

7.2 Protocol Objective

The objective of the protocol is to evaluate the relative efficacy of Drug T as adjunctive therapy to standard therapy (ST) alone in the prevention of AKI in gram-negative sepsis hospitalized patients.

7.3 Efficacy Data Collected and Protocol Schema

Possibly prognostic data relating to efficacy consists of demographic characteristics (age, sex, race, or ethnicity) and disease characteristics (chronic kidney insufficiency), admission type (medical or surgical), or reason for admission (trauma, cardiovascular, neurological, gastrointestinal, malignant, or pulmonary disease). Efficacy data collected in the trial to be summarized

TABLE 7.1

Protocol Schema

	Protocol Day					
Assessment	0	1	2	Exit ICU	28	56
Demography	X					
Disease characteristics	X					
Glomerular filtration rate	X	X	X	X	X	X
Urine output	X	X	X	X	X	X
RIFLE	X	X	X	X	X	X
SOFA	X	X	X	X	X	X
Mortality	X	X	X	X	X	X
Protocol treatment administration		X	X			

and/or statistically analyzed are the risk, injury, failure, loss, and end-stage kidney (RIFLE) classification [2], the sepsis organ failure assessment (SOFA) score [3], and mortality, per the schedule (baseline = day 0) in the protocol schema (Table 7.1).

7.4 Primary and Secondary Efficacy Endpoints

7.4.1 Primary Efficacy Endpoint

The primary efficacy measure in this protocol is the percent of patients who do not progress to AKI by protocol day 28. A patient is said to experience AKI if according to the RIFLE [2] criteria the patient is classified (Table 7.2) as Risk (R), Injury (I), or Failure (F).

TABLE 7.2

Risk, Injury, Failure, Loss, and End-Stage Kidney (RIFLE) Classification

Class	Glomerular Filtration Rate Criteria	Urine Output Criteria
Risk	Serum creatinine × 1.5	<0.5 mL/kg/h × 6 h
Injury	Serum creatinine × 2	<0.5 mL/kg/h × 12 h
Failure	Serum creatinine × 3, or serum creatinine ≥4 mg/dL with an acute rise >0.5 mg/dL	<0.3 mL/kg/h × 24 h, or anuria × 12 h
Loss	Persistent acute renal failure = complete loss of kidney function >4 weeks	
End-stage kidney disease	End-stage kidney disease >3 months	

RIFLE class is based on the worst of either glomerular filtration or urine output criteria. Glomerular filtration criteria are calculated as an increase of serum creatinine above baseline serum creatinine level. AKI should be both abrupt (within 1–7 days) and sustained (more than 24 h). If baseline serum creatinine is unknown and patients are without a history of chronic kidney insufficiency, a baseline serum creatinine using the modification of diet in renal disease equation for assessment of kidney function, assuming a glomerular filtration rate of 75 mL/min/1.73 m^2 should be calculated. When the baseline serum creatinine is elevated, an abrupt rise of at least 0.5 mg/dL to more than 4 mg/dL alone is sufficient to achieve class Failure [2].

7.4.2 Secondary Efficacy Endpoints

Secondary efficacy endpoints in this protocol are

1. The percent of patients who do not progress to AKI by protocol day 56
2. The cumulative percent of patients still alive at day 56
3. The SOFA score at day 28
4. The SOFA score at day 56

7.5 Objectives, Translated as Statistical Hypotheses

7.5.1 Primary Efficacy Objective as a Statistical Hypothesis

The primary efficacy objective of the protocol is framed as the alternative hypothesis H_a of the hypothesis-testing construct

$$H_0: P_{stt} = P_{st} \quad \text{versus} \quad H_a: P_{stt} < P_{st},$$

where P_{stt} and P_{st} represent the true proportions of patients treated with Drug T plus ST or ST alone, respectively, who experience AKI by study day 28. In words, the null hypothesis H_0 says that there is no difference in the proportions of patients experiencing AKI by study day 28 between the Drug T plus ST and ST alone groups (i.e., Drug T provides no benefit above ST alone); and H_a says that the study day 28 AKI rate in the Drug T plus ST group is less than that in the group receiving ST alone (i.e., Drug T provides benefit above ST alone).

7.5.2 Secondary Efficacy Objectives as Statistical Hypotheses

There are four univariate secondary statistical hypotheses. These reflect the endpoints defined in Section 7.4.2.

7.5.2.1 Percent of Patients with Acute Kidney Injury by Study Day 56

The first secondary efficacy objective is framed as the alternative hypothesis
H1a of the hypothesis-testing construct

$$H1_0: P1_{stt} = P1_{st} \quad \text{versus} \quad H1_a: P1_{stt} < P1_{st},$$

where $P1_{stt}$ and $P1_{st}$ represent the true proportions of patients treated with
Drug T plus ST or ST alone, respectively, who experience AKI by study
day 56. In words, the null hypothesis H_0 says that there is no difference in
the proportions of patients experiencing AKI by study day 56 between the
Drug T plus ST and ST alone groups (i.e., Drug T provides no benefit above
ST alone); and H_a says that the study day 56 AKI rate in the Drug T plus ST
group is less than that in the group receiving ST alone (i.e., Drug T provides
benefit above ST alone).

7.5.2.2 Cumulative Percent of Patients Surviving by Study Day 56

The second secondary efficacy objective is framed as the alternative hypothesis $H2_a$ of the hypothesis-testing construct

$$H2_0: P2_{stt} = P2_{st} \quad \text{versus} \quad H2_a: P2_{stt} > P2_{st},$$

where $P2_{stt}$ and $P2_{st}$ represent the true survival proportions of patients
treated with Drug T plus ST or ST alone, respectively, who survive from
any cause by study day 56. In words, the null hypothesis H_0 says that there is
no difference in the cumulative proportions of patients surviving by study
day 56 between the Drug T plus ST and ST alone groups (i.e., Drug T provides
no benefit above ST alone); and H_a says that the cumulative proportion
surviving by study day 56 in the Drug T plus ST group is greater than that
in the group receiving ST alone (i.e., Drug T provides benefit above ST alone).

7.5.2.3 SOFA Score at Study Day 28

The third secondary efficacy objective is framed as the alternative hypothesis
$H3_a$ of the hypothesis-testing construct

$$H3_0: \mu3_{stt} = \mu3_{st} \quad \text{versus} \quad H3_a: \mu3_{stt} < \mu3_{st}$$

where $\mu3_{stt}$ and $\mu3_{st}$ represent the true means of the distributions of SOFA
scores at day 28 of patients treated with Drug T plus ST or ST alone, respectively.
In words, the null hypothesis $H3_0$ says that there is no difference in day 28
mean SOFA scores between the Drug T plus ST and ST alone groups (i.e., Drug
T provides no benefit above ST alone); and $H3_a$ says that the day 28 mean
SOFA scores in the Drug T plus ST group is less than (note that smaller scores
represent less severity of the condition than larger scores) that in the group
receiving ST alone (i.e., Drug T provides benefit above ST alone).

7.5.2.4 SOFA Score at Study Day 56

The fourth secondary efficacy objective is framed as the alternative hypothesis $H4_a$ of the hypothesis-testing construct

$$H4_0: \mu4_{stt} = \mu4_{st} \quad \text{versus} \quad H4_a: \mu4_{stt} < \mu4_{st}$$

where $\mu4_{stt}$ and $\mu4_{st}$ represent the true means of the distributions of SOFA scores at day 56 of patients treated with Drug T plus ST or ST alone, respectively. In words, the null hypothesis $H4_0$ says that there is no difference in day 56 mean SOFA scores between the Drug T plus ST and ST alone groups (i.e., Drug T provides no benefit above ST alone); and $H4_a$ says that the day 56 mean SOFA scores in the Drug T plus ST group is less than (note that smaller scores represent less severity of the condition than larger scores) that in the group receiving ST alone (i.e., Drug T provides benefit above ST alone).

7.6 Protocol Design Features

The protocol is a randomized, ST-controlled, longitudinal, multicenter clinical trial designed to evaluate the efficacy of Drug T in the prevention of AKI in gram-negative sepsis hospitalized patients.

7.6.1 Experimental Design

In statistical experimental design nomenclature, the protocol will utilize a completely randomized design (CRD), with patients being centrally randomized to protocol treatment groups sequentially in time across all investigational sites. Although this design is typical in oncology clinical trials, in the vast majority of prospective clinical trials, investigational sites represent a constraint to randomization; i.e., patients are randomized to treatment groups within each investigational site, using a randomization schedule specific for each site. However, a centrally administered randomization is preferred in the study of diseases where one cannot be assured of relatively large numbers of patients at individual sites.

7.6.2 Treatment or Intervention Groups

There are two treatment or intervention groups:

ST = standard therapy for treating gram-negative sepsis patients

T + ST = standard therapy for treating gram-negative sepsis patients plus one or two (if needed) treatments with Drug T

7.6.3 Randomization

Male or female patients, age 18 years or older, who undergo screening and qualify for the protocol will be randomly assigned to either the ST group or to the T + ST group in a 1:1 ratio. The randomized assignment to protocol treatment groups will be made using a centrally administered interactive voice response system (IVRS). The randomization schedule will be generated by an independent data center.

7.6.4 Blinding

It is not possible to double-blind treatment medications. Efficacy and safety data will be collected on standardized data collection forms (DCFs). Each DCF will be verified against the patient's medical record by a study monitor and reviewed by a medical monitor, both of whom will be blinded to treatment group identity. Adverse events will be independently reviewed by an independent data safety monitoring committee (DSMC).

7.6.5 Number of Patients

From a fixed-sample-size point of view, approximately 480 patients (240 in the ST group and 240 in the T + ST group) are to be enrolled in the protocol. Two-hundred forty (240) patients per treatment group was determined on the basis of a statistical power of 95% and a one-sided [4] false-positive rate of 5%, to detect a clinically significant difference of 15 percentage points in AKI rates between the ST group (45%) and the T + ST group (30%) at protocol day 28 (primary endpoint). This sample size is somewhat conservative as the worst case of the Bernoulli variance is assumed.

7.6.6 Number of Protocol Centers

The number of centers to be recruited to participate in this multicenter protocol is expected to be 25–30, located either in the United States or Canada.

7.7 Statistical Analyses

All data collected in the trial and all endpoints defined on such data will appear in data listings in the clinical protocol report. Such listings will reflect treatment group and time of data collection. In addition, all data collected and endpoints will be descriptively summarized and presented by treatment group. Summary presentations include graphs where appropriate, the descriptive statistics (mean, standard deviation) and number of patients, or frequency distributions. In addition, the T + ST group will be described in terms of the number of patients requiring only one and two treatments courses of Drug T.

Inferential analyses comparing the **T + ST** and **ST** groups will be performed, with *P*-values providing the basis for inference for planned efficacy comparisons. *P*-values for efficacy comparisons will be one-sided and judged to be indicative of nominal statistical significance if the one-sided *P*-value is less than or equal to 0.05—provided no interim analyses are performed that require adjustment to the Type I error.

All listings, descriptive summaries, and inferential analyses will be generated using procedures of the statistical analysis system (SAS).

7.7.1 Trial Populations for Statistical Analyses

Four populations based upon the patients who qualified for the trial are defined for statistical analyses purposes. These are

1. The intent-to-treat (ITT) population, which consists of all patients who were randomized to protocol medications.
2. The beginning treatment (BT) population, which consists of all randomized patients who began protocol treatment (note that some patients may be withdrawn prior to beginning treatment with protocol medications).
3. The one-course treatment (OCT) population, which consists of all randomized patients who completed one protocol treatment course.
4. The two-course treatment (TCT) population, which consists of all randomized patients who completed two protocol treatment courses.

7.7.2 Demographics, Baseline Characteristics, Eligibility, and Disposition

Demographic and baseline disease characteristics, including age, gender, race, weight, chronic kidney insufficiency, admission type (medical or surgical), and reason for admission (trauma, cardiovascular, neurological, gastrointestinal, malignant, or pulmonary disease), will be summarized by treatment group using descriptive statistical techniques.

The number of patients screened, the number of patients enrolled, and the number of patients completing will be summarized by investigational site and across sites. For patients randomized, the number completing and the number of dropouts will be summarized by treatment group, by investigational site, and across sites. Exclusions from the protocol (dropouts and protocol deviations) will be listed and the reasons for the exclusion identified.

Treatment groups, across sites, will be inferentially compared, in terms of demographic and baseline disease characteristics, using two-sided *P*-values as a check on the success of the randomization. A one-way analysis of variance (ANOVA) using the general linear models procedure (PROC GLM) of SAS will be used for continuous variables. PROC FREQ of SAS will be used for categorical variables. Data on patients in the ITT population will be used in these analyses.

7.7.3 Efficacy Analyses

7.7.3.1 Primary Efficacy Analyses

The treatment groups will be compared in terms of the primary efficacy endpoint, proportion of patients with AKI by protocol day 28, using PROC FREQ of SAS, with both the Fisher's exact test (FET) and the Cochran–Mantel–Haenszel (CMH) options. If no interim analyses are performed that require adjustment to the Type I error, a difference between treatment groups in terms of the percentage of patients with AKI by protocol day 28, favoring $T + ST$, and a corresponding one-sided P-value less than or equal to the nominal 0.05, will be indicative of demonstrating Drug T to be effective, statistically.

These analyses will be performed on the ITT, BTE, OCT, and TCT populations, with the results based on the ITT population providing the primary basis for inference.

7.7.3.2 Secondary Efficacy Analyses

The treatment groups will be compared in terms of the secondary efficacy endpoints: the proportion of patients with AKI by day 56, the cumulative proportions of patients surviving by day 56, and the SOFA Scores at protocol days 28 and 56, using PROC FREQ of SAS, with either the FET or the CMH options. The FET option will be used for analysis of the dichotomous endpoint: cumulative AKI by day 56. The cumulative proportion surviving by day 56 will be analyzed using CMH time-to-death methods. The cumulative proportion surviving will also be analyzed. The mean scores feature of the CMH option will be used for the ordinal endpoints: SOFA scores at day 28 and day 56.

Analysis results of secondary endpoints, favoring Drug T which have an associated P-value less than or equal to the stated nominal Type I error level, may be regarded as supportive of the efficacy of Drug T. More specifically, differences between treatment groups in terms of the percentage of patients, or in terms of mean scores, if favoring Drug T, with a corresponding one-sided P-value less than or equal to 0.05, will be a signal of the possible statistical efficacy of Drug T. Ninety percent confidence intervals will also be provided.

Analyses of secondary endpoints will be performed on the ITT, BT, OCT, and TCT populations, with the results based on the ITT population providing the basis for inference.

7.7.3.3 *Analyses of Generalizability across Subpopulations*

Although a centrally administered randomization schedule does not argue for assessing the generalizability of treatment group results across investigational sites, results of analyses of primary and secondary endpoints will be explored for generalizability over levels of various factors: investigational site (if possible; or country due to the expected small numbers of patients per site), age, sex, race or ethnicity, and baseline disease characteristics. For dichotomous endpoints, the Breslow–Day test for interaction will be used. Since CMH analyses and GLM analyses of ordinal data produce similar results for moderate to large sample sizes, PROC GLM, with a linear model that regresses the endpoints on the fixed effects (treatment group, factor, and treatment-group-by-factor interaction), will be used to assess generalizability of treatment group differences in terms of ordinal endpoints. In these analyses, the focus is on the P-value for the interaction term. An associated P-value less than 0.10 will be interpreted as providing some evidence that treatment group differences may not be generalizable over levels of the factor.

7.7.4 Interim Analyses

Data related to patient outcome will be reviewed periodically by the DSMC. Following each review, the DMSC will make a recommendation to the company as to whether the trial should be terminated or continued in terms of best interests of patients. For company administrative planning purposes, an interim efficacy review may also occur when approximately 240 randomized patients finish day 28 assessments. The purpose of this review is primarily to assess whether the design difference of 15% is approximately 1/3 of the ST control group rate. The company will have the option of adjusting the sample size upward at this time and continuing the trial without Type I error penalty, stopping the trial, or statistically comparing the **T + ST** and **ST** groups. If a statistical test is performed during the interim efficacy review, a statistical alpha level of 0.005 will be used so that the final primary efficacy analysis will have an alpha level of 0.048, per O'Brien and Fleming [5].

7.8 Concluding Remarks

The purpose of this chapter is to identify key components that should be included in a statistical analysis plan accompanying a well-designed protocol. These components are objectives as stated in the protocol; efficacy data to be collected in the clinical trial of the protocol; primary and secondary efficacy endpoints as functions of the data to be collected; translation of protocol objectives into statistical hypotheses; protocol design features, including sample size determination, and statistical characteristics and plans for conducting statistical analyses. Formulating the key components and details of the planned statistical analyses were illustrated by providing a statistical analysis plan for a protocol in AKI prevention.

References

1. Specific Protocol to be supplied by the developer of the Statistical Analysis Plan.
2. Hoste EAJ, Clermont G, Kersten A, Venkataraman R, Angus DC, De Bacquer D, Kellum JA (2006): RIFLE criteria for acute kidney injury are associated with hospital mortality in critically ill patients: A cohort analysis. *Critical Care*; **10**: R73–R82.
3. Vincent JL, Moreno R, Takala J, Willatts S, De Mendonça A, Bruining H, Reinhart CK, Suter PM, Thijs LG (1996): SOFA (sepsis-related organ failure assessment) score to describe organ dysfunction/failure working group on sepsis-related problems of the European Society of Intensive Care Medicine. *Intensive Care Medicine*; **22**: 707–710.
4. Peace KE (1991): One-sided or two-sided p-values: Which most appropriately address the question of drug efficacy? *Journal of Biopharmaceutical Statistics*; **1**(1): 133–138.
5. O'Brien PC, Fleming TR (1979): A multiple testing procedure for clinical trials. *Biometrics*; **35**: 549–556.

8

Pooling of Data from Multicenter Clinical Trials

8.1 Introduction

Phase I clinical trials are almost always conducted at a single investigational site. Many Phase II clinical trials are conducted at two or more investigational sites or centers. Virtually all Phase III clinical trials have to be conducted at several investigational sites in order to accrue the number of patients required by the protocol.

The analyses of multicenter clinical trials pose challenges in terms of what are the most appropriate analyses of the data collected. Some analysts believe that the proper analysis of a multicenter clinical trial is based on an analysis of variance Model (1) with fixed effects of treatment and center, and then follow this analysis with the Model (2) that contains fixed effects of treatment, center, and center-by-treatment interaction to assess the significance of the interaction term. If the interaction term is not statistically significant, then treatment effects from Model (1) are reported and considered generalizable across centers. If the interaction term is significant, some analysts report the treatment effect from Model (1) with the caveat that the treatment effect is inconsistent across centers.

Other analysts aver that the proper analysis derives from Model (2), and if there is a statistically significant treatment-by-center interaction, there should be no overall pooled analysis of the data. Further, if the treatment-by-center interaction is statistically significant, some analysts test treatment effect from Model (2) and base an inference on the difference in treatment group means adjusted for differences between centers and (treatment-by-center interaction).

To get around the interaction problem, other analysts suggest that the proper analysis derives from an analysis of variance Model (3) with fixed treatment effects and random center and treatment-by-center effects, and base the test for treatment effect on the ratio of mean square for treatment divided by the mean square for treatment-by-center interaction. The main criticism of this latter strategy is that centers or investigators do not represent a random sample from some population of centers or investigators. Further, the power of the test for treatment effect from this strategy would be reduced (as compared to Model (1) or Model (2)), particularly in multicenter clinical trials that have few centers.

The main focus of this chapter is to discuss design-based and model-based approaches in the analysis of multicenter trials and to argue that a pooled analysis should be performed for every quality designed and conducted multicenter clinical trial.

8.2 Multicenter Clinical Trial Experimental Setting

In the typical multicenter clinical trial, patients who satisfy protocol inclusion criteria are randomized to treatment groups within each investigational center or site. That is, separate randomization schedules are generated for each center. Therefore, centers represent a constraint on randomization. Usually the design of a multicenter trial follows the completely randomized block design (CRBD) in the experimental design literature with centers as blocks (except there is no monotonic ordering of centers as there often is in applying a CRBD in other applied areas; for example, in the study of agricultural crop yield).

It is noted in passing that there are exceptions to the multicenter CRBD. For example, many clinical trials of rare diseases (and in some instances cancer) do not block on centers and use a centrally administered randomization schedule for a completely randomized design (CRD). This is due primarily to the paucity of patients at individual centers and/or to the difficulties and costs associated in supplying clinical trial medications for each center. Such trials pose even more difficult analytical problems in performing a (post hoc) pooled analysis of treatment effect across the investigational centers that enroll patients.

In a multicenter clinical trial of a drug (D) to a control (P = Placebo, say) following a CRBD, it is important to remember that there is only **one protocol** with **one objective**; that is, assess the efficacy or safety of the drug as compared to the control. Therefore, the data collected on patients randomized to drug or control at each investigational site represent to some extent convenience samples. Each provides an estimate of the efficacy or safety of the drug as compared to control at each center. Whereas randomization to drug or control within each center ensures valid estimates of treatment effect within centers, such trials are not designed to permit meaningful inferential statistical tests of treatment effects within centers (sample size estimation yields the number of patients to be entered in the protocol—across centers, rather than within centers). The analysis challenge is how to combine the estimates across centers to permit a valid inference (pooled) on treatment effect across centers.

8.3 Pre-Study Planning

To some extent, the protocol for a multicenter clinical trial ensures that patients who enter the protocol are similar across centers at entry. Patients who enter have the same disease. The same inclusion/exclusion criteria are applied across centers. The same prescreening procedures, including diagnostic workup, are followed across centers. And although the severity of disease may differ across individual patients and centers, there is usually a minimum severity required to enter the protocol.

In addition, investigator and center selection attempts to ensure that participating investigators are reasonably homogeneous. For example, principal investigators at the centers are usually board certified in treating the disease for which the drug is being developed. Therefore, they have similar knowledge, medical training, and expertise in treating the disease under study. And they often have a proven track record of conducting quality clinical investigations.

Further, the drug sponsor conducts investigator educational and training meetings prior to any patient being enrolled into the protocol. Both the primary investigator and his or her head research nurse (or assistant) attend these meetings. At these meetings, details of the protocol, the data collection form, and expectations of center personnel are presented under "one roof." The drug sponsor's medical monitors also conduct initiation visits at each center to further review the protocol, data collection form, and center expectations prior to the first patient being entered. The point is that all that can be done to ensure that all centers follow the protocol and use similar measurement procedures is done prior to the trial beginning.

8.4 Multicenter Clinical Trial Conduct

During the conduct of the clinical trial, medical monitoring personnel frequently monitor all participating centers. This is to ensure that all centers adhere to the protocol and federal regulations (e.g., *Good Clinical Practice Guidelines*), and that the data recorded on the data collection forms and patient records are accurate and of good quality. In general, monitoring visits during the conduct of the trial attempt to ensure that the study is being conducted per protocol and similarly in a quality manner across centers.

Through quality design and development of the protocol, planning, training, execution, and monitoring, practically all that can be done to ensure homogeneous patient populations, patient treatment and assessment, and measurement methodology across investigational centers, is done. Therefore, there is an a priori basis for pooling the estimates of treatment effect at each center across centers.

8.5 Biostatistical Analysis

Prior to beginning biostatistical analyses, it is helpful to recall what the null and alternative (protocol objective) hypotheses (see Sections 6.2 and 6.4.1) are:

H_0: Effect of drug (D) is no different from that of control (placebo = P)
H_a: Effect of D is better than that of P

or symbolically

$$H_0: \mu_d - \mu_p = 0$$

$$H_a: \mu_d - \mu_p > 0,$$

where μ_d and μ_p are the true within-trial effects of drug and placebo, respectively. Further, H_0 and H_a are the same for each center. Randomization of patients to treatment groups within centers guarantees valid, unbiased estimates of treatment effect within centers.

It is noted that many statisticians formulate H_a as two-sided. For a trial designed to provide proof of efficacy, there should be little doubt that the question of efficacy is one-sided, particularly for placebo controlled trials [1]. In fact, the first author has designed positive control trials as one-sided for more than 30 years. The idea is that the new drug could be slightly inferior to the active control but not so much as to be clinically meaningful. Positive control trials are what clinical trials of a new drug (test) versus a drug already marketed (standard) were called in 1970s. Such trials were referred to as Active Control Equivalence Studies (ACES) [2] in the mid-1980s. Now they are called noninferiority trials [3].

8.5.1 Design-Based Analysis Strategy

A design-based analysis strategy for a multicenter clinical trial begins with combining the estimates of treatment effect across centers in a manner consistent with the design of the trial and behavior of the data. Fundamentally, a design-based analysis strategy is no different than a meta-analysis of the treatment effect estimates across the centers [4]. That is, first compute the estimates (taken here as the difference in treatment group means) of treatment effect ($\hat{\delta}_i = \overline{T}_i - \overline{P}_i$) and the variance ($\hat{\sigma}_i^2$) of treatment effect at each center i ($i = 1, \ldots, c$), and then meta-analyze the $\hat{\delta}_i$ across centers.

8.5.1.1 Weighted Means and Variances

Weight (W_i) the estimates ($\hat{\delta}_i$) of treatment effect at each center as appropriate, then compute the **weighted mean or pooled estimate** ($\hat{\delta}$) of treatment effect, and estimate **its variance** ($\hat{\sigma}^2$), where

$$\hat{\delta} = \sum_{i=1}^{c} W_i \hat{\delta}_i \tag{8.1}$$

$$\hat{\sigma}^2 = \text{Var}(\hat{\delta}) = \sum_{i=1}^{c} W_i^2 \text{Var}(\hat{\delta}_i) = \sum_{i=1}^{c} W_i^2 \hat{\sigma}_i^2 + 2 \sum_{\substack{i,j=1 \\ i \neq j}}^{c} W_i W_j \hat{\sigma}_{ij} \tag{8.2}$$

$$= \sum_{i=1}^{c} W_i^2 \hat{\sigma}_i^2 \quad \text{(under independence of centers)} \tag{8.3}$$

and where $\overline{T}_i$ and $\overline{P}_i$ are the means of the data being analyzed over the patients in the D and P groups, respectively, $\hat{\sigma}_i^2$ is the estimate of the variance of $\hat{\delta}_i$, $\hat{\sigma}_{ij}$ is the estimate of the covariance between $\hat{\delta}_i$ and $\hat{\delta}_j$, and $\sum_{i=1}^{k} W_i = 1$. Note that for Equations 8.2 and 8.3 to hold, the W_i have to be regarded as constants. Typical choices of W_i are

$$W_i = \frac{1}{c}, \tag{8.4}$$

where c is the number of centers (fixed)

$$W_i = \frac{N_i}{N}, \tag{8.5}$$

where N_i is the number of patients at center i, and $N = \sum_{i=1}^{c} N_i$;

$$W_i = N_{id} N_{ip} / (N_{id} + N_{ip}) / W, \quad \text{where } W = \sum_{i=1}^{c} \frac{(N_{id} N_{ip})}{(N_{id} + N_{ip})} \tag{8.6}$$

and where N_{id} and N_{ip} are the numbers of patients in the D and P groups respectively at center i; or

$$W_i = \frac{\left(\frac{1}{\hat{\sigma}_i^2}\right)}{W}, \tag{8.7}$$

where $W = \sum_{i=1}^{c} \left(\frac{1}{\hat{\sigma}_i^2}\right)$.

The choice of weights in Equation 8.4 yields the arithmetic average or unweighted mean of the estimates of treatment effect across centers.

The choice of weights in Equation 8.5 yields the average of the estimates of treatment effect across centers weighted according to the number of patients at each center. Note that Equation 8.5 reduces to Equation 8.4 if there is balance across centers.

The choice of weights in Equation 8.6 yields the average of the estimates of treatment effect across centers weighted to allow treatment group imbalance at each center. Note that Equation 8.6 reduces to Equation 8.4 if treatment groups are balanced across centers.

The choice of weights in Equation 8.7 yields the average of the estimates of treatment effect across centers weighting the estimates inversely to their variance. Note that Equation 8.7 reduces to Equation 8.4 if the $\hat{\sigma}_i^2 (> 0)$ are the same (homogeneous) across centers. The traditional treatment of the weights given in Equation 8.7 replaces the $\hat{\sigma}_i^2$ by σ_i^2 and the σ_i^2 are considered known. This greatly simplifies inference using $\hat{\delta}$ given in Equation 8.1. However, to consider the $\hat{\delta}_i$ as random variables and not consider the $\hat{\sigma}_i^2$ as random variables seems a bit illogical.

8.5.1.2 *Inference on Treatment Effect*

To test the null hypothesis $H_0: \delta = \mu_d - \mu_p = 0$ versus $H_a: \delta = \mu_d - \mu_p > 0$, first standardize $\hat{\delta}$, to produce T, where

$$T = \frac{\{(\hat{\delta} - E(\hat{\delta}))\}}{\sqrt{\hat{\sigma}^2}}, \tag{8.8}$$

or

$$T = \frac{\{(\hat{\delta} - \delta)\}}{\sqrt{\hat{\sigma}^2}}, \quad \text{if the expected value of } \hat{\delta} \text{ is } \delta. \tag{8.9}$$

It is clear that the expected value of $\hat{\delta}\{E(\hat{\delta})\}$ given in Equation 8.1 is δ (which is 0 under H_0) if the W_i are constants. Obviously $E(\hat{\delta}) = \delta$ for the choice of W_i given by Equation 8.4.

$E(\hat{\delta}) = \delta$ for the choice of W_i given in Equation 8.5 if the N_i are regarded as fixed rather than random variables, except when the N_i are the same, in which case it would not matter whether the N_i are fixed or random. $E(\hat{\delta}) = \delta$ for the choice of W_i given in Equation 8.6 if the N_{id} and N_{ip} are regarded as fixed, rather than random variables, except when $N_{id} = N_{ip}$, in which case it would not matter whether N_{id} and N_{ip} are fixed or random. In practice, the frequentist analysis approach conditions on the number of patients entered (or completed), and therefore regards the N_i, N_{id}, and N_{ip} as fixed.

$E(\hat{\delta}) = \delta$ for the choice of weights given in Equation 8.7 if the $\hat{\sigma}_i^2$ are homogeneous, in which case the weighted mean in Equation 8.7 reduces to the arithmetic mean in Equation 8.4. If the $\hat{\sigma}_i^2$ are not homogeneous, then $E(\hat{\delta}) = \delta$ if the W_i are constant or if $\sum_{i=1}^{c} E(W_i) = 1$ and if the $\hat{\delta}_i$ and W_i are independent.

In inferential analyses, many replace the $\hat{\sigma}_i^2$ in Equation 8.7 with $\left(s_{id}^2/N_{id} + s_{ip}^2/N_{ip}\right)$, where s_{id}^2 and s_{ip}^2 are the computed sample variances and N_{id} and N_{ip} are the sizes of the drug and placebo groups at the ith center, respectively. Then compute T, and make an inference regarding H_0 using an extension of Satterthwaite's [5] or Welch's [6] formula to approximate the degrees of freedom of the t-test. Hundreds of statistical texts take this approach in comparing two group means when the group variances are unknown and are not homogeneous; that is, the Behrens–Fisher problem [7]. This is not unreasonable in the analysis of clinical trials where patients are entered by selection rather than being chosen at random from some population of patients with the disease under study. In this analysis setting, the W_i are considered constants (conditioning on the data available on the patients who participated in the trial); the inference there from being regarded as local—pertaining to the patients entered.

However, if the $\hat{\sigma}_i^2$ are not homogeneous, then $E(\hat{\delta}) = \delta$, where the W_i are given in Equation 8.7, provided the variation among the $\hat{\delta}_i$ is random about a mean of 0. To see this, suppose $\hat{\delta}_i = \delta + \xi$, where the ξ_i have some distribution with mean 0 and variance σ_i^2, and consider

$$\hat{\delta} = \sum_{i=1}^{c} W_i \hat{\delta}_i = \sum_{i=1}^{c} W_i \delta + \sum_{i=1}^{c} W_i \xi_i = \delta \sum_{i=1}^{c} W_i + \sum_{i=1}^{c} W_i \xi_i = \delta + \sum_{i=1}^{c} W_i \xi_i;$$

so

$$E(\hat{\delta}) = \delta + \sum_{i=1}^{c} E(W_i \xi_i) = \delta + \sum_{i=1}^{c} E(W_i) E(\xi_i) = \delta + 0 = \delta, \tag{8.10}$$

providing also that the W_i and ξ_i are independent (which holds under the assumption of normality).

Under the conditions of Sections 8.2 through 8.4, there is an a priori basis for considering each of the $\hat{\delta}_i$ as an unbiased estimate of δ. Therefore, a reasonable pooled, design-based analysis (either as a significance test or as a confidence interval) may be based on T given in Equation 8.9. For a choice of weights W_i for which $E(\hat{\delta}) \neq \delta$, a pooled analysis of the data may be based on Equation 8.8. Here, the inference would be on $E(\hat{\delta})$, rather than on δ—which is not the question the multicenter trial was designed to answer. One might thus question whether the results may be regarded as confirmatory. It is therefore crucial to examine the $\hat{\delta}_i$ and assess whether they reflect random variation about some constant.

It is noted that for dichotomous response data, the data at each center may be summarized by a two-by-two table of responders versus nonresponders by treatment group. Let O_i denote the number of responders in the pivotal cell of each two-by-two table, and $E(O_i)$ and $Var(O_i)$ denote the expected value and variance of O_i, respectively, computed from the hypergeometric distribution. The square of Equation 8.8 then becomes the Mantel–Haenszel statistic [8] for addressing association between treatment and response across centers. It is well known that the Mantel–Haenszel test is a valid test regardless of whether there is treatment-by-center interaction. In fact, interaction may be regarded as a component of the alternative hypothesis [9,10].

The Mantel–Haenszel test should be followed by a test for interaction, such as the Breslow–Day test [11] to temper the interpretation of the results. It is noted that since the Mantel–Haenszel statistic represents a minor modification to the χ^2 statistic proposed by Cochran [12], the Mantel–Haenszel statistic is commonly referred to as the Cochran–Mantel–Haenszel statistic.

Thus, for continuous data, a test based on Equation 8.8 may be regarded as a parametric analogue of the Cochran–Mantel–Haenszel test, and produces a valid test on $E(\hat{\delta})$ regardless of whether there is a treatment-by-center interaction. For consistency of analysis approach, the results of the test should be followed with a test for interaction to aid in the interpretation of the inference on $E(\hat{\delta})$.

8.5.2 Model-Based Analysis Strategies

8.5.2.1 Fixed Center and Treatment Effects: No Interaction or No Significant Interaction

Run the no interaction ANOVA Model (1) and provide an inference (significance test or confidence interval) on the treatment effect:

$$Y_{ijk} = \mu + C_i + T_j + \xi_{ijk}, \qquad \text{(Model 1)}$$

where
C_i is the fixed effect of the ith center
T_j is the fixed effect of the jth treatment
Y_{ijk} is the response of the kth patient in jth treatment group at the ith center
ξ_{ijk} is the random measurement error in observing Y_{ijk}
μ is a constant effect common to all responses
the ξ_{ijk} are independent and follow a normal distribution with mean 0 and variance σ_i^2, and where $i = 1, \ldots, c; j = 1, \ldots, t;$ and $k = 1, \ldots, n_{ij}$

To aid in the interpretation of the inference from Model (1), Model (2) is then run:

$$Y_{ijk} = \mu + C_i + T_j + (CT)_{ij} + \xi_{ijk}, \qquad \text{(Model 2)}$$

where $(CT)_{ij}$ is the fixed interaction effect between the ith center and jth treatment, and interest from the ANOVA is **only on the statistical significance of the interaction term**. If the interaction term is not statistically significant, then the inference on treatment effect from Model (1) is reported and the estimate of treatment effect is considered generalizable across centers. A point to be made here is that Model (2) is run after running Model (1) solely for interpretation of the treatment effect from Model (1).

8.5.2.2 Center and Treatment as Fixed Effects: Significant Interaction

If the interaction term in Model (2) is significant, some analysts report the treatment effect from Model (1) with the caveat that the treatment effect is inconsistent across centers, and rank the estimates of treatment effect at each center to illustrate the range across centers. This display may be followed by a graphical presentation of confidence intervals based on the estimates of treatment effect at the individual centers. Parenthetically, since the estimate of treatment effect from Model (1) is based on an average of the treatment effects at individual centers, one expects intuitively that not all treatment effects across centers are the same. If any center for which the estimate of treatment effect is clearly higher (or lower) than others, the center and data from the center should be investigated to assess whether there are explanations for the discrepancy.

Other analysts do not run Model (1) first and aver that the proper analysis derives from Model (2), and if there is a statistically significant treatment-by-center interaction, there should be no overall pooled analysis of the data. Further, if the treatment-by-center effect is statistically significant, some analysts base inference on from Model (2), with the estimate of treatment effect adjusted for differences between centers and treatment-by-center interaction. However, this adjusted treatment effect would not in general provide an unbiased estimate of the treatment effect $(\mu_d - \mu_p)$ explicit in the protocol objective (H_a of Section 8.5).

8.5.2.3 Random Center and Fixed Treatment Effects

To get around the interaction problem, other analysts suggest that the proper analysis derives from an analysis of variance Model (3):

$$Y_{ijk} = \mu + C_i + T_j + (CT)_{ij} + \xi_{ijk}, \qquad \text{(Model 3)}$$

where the terms in Model (3) are identical to those in Model (2), except that the C_i are random, independently, and identically distributed with mean 0 and common variance that are independent of the ξ_{ijk}; and base the test for treatment effect on the ratio of mean square for treatment divided by the mean square for treatment-by-center interaction. The main criticism of this latter strategy is that centers or investigators do not represent a random sample from some population of centers or investigators. Further, the power of the test for treatment effect from this strategy would be reduced (as compared to those based on Model (1) or Model (2)), particularly in multicenter clinical trials that have few centers.

8.6 Concluding Remarks

The main focus of this chapter is to discuss design-based and model-based approaches in the analysis of multicenter trials and to argue that a pooled analysis should be performed for every quality designed and conducted multicenter clinical trial. Through quality design and development of the protocol, planning, training, execution, and monitoring, practically all that can be done to ensure homogeneous patient populations, patient treatment and assessment, and measurement methodology across investigational centers, is done. There is therefore an a priori basis for pooling the estimates of treatment effect at each center across centers.

8.6.1 Design-Based Inference

Under the conditions of Sections 8.2 through 8.4, there is an a priori basis for considering each of the $\hat{\delta}_i\{=(\overline{T}_{i\cdot} - \overline{P}_{i\cdot})\}$ as an unbiased estimate of $\delta\{=(\mu_d - \mu_p)\}$. Therefore, a reasonable pooled, design-based analysis (either as a significance test or as a confidence interval) may be based on T:

$$T = \frac{\{(\hat{\delta} - E(\hat{\delta}))\}}{\sqrt{\hat{\sigma}^2}},$$

where $\hat{\delta} = \sum_{i=1}^{c} W_i \hat{\delta}_i$, $\hat{\sigma}^2$ is the variance of the $\hat{\delta}$, and the W_i are an appropriate choice of weights; for example, given in Equations 8.4 through 8.7. The choice of weights in Equation 8.4 yields the arithmetic average of the estimates of treatment effect across centers. The choice of weights in Equation 8.5 reduces to Equation 8.4 if there is balance across centers. The choice of weights in Equation 8.6 reduces to Equation 8.4 if treatment groups are balanced across centers. The choice of weights in Equation 8.7 reduces to Equation 8.4 if the variances ($\hat{\sigma}_i^2$) of the $\hat{\delta}_i$ are homogeneous across centers. Cox [13] notes that the weighted average of the $\hat{\delta}_i$ for the choice of weights specified in Equation 8.7 is "best" when the variances $\hat{\sigma}_i^2$ are known.

In order for the inference based on T of Equation 8.8 to provide an inference of the hypothesized treatment effect, it is crucial for the analyst to verify that expected value of $\hat{\delta}$ is δ. If not (which could reflect a treatment-by-center interaction), and if the test based on T of Equation 8.8 is statistically significant, one may conclude evidence of an overall treatment effect, but the treatment effect may not generalize across centers. In this case, the analyst is compelled to communicate the magnitude of the treatment effect at individual centers. If there is a subset of centers for which the expected value of $\hat{\delta}$ is δ, it is reasonable to report the combined treatment effect for these centers along with the treatment effects for outlying centers.

Finally, if central limit theory may not be drawn upon regarding inference based on T, resampling-based methods may be used.

8.6.2 Model-Based Inference

My practice has been to run Model (1) for providing inference on treatment effect, then run Model (2) to assess treatment-by-center interaction and report accordingly. If the interaction is nonsignificant, then the estimate of treatment effect is considered generalizable across centers. If the interaction is significant, then the estimate of treatment effect may not be generalizable across centers, and descriptive summaries and graphical displays of the per center estimates of treatment effect should be presented to convey the nature of the interaction. Since the multicenter clinical trial is not designed from a power perspective to detect interaction, many analysts, for example Fleiss [14], use a significance level of 0.10 to judge the significance ($P \leq 0.10$) of the test for interaction.

To better understand the data and broader nature of the inference on treatment effect, Model (2) may also be run to explore generalizability of treatment effect across factors other than centers. Factors to be considered are demographic characteristics (e.g., age, sex, race, or ethnicity) and disease characteristics (e.g., baseline severity) so that the interpretation of the effect may be appropriately tempered. In these analyses, interest is solely on the significance of the treatment-by-factor interaction. Results of this exploration may be helpful in generating the drug product label.

Lack of homogeneity among centers in a multicenter clinical trial can demonstrably impact the statistical detection of treatment effects [15]. A goal of a quality designed and quality conducted multicenter clinical trial is to strive for homogeneity among centers. In order to accomplish or come close to accomplishing, this goal requires ownership and commitment from all personnel having some responsibility in the design, conduct, monitoring, data management, statistical analysis, and reporting of the trial.

It may be that modifying the typical design of multicenter trials to account for biological variation in terms of how patients metabolize the drug may lead to greater homogeneity of treatment effect across centers. For example, after patients qualify for the protocol but prior to randomization, give them a single dose of the drug, obtain sufficient blood samples to estimate the maximum concentration C_{MAX}, and then stratify before randomization on levels of C_{MAX} [16].

References

1. Peace KE (1991): One-sided or two-sided *p*-values: Which most appropriately address the question of drug efficacy? *Journal of Biopharmaceutical Statistics;* **1**(1): 133–138.
2. Makuch RW, Pledger G, Hall DB, Johnson MF, Herson J, Hsu JP (1990): Active control equivalence studies. In: *Statistical Issues in Drug Research and Development*, Peace, KE (ed.), Marcel Dekker, Inc., New York, Chap. 4, pp. 225–262.
3. Snappin S (2000): Noninferiority trials. *Current Controlled Trials in Cardiovascular Medicine;* **1**(1): 19–21.

4. Peace KE, Dickson B (1987): A meta-analysis of duodenal ulcer relapse using actual patient data: A comparison of the effect of acute treatment with cimetidine, misoprostol and placebo. *Gastroenterology*; **95**: 1370.

5. Satterthwaite FE (1946): An approximate distribution of estimates of variance components. *Biometrics*; **2**: 110–114.

6. Welch BL (1938): The significance of the difference between two means when the population variances are unequal. *Biometrika*; **29**(3–4): 350–382.

7. Cochran WG (1964): Approximate significance levels of the Behrens–Fisher test. *Biometrics*; **20**(1): 191–195.

8. Mantel N, Haenszel W (1959): Statistical aspects of the analysis of data from retrospective studies of disease. *Journal of the National Cancer Institute*; **22**(4): 719–748.

9. Landis JR, Heyman ER, Koch GG (1978): Average partial association in three way contingency tables: A review and discussion of alternative tests. *International Statistical Reviews*; **46**: 237–254.

10. Landis JR, Heyman ER, Koch GG (1978): An application of the generalized Cochran–Mantel–Haenszel procedure to multicenter clinical trial data with two attachments. In: *Annual Meeting of the Biostatistics Subsection Meeting of the Pharmaceutical Manufacturers Association*, Crystal City, VA.

11. Breslow NE, Day NE (1980): *Statistical Methods in Cancer Research: Vol. I—The Analysis of Case-Control Studies*, International Agency for Research on Cancer, Lyon.

12. Cochran WG (1954): Some methods for strengthening the common χ^2 tests. *Biometrics*; **10**: 417–451.

13. Cox DR (1982): Combination of data. In: *Encyclopedia of Statistical Science*, Vol. 2, Kotz, S, Johnson, NL (eds.), Wiley, New York, pp. 45–53.

14. Fleiss JL (1986): Analysis of data from multiclinic trials. *Controlled Clinical Trials*; **7**: 267–275.

15. Peace KE (1992): The impact of investigator heterogeneity in clinical trials on detecting treatment differences. *Drug Information Journal*; **26**: 463–469.

16. Peace KE (1994): To pool or not (to pool). In: *Annual Meeting of the American Statistical Association*, August, 1994, Toronto, Ontario, Canada; #1217.

9

Validity of Statistical Inference

9.1 Introduction

Nearly six decades have elapsed since the MRC Tuberculosis Research Unit conducted the first randomized controlled clinical trial [1–3]. It is widely held [4,5] that the randomization and control design aspects of the trial were the brainchildren of Sir Austin Bradford Hill, Director of the MRC Statistical Research Unit. The 1962 Kefauver–Harris (K–F) Amendments [6] to the Federal Food, Drug and Cosmetics Act of 1938 represented a watershed event in the evolution of evidence to support drug claims. This landmark legislation required that all drugs thereafter be proven effective prior to being approved by the Food and Drug Administration (FDA) for marketing in the United States. The authors and others have often referred to the K–F Amendments as *the full employment act of biostatisticians in the pharmaceutical industry*.

Much progress has been made in strengthening evidence to support claims deriving from clinical trials since the first randomized control clinical trial (RCCT). The FDA has been a major player in advancing the need for better quality clinical trials, as well as evolving evidentiary methodological standards to accomplish (see comments by Temple and O'Neill [6]). The double blind (DB) RCCT is now considered the gold standard for evidentiary medicine.

Strengthening the evidence to support claims deriving from clinical trials is the result of, first, recognizing the need for improvement and, second, the collective desire to improve quality in all aspects of such investigations [7–9]. Improving the experimental design of the investigation is one aspect, and this includes ensuring an adequate number of participants [10–13]. Improving the quality of reporting the investigation [14–18] is another aspect.

Recognizing that clinical drug trials don't necessarily mimic clinical practice has spawned the relatively new area of translational research [19]. "Translational medicine is a branch of medical research that attempts to more directly connect basic research to patient care. Translational medicine is growing in importance in the healthcare industry, and it is a term whose precise definition is in flux. In the case of drug discovery and development, translational medicine typically refers to the 'translation' of basic research into real therapies for real patients. The emphasis is on the linkage between the laboratory and the patient's bedside, without a real disconnect. This is often called the 'bench to bedside' definition." [20].

All of these settings require the design of an investigational protocol, conducting the investigation per the protocol and collecting the data, statistically analyzing the data, making valid inferential conclusions relative to the objectives of the protocol, and reporting the results. When considering the validity of statistical inferences from clinical trials, many will restrict attention to whether the statistical methodology used to analyze the data is appropriate for the type of data and whether the assumptions underlying the methodology hold for the data. This is necessary for an inference from a statistical analysis to be valid, but it is not sufficient. Valid inferences derive from well-planned, well-conducted, and properly analyzed investigations.

All aspects of an investigation, whether in the clinical drug development area, in the medical university research area, in the public health intervention area, or in the basic laboratory research area, should be documented to permit an audit of "what was to be done," "what was done," and how differences might affect conclusions or inferences. Planning activities culminate in a protocol [7,11] for the investigation. The protocol starts with a well-defined question or objective that requires an investigation to answer [9]. The data or endpoints needed to provide an answer are identified. The question is then formulated within a hypothesis testing framework. The number of subjects required to address the question is determined. Procedures for conducting the experimental investigation that produces the required data are developed. Methods for collecting, computerizing, and quality assuring the data are specified. Statistical methods for analyzing the data addressing the question are described.

9.2 Planning the Investigation

9.2.1 Research Question and Endpoints

The research question of the investigation should be defined so that it is unambiguous. For example, in an investigation about the antihypertensive efficacy of drug D in some defined population, the statement, "The objective of this investigation is to assess the efficacy of drug D," although providing general information as to the question ("Is D efficacious?"), is ambiguous. The statement, "The objective of this investigation is to assess whether drug D is superior to placebo P in the treatment of hypertensive patients with diastolic blood pressure (DBP) between 90 and 100 mmHg for 6 months" is better—as the hypertensive population to be treated and what is meant by efficacious in a comparative sense are specified. However, the data or endpoint(s) upon which antihypertensive efficacy will be based is not specified. DBP is stated, but how will it be measured?—Using a sphygmo-manometer or a digital monitor? Will DBP be measured in the sitting, standing, or supine position? Further, what function of the DBP will be used?—The change from baseline to the end of the treatment period? Or whether the patient achieves a therapeutic goal of normotensive (DBP $\leq$ 80 mmHg) by the end of the treatment period?

9.2.2 Hypothesis Testing Framework

Reformulating the question within a hypothesis testing framework adds clarity [7,9]. The question regarding the efficacy of D as an antihypertensive is the alternative hypothesis: H_a: $\mu_D - \mu_P = \delta = \delta_a > 0$ versus the null hypothesis, H_0: $\delta = 0$, where δ is the difference between the true effects of D and P, and δ_a is the specified value of δ reflecting the magnitude of comparative efficacy of D desired to be detected in the planned investigation. It should be noted that H_a has to be one-sided [21] to capture the question of the efficacy of D (as compared to P).

There are many who disagree that the question of efficacy is one-sided, and the references in the first author's paper [21] may be seen for some of those views. Those who work in drug development in the pharmaceutical industry are aware that the FDA routinely request two-sided *P*-values. The authors' arguments in support of one-sided *P*-values to address efficacy, particularly for Phase III, placebo-controlled clinical trials, are logical and scientifically defensible and clearly articulated [21].

9.2.3 The Number of Subjects

The number of subjects required to provide a valid inference must be determined prior to beginning the investigation [12, see also Chapter 4]. It requires specifying the difference δ_a between interventions, reflecting similarity or superiority, the magnitude of the Type I error α, the statistical power $1 - \beta$ or degree of certainty required to detect δ_a, and an estimate of variability of the data or endpoint reflecting the question. The difference δ_a reflects the minimum difference between regimens in order to conclude superiority of one regimen (if the question is superiority), and reflects the maximum difference between regimens to conclude similarity or non-inferiority (if similarity or non-inferiority is the question). Sample size determination is not a cookbook exercise and should not be taken lightly [12,22–24]. In clinical trials, the specification of δ_a is the responsibility of the project clinician and requires careful thinking and exploration by both the statistician and the project clinician. A δ_a too large may lead to failure to answer the question due to too small a sample. A δ_a too small would increase costs of conducting the investigation and may not be accepted as clinically meaningful.

One of the reasons we began recommending a power of 95% to detect a difference of δ_a with a false positive rate of 5% in Phase III placebo-controlled clinical trials was because experience had taught us that clinicians usually overestimate the efficacy of a drug at the design stage. If one designs a trial with these levels of Type I and Type II errors, one will be able to detect a difference as small as $1/2\ \delta_a$ as statistically significant ($P \leq 0.05$) at the analysis stage (see Table 4.3). Strictly speaking, this requires the number of patients in the analysis to be equal to the number of patients at the design stage and that the variance in the analysis for analyzing efficacy to be equal to the estimated variance at the design stage. Analyses based on the intention-to-treat philosophy would satisfy the sample size requirement. Further, for dichotomous response, using the worst case binomial variance at the design stage will guarantee that the variance requirement at the analysis stage is met; in fact, using the variance inherent in the data analyzed will produce statistical significance if the observed estimate of efficacy is slightly less than $1/2\ \delta_a$.

Many choose an 80% power when designing Phase III clinical trials. Whereas 80% is better than any lower power, we consider it too low. A clinical trial designed with an 80% power is roughly 57% as large (see Table 4.1) as one designed with 95% power. Determining sample size for Phase III pivotal proof-of-efficacy trials has an efficacy imperative. It is the professional responsibility of the biostatistician supporting such trials to ensure at the design stage that adequate numbers of patients are studied so that if the drug is truly effective, it will be detected as such at the analysis stage. Designing Phase III efficacy trials with 95% power rather than 80% will enable the clinical safety profile of the drug to be better described and estimated. Thus, not only is there an efficacy imperative attendant to designing Phase III clinical trials, there is an ethical imperative as well.

9.2.4 Procedures for Conducting the Investigation

Procedures for conducting the investigation are crucial to the success of the investigation. All procedures or methods pertinent to how subjects are selected and treated, the data measurement process, elimination or reduction of bias, visit scheduling, patient and investigator expectations, handling of adverse events, problem management, and so on should be specified (see Section 6.3.2.5). Failure to minimize sources of variability [8] other than true inter- and intra-subject variability may lead to failure to reach the desired conclusion (see Chapter 8).

9.2.5 Data Collection, Computerization, and Quality Assurance

Data collection, computerization, and quality assurance methods for the data should be specified prior to beginning the investigation. Fundamental to any valid inference is the integrity of the data analyzed. One must have assurance that the data analyzed are the data collected—and that the data collected accurately reflect the condition being studied.

There are three general phases in data collection and management prior to statistical analyses. The first is to ensure that the data recorded at the investigational site is accurate. Such data are recorded in the investigator's patient file (or record) and also on the data collection form (DCF) provided by the drug sponsor for the particular clinical trial. There must be assurance that data in the patient record is the same as on the DCF. The second is to enter the data from the DCFs into the sponsor's computerized database for the clinical trial. This entry process must be quality assured so that the data in the database is the same as that on the DCFs. The third is to release the quality assured database to the biostatistician for statistical analyses. Usually the data set provided to the biostatistician contains endpoints computed on the actual data. One must have the assurance that such endpoints are correctly computed.

Assurance of the first step is the responsibility of the sponsor's medical monitor for the investigational site and is accomplished by thorough and frequent monitoring visits and interaction with site personnel. Data management personnel often discover data inconsistencies or data elements that need to be queried in the entry and quality assurance processes and will forward these to the site for resolution. The biostatistician may further find data elements during the analysis process that need to be resolved by the site.

Assurance of the second step is the responsibility of the data management department. Many pharmaceutical companies double enter data (by different data entry personnel) from the DCFs, then cross-check the two databases and print out mismatches and verify. This leads to one database that is relative free of entry errors. Further, key efficacy and safety data are printed out and verified against the DCFs to ensure no errors in entry of these data. The remaining data is usually quality assured by random sampling schemes applied to the database and checked against the DCFs. Any entry errors are corrected in the database, and the sampling process repeated until an acceptable database error rate is obtained.

Assurance of the third step is the joint responsibility of database management personnel and the biostatistician. Database management personnel assure that the data in the analysis data set is identical with that in the database. The biostatistician assures that the computation of the endpoints from the actual data is correct. If not, then he or she works with data management personnel to ensure the correct computations.

9.2.6 Statistical Methods

Statistical methods for analyzing the data must be identified and described prior to beginning the investigation and included in the statistical analysis plan [11, see also Sections 6.4 and 7.7]. In order for an inference from a statistical analysis to be scientifically valid, there must be an a priori commitment to the question and methods of analysis—subject to assumptions underlying the methods being satisfied by the data.

9.3 Conducting the Investigation

The investigation per the scientific plan or protocol and procedures must be conducted in a quality and unbiased manner. The investigation should be carefully monitored to ensure adherence to the protocol and any institutional or regulatory requirements. For multi-investigator studies, an additional goal of monitoring is to reduce inter-investigator heterogeneity [8].

9.4 Statistical Analyses, Interpretation, and Inference

Once the data collected are computerized and quality assured, planned statistical analyses may begin. Assumptions underlying the validity of the analysis methods specified in the protocol should be checked to see if they hold for the data being analyzed.

For example, analysis of variance (ANOVA) methods of treatment groups require that measurement errors are independent and normally distributed with mean zero and homogeneous variance across the groups. When data are measured on different patients, independence is usually assumed. Normality may be assessed by the Shapiro–Wilk test [25]. Levene's test [26] may be used to assess homogeneity of variances. These tests are applied to the residuals from the model and require the user to output residuals to a user-defined data set. Various plots (e.g., histogram, normal probability plot) of the residuals as well as descriptive statistics of the residuals are also helpful. If the normality assumption doesn't hold, then transformations of the data that lead to the assumptions being satisfied or nonparametric methods may be performed. If variances are heterogeneous, Satterthwaite's procedure [27] may be used to approximate the degrees of freedom.

As another example, analysis of covariance (ANCOVA) methods require the additional assumptions that the covariate is independent of the influence of the treatment received in the treatment groups and that the regressions of response on the covariate within each treatment group are parallel across the treatment groups. This assumption may be easily checked by assessing the statistical significance of the interaction term in the ANCOVA model:

$$Y_{ij} = \mu + T_i + \beta X_{ij} + \gamma(T_i * X_{ij}) + \varepsilon_{ij}$$

where

Y_{ij} is the response on the jth patient in the ith treatment group

μ is a constant common to all patients

X_{ij} is the covariate on the jth patient in the ith treatment group

β is the slope of the common linear regression over groups

$T_i {}^* X_{ij}$ is the interaction term between treatment group and the covariate

γ is the interaction parameter

ε_{ij} is the measurement error in observing Y_{ij}

ε_{ij} are assumed to be identically, independently, and normally distributed with mean 0 and common variance σ^2; $i = 1, \ldots, k$ and $j = 1, \ldots, n_i$

Statistical significance for the interaction effect is often assessed using a P-value larger than 0.05 (since the power is typically low), say 0.10. A statistically significant interaction effect signals a treatment effect, and that the effect of treatment is not constant over the range of the covariate. Therefore, the reduced model obtained by dropping the interaction effect from the ANCOVA model should not be used for inference. Alternatively, one may fit separate linear regressions within each treatment group, estimate the treatment effect (adjusted for the covariate) at various values (low, middle, high) of the covariate range, and provide confidence intervals of the adjusted treatment effect at covariate values.

Rarely does an investigation finish with complete data on the planned number of subjects. There are numerous reasons for this: dropouts due to adverse experiences or lack of efficacy, missed visits due to brief illnesses or a variety of logistical reasons, relocation, and so on. The reasons for missing data should be thoroughly investigated, and if the data are missing at random, procedures [28] exist that permit a valid statistical analysis. However, whether the inference is credible and generalizable will depend on the amount of missing data.

Crucial to the validity of an inference is the integrity of the Type I error. On the simplest level, a valid analysis produces an estimate of comparative effect of interventions and a corresponding P-value. The estimate may be regarded as a real comparative effect, provided the P-value is small (<0.05) and is correctly determined. Parenthetically, conclusions about the comparative effect should not be based on the P-value alone, but also on the size of the effect. There is not much utility in statistical significance of findings in the absence of their clinical significance or relevance. Analyses of multiple end-points or multiple analyses of the same endpoint lead to chance findings when no effects exist. This is easily seen by writing the equation for the probability of at least one statistically significant result out of k independent analyses when none exist: $P[\text{at least 1 significant result} \mid \text{none are}] = 1 - (1 - \alpha)^k$, when testing at the α level of significance. This probability is 0.401 if $k = 10$ and $\alpha = 0.05$. Thus, out of 10 independent analyses each at a Type I error rate of 5%, there is a 40% chance of declaring at least one statistically significant when in fact no differences exit (i.e., the null hypothesis is true).

9.5 Reporting Results of Investigations

One goal of reporting results of clinical investigations is to permit translating such investigations into practice. Attempts at translating investigations into practice have been reported in many areas. Some are AIDS [29], cancer [30], Epoetin use [31], genital herpes [32], heart failure [33], hypertension [34], internal medicine [35], and obstetrics [36]. If the results of investigations are to be translated into practice, reporting the implementation aspects of the investigation must be improved [37].

9.6 Concluding Remarks

When considering whether an inferential conclusion from an investigation is valid, consider these questions: (1) Was there an a priori commitment to the question? (2) Was (were) the endpoint (s) appropriate for the question (s)? (3) Was the experimental design appropriate for the condition being studied? (4) Was the investigation conducted in a quality manner to eliminate bias and to ensure accuracy of the data? (5) Were steps taken to preserve the integrity of the Type I error? (6) Were the statistical methods for analyses valid (assumptions checked, dropouts appropriately handled, correct variance term, etc.)? (7) Were the results of statistical analyses properly interpreted (the correct inferred population, impact of multiple endpoints or analyses, etc.)?

In over 30 years of supporting research and clinical development of pharmaceuticals and public health intervention programs, the first author has had the opportunity to analyze data from, and evaluate hundreds of clinical trials and intervention programs. In many cases, the first author has developed innovative analysis methods. While valid data analyses are necessary and important, it is the authors' belief based on experience and observation that advances in science, advances in the treatment of patients, and improvements in public health derive from well-planned and well-conducted investigations more so than from esoteric analyses of data. As Dr. Lewis Thomas said so eloquently [13] "From here on, as far ahead as one can see, medicine must be building as a central part of its scientific base a solid underpinning of biostatistical and epidemiological knowledge. Hunches and intuitive impressions are essential for getting the work started, but it is only through the **quality of numbers at the end that the truth can be told.**" The authors add that no analysis of data can salvage a poorly designed or poorly conducted investigation. To put it simply, there is no statistical fix.

References

1. MRC Streptomycin in Tuberculosis Trials Committee (1948): Streptomycin treatment of pulmonary tuberculosis. *British Medical Journal*; **ii**: 769–783.
2. Landsborough TA (1975): *Half a Century of Medical Research*, Her Majesty's Stationary Office, London, U.K., pp. 238–239.
3. Sutherland I (1998): Medical research council streptomycin trial. In: *Encyclopedia of Biostatistics*, Wiley, Chichester, U.K., pp. 2559–2567.
4. Bradford Hill A (1990): Memories of the British streptomycin trial in tuberculosis. *Controlled Clinical Trials*; **11**: 77–90.
5. Armitage P (1992): Bradford Hill and the randomised controlled trial. *Pharmaceutical Medicine*; **6**: 23–37.
6. Bren L (2007): The advancement of controlled clinical trials. *FDA Consumer Magazine*; http://www.fda.gov/fdac/features/2007/207_trials.html
7. Peace KE (1991): Shortening the time for clinical drug development. *Regulatory Affairs Professionals Journal*; **3**: 3–22.
8. Peace KE (1992): The impact of investigator heterogeneity in clinical trials on detecting treatment differences. *Drug Information Journal*; **26**: 463–469.
9. Peace KE (2006): Importance of the research question relative to analysis. *Philippine Statistical Association Newsletter*; **1**(1): 7–9.
10. Peace KE (1991): Sample size considerations of clinical trials pre-market approval (invited presentation). In: 27th *Annual Meeting of the Drug Information Association*, Washington, DC.
11. Peace KE (2005): Statistical section of a clinical trial protocol. *The Philippine Statistician*; **54**(4): 1–8.
12. Peace KE (2006): Sample size considerations of clinical trials pre-market approval. *The Philippine Statistician*; **55**(2): 1–27.
13. Thomas L (1977): Memorial Sloan–Kettering cancer center. *Science*; **198**: 675.
14. Bailar JC III, Mosteller F (1988): Guidelines for statistical reporting in articles for medical journals: Amplifications and explanations. *Annals of Internal Medicine*; **108**: 266–273.
15. Begg C, Cho M, Eastwood S, Horton R, Moher D, Olkin I, Pitkin R, Rennie D, Schulz KF, Simel D, Stroup DF (1996): Improving the quality of reporting of randomized controlled trials: The CONSORT statement. *Journal of the American Medical Association*; **276**: 637–639.
16. Moher D, Cook DJ, Eastwood S, Olkin I, Rennie D, Stroup DF (1999): Improving the quality of reports of meta-analyses of randomised controlled trials: The QUOROM statement. *The Lancet*; **354**: 1896–1900.
17. Peace KE (1984): Data listings and summaries should also reflect experimental structure. *Biometrics*; **40**(1): 256.
18. Stroup DF, Berlin JA, Morton SC, Olkin I, Williamson GD, Rennie D, Moher D, Becker BJ, Sipe TA, Thacker SB, for the Meta-analysis of Observational Studies in Epidemiology (MOOSE) Group (2000): Meta-analysis of observational studies in epidemiology: A proposal for reporting. *Journal of the American Medical Association*; **283**: 2008–2012.
19. Pizzo P (2002): Letter "Comments re Translational Medicine," http://mednews.stanford.edu/stanmed/2002fall/letter.html

20. Wikipedia, the free encyclopedia (redirected from Translational Medicine: 2007); http://en.wikipedia.org/wiki/Translational_medicine
21. Peace KE (1991): One-sided or two-sided p-values: Which most appropriately address the question of drug efficacy? *Journal of Biopharmaceutical Statistics*; **1**(1): 133–138.
22. Lwanga SK, Lemeshow S (1991): *Sample Size Determination in Health Studies: A Practical Manual (Paperback)*, World Health Organization, Geneva, Switzerland, 80pp.
23. Lenth RV (2001): Some practical guidelines for effective sample size determination. *The American Statistician*; **55**: 187–194.
24. Brasher PMA, Brant RF (2007): Sample size calculations in randomized trials: Common pitfalls. *Canadian Journal of Anesthesia*; **54**: 103–106.
25. Shapiro SS, Wilk MB (1965): An analysis of variance test for normality. *Biometrika*; **52**(3): 591–599.
26. Levene, H (1960): In: *Contributions to Probability and Statistics: Essays in Honor of Harold Hotelling*, I. Olkin et al. (eds.), Stanford University Press, Stanford, CA, pp. 278–292.
27. Satterthwaite FE (1946): An approximate distribution of estimates of variance components. *Biometrics*; **2**: 110–114.
28. Ibrahim JG, Molenberghs G (2009): Missing data methods in longitudinal studies: A review. *Test*; **18**(1): 1–43.
29. Turner BJ, Newschaffer CJ, Zhang D, Fanning T, Hauck WW (1999): Translating clinical trial results into practice: The effect of an AIDS clinical trial on prescribed antiretroviral therapy for HIV-infected pregnant women. *Annals of Internal Medicine*; 15 June; **130**(12): 979–986.
30. Jatoi I, Proschan MA (2006): Clinical trial results applied to management of the individual cancer patient. *World Journal of Surgery*; **30**(7): 1184–1189.
31. Cotter D, Thamer M, Narasimhan K, Zhang Y, Bullock K (2006): Translating epoetin research into practice: The role of government and the use of scientific evidence. *Health Affairs*; **25**(5): 1249–1259.
32. Hook EW, Leone P (2006): Time to translate new knowledge into practice: A call for a national genital herpes control program. *The Journal of Infectious Diseases*; **194**: 6–7.
33. Patel P, White D, Deswal A (2007). Translation of clinical trials results into practice: Temporal patterns of beta-blocker utilization for heart failure at hospital discharge and during ambulatory follow-up. *American Heart Journal*; **153**(4): 515–522.
34. Goldstein MK, Coleman RW, TU SW, Shankar RD, O'Connor MJ, Musen MA, Martins SB, Lavori PW, Shlipak MG, Oddone E, Advani AA, Gholami P, Hoffman BB (2004): Translating research into practice: Organizational issues in implementing automated decision support for hypertension in three medical centers. *Journal of American Medical Information Association*; June 7; **11**: 368–376.
35. Julian DG (2004): Translation of clinical trials into clinical practice. *Journal of Internal Medicine*; **255**: 309–316.
36. Jesse DE (2007): Translating POP (Psychosocial Obstetrical Profile) research results into practice and policy. In: *The 18th International Nursing Research Congress Focusing on Evidence-Based Practice*, Vienna, Austria, 11–14 July.
37. Mayo-Wilson E (2007): Reporting implementation in randomized trials: Proposed additions to the consolidated standards of reporting trials statement. *American Journal of Public Health*; **97**: 630–633. doi:10.2105/AJPH.2006. 094169.

10

Bioequivalence Clinical Trials

10.1 Introduction

A bioequivalence clinical trial is a clinical trial that follows a protocol whose objective is to demonstrate that two (or more) formulations of the same drug are "bioequivalent." Two formulations of the same drug are said to be bioequivalent if they have identical or comparable bioavailability. Bioavailability is thought of as the extent and rate to which the active drug (or active metabolite) gets into the bloodstream and is hence made available to tissue and the target organ.

10.2 Absorption, Distribution, Metabolism, and Excretion (ADME)

When a drug gets into the body it is absorbed into the bloodstream and distributed throughout the body where it undergoes metabolism and elimination.

Absorption (A) refers to the process of the drug getting into the bloodstream, from where it gets to the site of action or target organ in the body. Absorption is dependent upon the route of administration as well as the formulation of the drug.

Distribution (D) pertains to the distribution of the drug throughout the body by the circulatory system or bloodstream.

Metabolism (M) occurs during distribution when the drug is acted on by enzymes that convert it into various metabolites as it passes through the liver. Metabolites are usually inactive. Some drugs exhibit a large *first-pass effect*. This refers to absorption via the portal vein to the liver and from there to the bloodstream, which results in extensive metabolism. For drugs that have a large *first-pass effect*, the active drug is rendered inactive quickly, and represents a problem with some drugs administered orally.

Elimination (E) refers to the removal of the active drug from the body. Some elimination occurs during metabolism, if the metabolites are inactive. The main route of elimination is renal as the drug gets to the kidney from the bloodstream and is eliminated in urine. Some of the drug is eliminated in fecal excretion. For drugs such as anesthetic gases some elimination occurs through the lungs.

10.3 Bioavailability

The bioavailability of a drug in a particular dosage form is not only the fraction of the active drug that gets into the bloodstream unchanged, but also the rate at which the active drug (or active metabolite) gets into the blood- stream and is hence made available to tissue and the target organ. To estimate bioavailability, a series of blood samples are needed following administration of the dosage form, from which concentrations of the drug in blood (more often plasma) are determined. These concentrations along with the corresponding times of sample collection may be plotted to produce a concentration-by-time curve (Figure 10.1)—reflecting oral dosing and 11 times of sample collection.

10.3.1 Basis for Estimating Bioavailability

The basis for estimating bioavailability (in terms of the amount of drug absorbed) derives from the well-known pharmacokinetic principal

$$A = \frac{AUC}{K_e V}, \tag{10.1}$$

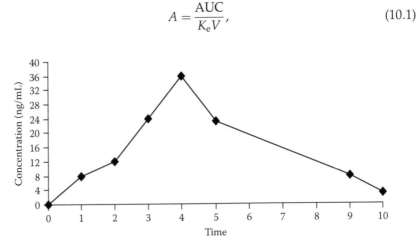

FIGURE 10.1
Blood/plasma concentration-by-time curve.

where
  A denotes the amount of drug absorbed
  AUC denotes the area under the blood or plasma concentration-by-time curve
  K_e is the elimination rate constant
  V is the volume of distribution
  K_eV is the clearance

Equation 10.1 assumes that elimination is solely from the "blood compart-ment" and that elimination follows linear kinetics.

10.3.2 Relative Bioavailability

Often the amount of the drug absorbed is expressed as a fraction of the dose administered; that is, *A* from Equation 10.1 is divided by the dose in the dosage form. If we wish to compare the bioavailability of a dose D1 to a dose D2 of a drug, then we compute the ratio of the fraction of dose D1 absorbed to the fraction of dose D2 absorbed. This ratio is said to represent the ***bioavailability of dose D1 relative to dose D2***. From Equation 10.1, if clearance remains constant (which is reasonable if subjects are given both doses separated by a washout during which the drug from the first dose is eliminated from the body) we obtain

$$\text{Relative bioavailability} = \frac{(\text{AUC})_{D1}(D2)}{(\text{AUC})_{D2}(D1)}, \tag{10.2}$$

where
  $(\text{AUC})_{D1}$ denotes the area under the blood/plasma concentration-by-time curve following administration of dose D1
  $(\text{AUC})_{D2}$ denotes the area under the blood/plasma concentration-by-time curve following administration of dose D2
  D1 denotes the amount of drug in dose D1
  D2 denotes the amount of drug in dose D2

10.3.3 Absolute Bioavailability

If the dose D1 is administered non-IV (intravenously) and the dose D2 is administered IV, then Equation 10.2 provides the absolute bioavailability of dose D1 relative to the IV administration. In this case, the amounts of drug in doses D1 and D2 would be the same:

$$\text{Absolute bioavailability of Dose D1} = \frac{(\text{AUC})_{D1}(\text{Dose IV})}{(\text{AUC})_{\text{DoseIV}}(D1)}. \tag{10.3}$$

If Dose D1 was also administered IV, then Equation 10.3 reduces to 1, so that the absolute bioavailability of an IV dose is 1, which is intuitively the case, since the drug is administered directly into a vein, which makes it 100% available to the bloodstream.

10.4 Factors That Affect Bioavailability

There are many factors that affect bioavailability. These are the formulation or dosage form of the drug, the route of administration, and the state of the biological system. The chemical form (e.g., salt, ester, acid, etc.) of the drug determines absorption potential.

10.4.1 Formulation or Dosage Form

Examples of dosage forms or formulations of drugs are tablet, capsule, caplet, salve or cream, transdermal patch, nasal spray, solution, or liquid suspension. A formulation of a drug contains the active drug but also contains inactive ingredients called excipients. Examples of excipients are fillers, binders, wetting agents, flavorings, stabilizers, etc., that have certain physical characteristics—hardness, coating, particle size, milling, micronizing, or compression. Excipients are needed to ensure desirable properties of the formulation. For example, an oral formulation (non-sustained release) must dissolve in the gut. However, the formulation must be stable enough so that it will retain the dose of the drug when it sits on pharmacy shelves. So dissolution properties of the formulation are important.

10.4.2 Routes of Administration

The bioavailability of a drug is also affected by the route of administration. The route of administration is largely determined by the formulation. Drugs may be injected into a vein (IV administration), into a muscle (intramuscularly—IM administration), or subcutaneously. Drugs may be administered orally (e.g., as a tablet, capsule, solution or liquid suspension, or sublingually). Some drugs are administered rectally in the form of a suppository. Other drugs such as testosterone and those aimed at the cessation of smoking may be administered as a transdermal patch. Others may be administered to the skin as a salve or cream, or just below the skin, subcutaneously. Some drugs are administered intranasally as a spray.

10.4.3 State of the Biological System

The state of the biological system into which a drug is administered may affect bioavailability. Since absorption and metabolism usually slows down with age, the bioavailability of a drug in young people may differ from that of old people. Gender, body fat, the type of disease, food, exercise, heart rate, all may affect the bioavailability of a drug. Other drugs may affect the bioavailability of a drug. In order to ensure proper labeling of a new drug, the drug company conducts clinical pharmacokinetic trials to assess the effect the factors mentioned above have on the bioavailability of the new drug.

When a drug is administered to a patient, the desire is to get the drug to the site of action, tissue, or target organ in therapeutic levels. Since the site of action is not accessible to direct sampling, we rely on blood level clinical trials to determine bioavailability.

10.5 Blood Level Clinical Trials

Blood level clinical trials are clinical trials in which blood samples are collected from volunteers for the purpose of addressing some objective that requires concentration levels of a drug in blood (or plasma) samples. Since the site of action is not accessible (or may be unethical to access) for direct sampling, blood level trials are needed to estimate ADME characteristics of the drug (in the particular formulation). In the simplest form, blood level trials provide a sequence of blood/plasma drug concentrations over time (corresponding to the times of sample collections) that delineates the progress of the drug through the circulatory system in each volunteer.

Blood level clinical trials are routinely conducted in the pharmaceutical industry. When a company wishes to change the formulation of their marketed product, a blood level trial has to be conducted that demonstrates bioequivalence between the new and marketed formulations. Even if the formulation is not changed, but the site of manufacturing is, a blood level trial has to be conducted that demonstrates the bioequivalence between the formulations manufactured at the two sites. The development of a generic formulation of a drug that is no longer under patent protection requires demonstration that the generic formulation is bioequivalent to the innovator formulation.

10.6 Bioequivalence

Strictly speaking bioequivalence of two formulations of the same drug implies equivalent bioavailability of the two formulations. This means the drug in the two formulations would enter the bloodstream at the same rate and in the same amount. Two formulations of the same drug may not have identical bioavailability yet still demonstrate therapeutic equivalence, and thus be considered bioequivalent. Formulations of drugs whose therapeutic index (ratio of the minimum toxic concentration to the median effective concentration) is wide would be expected to be therapeutically equivalent. That is, the efficacy and safety of such formulations are not usually affected by small to moderate differences in bioavailability. In contrast, for drugs with a relatively narrow therapeutic index, differences in bioavailability may cause substantial therapeutic nonequivalence [1].

10.6.1 Bioavailability Parameters or Endpoints Needed for Bioequivalence

Parameters needed in the statistical assessment of bioequivalence are area under the blood/plasma concentration-by-time curve (AUC), maximum concentration (CMAX), and time required to reach maximum concentration (TMAX). Theoretically, CMAX occurs when the absorption rate equals the elimination rate.

These parameters are illustrated in Figure 10.2 for a test (T) and a reference (R) formulation of a drug administered orally. Note that $T\_Max(T) < T\_Max(R)$, $C\_Max(T) > C\_Max(R)$, and $AUC(T) > AUC(R)$. In addition, $AUC_{0-4}(T) > AUC_{0-4}(R)$, where $AUC_{0-4}(T)$ and $AUC_{0-4}(R)$ are the partial areas under the concentration-by-time curves at the time formulation T reaches its maximum concentration. Thus, the drug in the test formulation reaches the bloodstream faster and in a greater amount in formulation T than in formulation R. If the differences between the two formulations in terms of these three parameters are statistically significantly different, one expects the bioavailability of

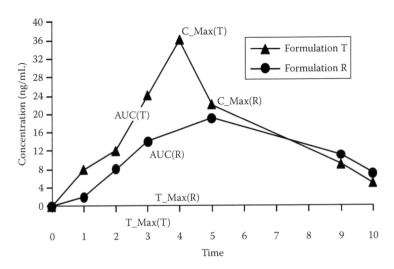

FIGURE 10.2
Plasma concentration-by-time curves of test and standard formulations.

formulations T and R to be different. Whether these differences are large enough to declare the formulations to be bioinequivalent depends on the decision criterion for concluding bioequivalence.

AUC computed from the data as in Figure 10.2 is typically symbolized as AUC_{0-t}, where t denotes the last time of sample collection. Other bioavailability parameters of interest that can be estimated from the blood/plasma concentration-by-time curve are

β_t = terminal elimination rate
$t_{1/2}$ = terminal half-life

and

$AUC_{0-\infty}$ = AUC extrapolated to infinity
AUC extrapolated to infinity is often called total exposure

It has been noted that bioavailability means the rate and extent to which the drug in a particular formulation reaches the bloodstream and that six endpoints or functions of the concentration-by-time curve data—AUC, CMAX, TMAX, β_t, $t_{1/2}$, and $AUC_{0-\infty}$—are of interest. From Equation 10.1, the analysis of AUC provides an inference as to the amount of drug absorbed. Yet none of the six endpoints is interpreted as the rate of absorption. The ratio of CMAX to TMAX approximates the average rate of absorption over the interval (0; TMAX). If the time to maximum concentration for formulation T is less than the time to maximum concentration for formulation R, to infer that the rate of absorption of formulation T is faster than the rate of absorption of formulation R requires the maximum concentration of formulation T to be at least as large as the maximum concentration of formulation R.

10.6.2 Decision Criterion for Concluding Bioequivalence

The FDA's Division of Biopharmaceutics has specified a decision criterion for concluding bioequivalence. The FDA considers a test formulation (e.g., a generic formulation) T of a drug to be bioequivalent to the reference formulation (innovator formulation) R of the same drug if the 90% confidence interval (CI) on the relative mean of T to R is between 80% and 125% for CMAX, $AUC_{(0-t)}$, and $AUC_{(0-\infty)}$ in both the fasting and fed states [2]. Although there are some exceptions to the fed state requirement, usually two blood level trials need to be conducted, one in the fasting state and one following the consumption of a meal.

The decision criterion for concluding bioequivalence is therefore

$$90\% \ CI = (LL; UL) \subseteq (0.80; 1.25), \qquad (10.4)$$

where (LL; UL) is a 90% CI on the ratio (μ_T/μ_R) of the mean (μ_T) of T to the mean of R (μ_R) for CMAX, $AUC_{(0-t)}$, and $AUC_{(0-\infty)}$. That is, the 90% CI must be contained in the decision interval.

When the decision interval for concluding bioequivalence was first proposed, it was the symmetric interval (0.80; 1.20). Westlake's [3] symmetric CI
methodology provided a natural inferential basis for concluding bioequivalence if analyzing bioavailability data on the original scales. Since such data
on the original scales do not often follow a normal distribution, but logarithmically transformed data do, the decision interval was changed so that
the upper limit became 1.25. It should be noted that if the endpoints of
the resulting interval are logarithmically transformed, a symmetric interval
(log 4 − log 5; log 5 − log 4) is obtained. So Westlake's symmetric CI still
provides an inferential basis for concluding bioequivalence.

As is indicated in Chapter 2, approval of generic formulations of drugs on
the basis of bioequivalence was established by the *Drug Price Competition and
Patent Term Restoration Act of 1984*, also known as the Hatch–Waxman Act.
This Act expedites the approval of less expensive generic formulations of
drugs by allowing FDA market approval without conducting costly clinical
trials of the generic formulation. The vehicle for submission of a request for
market approval of a generic formulation to the FDA is the *abbreviated new
drug application* (ANDA); *abbreviated* since if the generic formulation is bioequivalent to the innovator formulation, preclinical studies and clinical trials
to establish safety and efficacy are not required.

10.7 Design of Bioequivalence Trials

Generally the design of a protocol for a bioequivalence trial follows that of
the design of a protocol for a clinical trial of efficacy (Chapter 6), except that
the objective is bioequivalence rather than effectiveness. This includes clearly
formulating the objective; choosing the most appropriate experimental
design, identifying the most appropriate endpoints to address the objective;
determining the sample size; assignment of participants to the formulations
and specifying steps to minimize bias; and developing the statistical analysis
section for the protocol.

10.7.1 The Objective of Bioequivalence

In clinical trials of efficacy, the efficacy objective is the alternative hypothesis
and the inefficacy objective is the null hypothesis. Anderson and Hauck [4,5]
formulated the objective of bioequivalence as the alternative hypothesis
versus the null hypothesis of bioinequivalence. The beauty of this formulation is that the conclusion of bioequivalence is reached by rejecting the
null hypothesis and provides an inferential framework for concluding

bioequivalence similar to that for concluding effectiveness. The null (H_0) and alternative (H_a) hypotheses are

H_0: Formulations T and R are bioinequivalent
H_a: Formulations T and R are bioequivalent

H_0 and H_a may be translated as

$$H_0: 0.80 > \frac{\mu_T}{\mu_R} \quad \text{or} \quad \frac{\mu_T}{\mu_R} > 1.25$$
$$H_a: 0.80 \le \frac{\mu_T}{\mu_R} \le 1.25. \tag{10.5}$$

Formulating the objective of bioequivalence as the interval under H_a leads to the use of CIs for inferential purposes.

Schuirmann [6] proposed specifying the hypothesis of bioequivalence as two separate one-sided alternative hypotheses

$$H_{01}: 0.80 > \frac{\mu_T}{\mu_R} \quad H_{02}: \frac{\mu_T}{\mu_R} > 1.25$$
$$H_{a1}: 0.80 \le \frac{\mu_T}{\mu_R} \quad H_{a2}: \frac{\mu_T}{\mu_R} \le 1.25, \tag{10.6}$$

and proposed conducting two one-sided tests, each at the 0.05 level of significance as an inferential basis for concluding bioequivalence. It is noted that the construction in (10.6) is the decomposition of the construction in (10.5). Here, both (10.5) and (10.6) are specified reflecting the endpoints of the decision interval for concluding bioequivalence. The methodologies of Anderson and Hauck and of Schuirmann hold if the decision interval is of the more general form $L \le \mu_T/\mu_R \le U$.

10.7.2 Experimental Design Considerations

In designing bioequivalence trials, attention should be given to the basis for the type of experimental design, the drug elimination interval, the times of blood sample collection, and specific experimental design considerations.

10.7.2.1 The Type of Experimental Design

A large source of variability in the observations of drug concentrations in blood or plasma is due to subjects. It may be due to size or difference in "volume of distribution," differing metabolic rates, differing amounts of tissue or protein binding, or absorption characteristics. A design that uses each subject more than once and therefore allows estimation and removal of intersubject variability from formulation comparisons is usually more efficient than a completely randomized design. Quoting from the FDA guidance for bioavailability and bioequivalence requirements [7], *A single-dose study should* *be **crossover in design**, unless a parallel design or other design is more appropriate for valid scientific reasons, and should provide for a drug elimination period.*

10.7.2.2 Drug Elimination Period

Unless some other approach is appropriate for valid scientific reasons, the drug elimination period should be either (i) at least three times the half-life of the active drug ingredient or therapeutic moiety, or its metabolite(s), measured in the blood or urine; or (ii) at least three times the half-life of decay of the acute pharmacological effect [7].

10.7.2.3 Times of Collection of Blood Samples

1. *When comparison of the test product and the reference material is to be based on blood concentration time curves, unless some other approach is more appropriate for valid scientific reasons, blood samples should be taken with sufficient frequency to permit an estimate of both (i) the peak concentration in the blood of the active drug ingredient or therapeutic moiety, or its metabolite(s), measured; and (ii) the total area under the curve for a time period at least three times the half-life of the active drug ingredient or therapeutic moiety, or its metabolite(s), measured.*

2. *In a study comparing oral dosage forms, the sampling times should be identical.*

3. *In a study comparing an intravenous dosage form and an oral dosage form, the sampling times should be those needed to describe both (i) the distribution and elimination phase of the intravenous dosage form; and (ii) the absorption and elimination phase of the oral dosage form [7].*

A sample should be taken just prior to dosing (at time = 0) in the first and second periods of the crossover design. The guidelines [7] indicate that the elimination period (called washout period in crossover designs) should be three half-lives for single-dose oral studies and five half-lives for multiple-dose oral studies. In deciding on the total number of samples taken, ethical considerations dictate that one considers the total amount of blood loss during the study. In multiple-dose studies, the minimum concentration (CMIN) should be taken during buildup to verify that steady state has been achieved.

10.7.2.4 Specific Experimental Designs

Specific design considerations involve choosing the most appropriate experimental design. There are some settings where a parallel design is used. More often, a crossover design is used.

10.7.2.4.1 Parallel Designs

Parallel designs may be used for bioequivalence trials for drugs with long half-lives, since using a crossover design would require an unreasonable length of time to complete. They may also be used for drugs with potential toxicities due to ethical reasons. Also for bioequivalence trials of many formulations simultaneously, it may be cheaper and more time efficient to conduct such trials using a parallel design rather than a crossover (or Latin square) design with many periods. Although bioequivalence trials are almost always conducted in normal volunteers (subjects), parallel blood level trials of a new drug may be conducted in very ill patients to study bioavailability of the drug in patients. This is often the case in the development of antineoplastic drugs. If a parallel design is used for a bioequivalence trial, each subject receives one and only one formulation of the drug in random fashion. Usually, formulation groups are balanced in terms of numbers of subjects. The design schema for a two-formulation, one-period, parallel design appears in Table 10.1.

TABLE 10.1

Two-Formulation Parallel Design

	Period 1
Group 1	Formulation R
Group 2	Formulation T

A one-way analysis of variance model that accounts for the design features is

$$Y_{ij} = \mu + \phi_l + \xi_{ij}, \tag{10.7}$$

where Y_{ijk} is the response (e.g., AUC) on the jth subject in the ith formulation group; $i = 1, 2; l = T, R; j = 1, 2, \ldots, N_i;$ μ is an effect common to all responses; ϕ_l is the direct effect of the lth formulation; and ξ_{ij} denotes measurement error in observing the response Y_{ij} and are usually assumed to be independent and identically distributed with mean 0 and variance σ_e^2.

10.7.2.4.2 Crossover Designs

A crossover design may be thought of as a blocked design where subjects are rows (blocks) and columns are periods of formulation administration, and where each subject receives more than one formulation in random fashion. In order to have "clean" estimates of the direct effects of formulations (rather than the effect of the formulation received in one period be contaminated by residual effect of the formulation received in the previous period), good design principles require washout intervals between periods of formulation administration.

An analysis of variance model that accounts for the design features is one that explains the total variation among responses as the additive sum of variation due to subjects (intersubject variation), variation due to periods, variation due to formulations, and residual error variation. Defining sequences as the distinct orders of formulation administration gives rise to an analysis of variance model that accounts for the design features in the following manner:

$$Y_{ijk} = \mu + S_i + S_{i(j)} + \pi_k + \phi_l + \xi_{ijk}, \tag{10.8}$$

where Y_{ijk} is the response (e.g., AUC) on the jth subject in the ith sequence in the kth period (receiving the lth formulation); $i = 1, 2; k = 1, 2; l = T, R; j = 1, 2, \ldots,$ N_i; μ is an effect common to all responses; S_i is the effect of the ith sequence, $S_{i(j)}$ is the effect of the jth subject in the ith sequence; π_k is the effect of the kth period; ϕ_l is the direct effect of the lth formulation; and ξ_{ijk} denotes measurement error (within subjects) in observing the response Y_{ijk} and are usually assumed to be independent and identically distributed with mean 0 and variance σ_e^2.

In this framework, subjects are randomly assigned to the distinct sequences of formulation administration, and variation due to subjects is partitioned into variation due to sequences and variation due to subjects within sequences. To test for sequence differences, the $S_{i(j)}$ are assumed to be independent and identically distributed with mean 0 and variance σ_s^2 and independent of the ξ_{ijk}, and may be tested using the F-ratio of mean square for sequences divided by mean square for subjects within sequences. So $S_{i(j)}$ and ξ_{ijk} are random components in Equation 10.8, whereas the effects of sequences, periods, and formulations are fixed effects.

Comparisons of differences in formulations are based on within-subject changes, and each subject serves as his or her own control. In bioequivalence, clinical trials crossover designs are the norm since variability between subjects is usually greater than variability within subjects. In addition, as long as the correlation between responses within subjects is positive (which is expected in quality conducted bioequivalence trials), a crossover design will require fewer subjects than a parallel design.

There are many types of crossover designs used in bioequivalence clinical trials. Examples are the two-sequence, two-period, two-formulation design [8–12], the four-sequence, two-period, two-formulation design [12–14]; the two-sequence, three-period, two-formulation design [12,14,15]; the three-sequence, three-period, three-formulation design; the six-sequence, three-period, three-formulation design [16]; and balanced incomplete block (BIB) designs [17]. There are many excellent textbooks on crossover designs such as those by Chow and Liu [12], Ratkowsky et al. [14], and Jones and Kenward [18]. The references here and in the reference section represent only a few of those available on crossover designs. A recent Google search on the topic "crossover designs" yielded 83,800 "hits."

10.7.2.4.2.1 Two-Sequence, Two-Period, Two-Formulation Crossover Design   The most frequently used design for bioequivalence clinical trials of a test formulation (T) against a reference formulation (R) is the two-sequence (TR, RT), two-period, two-formulation crossover design. As is indicated in Section 10.7.2.1, using this design is consistent with FDA recommendations. The schema reflecting this design appears as Table 10.2.

Bioequivalence clinical trials are designed to include an adequate washout interval between formulation administration, and samples are collected at time 0 just prior to administering the formulation in each period. Therefore, one does not expect carryover effects into the second period from the formulations

TABLE 10.2

Two-by-Two-by-Two Crossover Design Schema

	Period 1	Period 2
Sequence 1	Formulation R	Formulation T
Sequence 2	Formulation T	Formulation R

given in the first period. Therefore, a reasonable analysis of variance model for this design is given in Equation 10.8, which allows a check on whether the randomization is successful by comparing sequences in terms of bioavailability endpoints and permits a valid test of direct formulation effects.

However, if one expects carryover effects, an appropriate analysis of variance model for the two-sequence, two-period, two-formulation crossover design is

$$Y_{ijk} = \mu + S_{i(j)} + \pi_k + C_l + \phi_l + \xi_{ijk}, \tag{10.9}$$

where Y_{ijk} is the response (e.g., AUC) on the jth subject in the ith sequence in the kth period; $i = 1, 2; k = 1, 2; l = T, R; j = 1, 2, \ldots, N_i$; μ is an effect common to all responses; $S_{i(j)}$ is the effect of the jth subject in the ith sequence; π_k is the effect of the kth period; C_l is the carryover effect from the drug in the lth formulation (T or R) received in the first period into the second period; ϕ_l is the direct effect of the lth formulation; and ξ_{ijk} denotes measurement error (within subject) in observing the response Y_{ijk}. The ξ_{ijk} are assumed to be independent and identically distributed with mean 0 and variance σ_e^2. The $S_{i(j)}$ are assumed to be independent and identically distributed with mean 0 and variance σ_s^2 and independent of the ξ_{ijk}.

Table 10.2 displays the means of the response (e.g., AUC) data following the model given in Equation 10.8 by sequence-and-period, by sequence and by period. Table 10.4 contains estimators of differential carryover and direct effects and their expected values from the model in terms of the means in Table 10.3. If the model given in Equation 10.9 is used, the estimator of the difference in direct effects ($\phi_T - \phi_R$) of formulations is biased (Table 10.4) by the presence of the differential carryover effect ($C_T - C_R$). Thus to address the question of bioequivalence of the two formulations in terms of direct formulation effects, one has to test first whether the differential carryover effect is 0

TABLE 10.3

Means by Sequence, Period, and Sequence and Period

	Period 1	Period 2	Period Margin
Sequence 1	$\overline{Y}_{11.}$	$\overline{Y}_{12.}$	$\overline{Y}_{1..}$
Sequence 2	$\overline{Y}_{12.}$	$\overline{Y}_{22.}$	$\overline{Y}_{2..}$
Sequence Margin	$\overline{Y}_{.1.}$	$\overline{Y}_{.2.}$	$\overline{Y}_{...}$

TABLE 10.4

Estimator/Expected Values of Effects

Effect	Estimator	Expected Value
Carryover	$(\bar{S}_1 - \bar{S}_2)^a$	$C_T - C_R$
Direct	$(\bar{Y}_T - \bar{Y}_R)^b$	$\phi_T - \phi_R + 1/2(C_R - C_T)$

$^a \quad \bar{S}_1 - \bar{S}_2 = \bar{Y}_{1..} - \bar{Y}_{2..} = (\bar{Y}_{11.} + \bar{Y}_{21.})/2 - (\bar{Y}_{12.} + \bar{Y}_{22.})/2$
$\qquad = (\bar{Y}_{11.} - \bar{Y}_{12.})/2 - (\bar{Y}_{22.} - \bar{Y}_{21.})/2$
$^b \quad \bar{Y}_T - \bar{Y}_R = (\bar{Y}_{11.} + \bar{Y}_{22.})/2 - (\bar{Y}_{21.} + \bar{Y}_{12.})/2$

(i.e., test H_0: $C_T - C_R = 0$). So the inference on the difference in direct formulation effects is conditional on the test for equality of carryover effects, and potentially raises the question whether the overall Type I error should be split?

If H_0: $C_T - C_R = 0$ is not rejected at some specified Type I error level, then data from the full crossover design may be used for inferences on direct formulation effects. However, if H_0 is rejected, then data from the first period only is used for comparison of direct formulation effects. Since the test of H_0 has lower power (the trial is not designed to test for differential carryover effects), usually the Type I error level of the test is chosen to be at least 0.10.

10.7.2.4.2.2 Four-Sequence, Two-Period, Two-Formulation Crossover Design A design that has increasingly gained use in bioequivalence clinical trials since it was proposed by Balaam [13] is the four-sequence, two-period, two-formulation design with schema given in Table 10.5. Sequences 1 and 2 are identical to those of the two-sequence, two-period, two-formulation crossover design. Sequences 3 and 4 have the same formulations in both periods. The estimator of the difference in direct formulation effects in this design is unbiased; i.e., it is not contaminated by the presence of differential carryover effects [12–14] as was the case in the two-sequence, two-period, two-formulation crossover design. Thus, inference on direct effects is not conditional on testing whether carryover effects are equal. Inferences on both the difference in direct formulation effects and the difference in carryover effects are based on within-subject linear contrasts. In addition, this design is optimal among crossover designs with two periods and two formulations [12].

TABLE 10.5

Four-by-Two-by-Two Crossover Design Schema

	Period 1	Period 2
Sequence 1	Formulation R	Formulation T
Sequence 2	Formulation T	Formulation R
Sequence 3	Formulation R	Formulation R
Sequence 4	Formulation T	Formulation T

The schema for the four-sequence (TR, RT, TT, RR), two-period, two-formulation crossover design is given in Table 10.5. In using this design, subjects would be randomized to the sequences of formulation administration and a washout interval of sufficient length (3–5 half-lives) would occur between periods of formulation administration.

An analysis of variance model appropriate for this design is

$$Y_{ijk} = \mu + S_i + S_{j(i)} + \pi_k + \phi_l + C_l + \xi_{ijk}, \tag{10.10}$$

where Y_{ijk} is the response (e.g., AUC) on the jth subject in the ith sequence in the kth period; $i = 1, 2; k = 1, 2; l = T, R; j = 1, 2, \ldots, N_i; \mu$ is an effect common to all responses; S_i is the effect of the ith sequence; $S_{i(j)}$ is the effect of the jth subject in the ith sequence; π_k is the effect of the kth period; C_l is the carryover effect from the drug in the lth formulation (T or R) received in the first period into the second period; ϕ_l is the direct effect of the lth formulation; and ξ_{ijk} denotes measurement error (within subject) in observing the response Y_{ijk}. The ξ_{ijk} are usually assumed to be independent and identically distributed with mean 0 and variance σ_e^2. The $S_{i(j)}$ are assumed to be independent and identically distributed with mean 0 and variance σ_s^2 and independent of the ξ_{ijk}.

In comparing the analyses of variance models for the two-sequence, two-period, two- formulation crossover design and the four-sequence, two-period, two-formulation crossover design given in Equations 10.9 and 10.10, respectively, one notices that they are identical with the exception that a term for sequence effects is added to the model in Equation 10.10. Sequence effects and carryover effects are confounded in the two-sequence, two-period, two-formulation crossover design, but not the four-sequence, two-period, two-formulation crossover design.

A variant of the four-sequence, two-period crossover design is often used in clinical trials of epilepsy [19] comparing the efficacy of two anti-epilepsy drugs (say A and B). In such applications, patients are randomized to the two drugs and treated for a period (1) of time. Those who do not respond (e.g., seizures are not controlled) are crossed over to the alternative drug and treated for an additional period (2) of time, whereas those who do respond continue for the additional period (2) of time on the drug to which they were randomized.

This produces four possible sequences of drug administration: AB, BA, AA, and BB. Note that patients are randomized to only sequences AA and BB. Whether a patient is in sequence AB or BA depends on whether the patient fails to respond to the drug to which he or she was randomized. In this application, there is usually no washout interval between periods as it is unethical to withdraw drug from epilepsy patients who are in a controlled state. Proponents of this design for this application argue that since the expected value of the contrast for differential drug effects does not contain carryover effects a washout interval between periods of drug administration is not needed.

TABLE 10.6

Two-by-Three-by-Two Crossover Design Schema

	Period 1	Period 2	Period 3
Sequence 1	Formulation R	Formulation T	Formulation T
Sequence 2	Formulation T	Formulation R	Formulation R

10.7.2.4.2.3 Two-Sequence, Three-Period, Two-Formulation Crossover Design   The schema for the two-sequence, three-period, two-formulation crossover design is given in Table 10.6. In using this design, subjects would be randomized to the sequences (RTT, TRR) of formulation administration and a washout interval of sufficient length (3–5 half-lives) would occur between periods of formulation administration.

An analysis of variance model appropriate for this design is

$$Y_{ijk} = \mu + S_i + S_{j(i)} + \pi_k + \phi_l + C_l + \xi_{ijk}, \tag{10.11}$$

where Y_{ijk} is the response (e.g., AUC) on the jth subject in the ith sequence in the kth period; $i = 1, 2$; $k = 1, 2, 3$; $l = T, R$; $j = 1, 2, \ldots, N_i$; μ is an effect common to all responses; S_i is the effect of the ith sequence; $S_{i(j)}$ is the effect of the jth subject in the ith sequence; π_k is the effect of the kth period; C_l is the carryover effect from the drug in the lth formulation (T or R) received in the first or second period into the following period (first-order carryover effects); ϕ_l is the direct effect of the lth formulation; and ξ_{ijk} denotes measurement error (within subject) in observing the response Y_{ijk}. The ξ_{ijk} are usually assumed to be independent and identically distributed with mean 0 and variance σ_e^2. The $S_{i(j)}$ are assumed to be independent and identically distributed with mean 0 and variance σ_s^2 and independent of the ξ_{ijk}.

In the balanced case (equal numbers of subjects within sequences), direct and residual effects are not confounded in this design. This means that inference on direct formulation effects is not conditional on carryover effects or vice versa. This design is also more efficient than its extension to four sequences in which subjects are crossed over in period 3 from the formulation received in period 2 (i.e., the sequences RTR and TRT are added) [15].

10.7.2.4.2.4 Six-Sequence, Three-Period, Three-Formulation Crossover Design   A design for bioequivalence clinical trials when there is interest in the simultaneous comparison of each of the two test formulations (T_1, T_2) against the reference (R) formulation is the six-sequence ($T_1 T_2 R, T_1 R T_2, T_2 T_1 R, T_2 R T_1, R T_1 T_2, R T_2 T_1$), three-period, three-formulation crossover design. The schema for this design is given in Table 10.7. In using this design, subjects would be

TABLE 10.7

Six-by-Three-by-Three Crossover Design Schema

	Period 1	Period 2	Period 3
Sequence 1	Formulation T_1	Formulation T_2	Formulation R
Sequence 2	Formulation T_1	Formulation R	Formulation T_2
Sequence 3	Formulation T_2	Formulation T_1	Formulation R
Sequence 4	Formulation T_2	Formulation R	Formulation T_1
Sequence 5	Formulation R	Formulation T_1	Formulation T_2
Sequence 6	Formulation R	Formulation T_2	Formulation T_1

randomized to the six sequences of formulation administration, and a washout interval of sufficient length (at least 3–5 half-lives) would occur between periods of formulation administration. This design is one of many originally proposed by Williams [20] that are balanced for carryover effects of formulations.

An analysis of variance model appropriate for this design is

$$Y_{ijk} = \mu + S_i + S_{j(i)} + \pi_k + \phi_l + C_l + \xi_{ijk}, \tag{10.12}$$

where Y_{ijk} is the response (e.g., AUC) on the jth subject in the ith sequence in the kth period; $i = 1, 2, 3, 4, 5, 6$; $k = 1, 2, 3$; $l = T_1, T_2, R$; $j = 1, 2, \ldots, N_i$; μ is an effect common to all responses; S_i is the effect of the ith sequence; $S_{i(j)}$ is the effect of the jth subject in the ith sequence; π_k is the effect of the kth period; C_l is the carryover effect from the drug in the lth formulation (T_1, T_2 or R) received in the first or second period into the following period (first-order carryover effects); ϕ_l is the direct effect of the lth formulation; and ξ_{ijk} denotes measurement error (within subject) in observing the response Y_{ijk}. The ξ_{ijk} are usually assumed to be independent and identically distributed with mean 0 and variance σ_e^2. The $S_{i(j)}$ are assumed to be independent and identically distributed with mean 0 and variance σ_s^2 and independent of the ξ_{ijk}.

Note that there are three direct formulation effects (ϕ_{T1}, ϕ_{T2}, and ϕ_R) and three first-order carryover formulation effects (C_{T1}, C_{T2}, and C_R). In the balanced case, direct and residual effects are not confounded in this design. This means that inference on direct formulation effects is not conditional on carryover effects or vice versa. Chow and Liu [12] provide an excellent discussion and methods for a proper analysis of data from this design, as well as other designs presented in this chapter.

10.7.2.4.2.5 Balanced Incomplete Block Designs Four different designs for conducting bioequivalence clinical trials of formulations have been considered thus far. Three involved two formulations. Two of these required two periods while one required three periods. The fourth involved three formulations and required three periods. A crossover design requires at least as many periods as there are formulations. If there are many formulations (as few of three), the time required to conduct a bioequivalence trial could be quite long. Not only must each period be long enough to adequately describe the elimination phase, but the washout intervals must also be sufficiently long to ensure that there is no residual drug in the bloodstream from one period at the beginning of the following period. For drugs that have long half-lives, the total time for periods and washout intervals could be enormous.

BIB designs offer a reasonable alternative (Westlake in Peace) to a full crossover (or Latin square) design when the desire is to reduce the number of periods. An example of a BIB design of six sequences, two periods, two test formulations (T_1 and T_2), and a reference formulation (R) appears in Table 10.8. The design is balanced since each formulation appears twice in each period. The first three sequences represent the three pairwise comparisons between the three formulations. The last three sequences represent the three pairwise comparisons in reverse order. Subjects would be randomized to sequences in blocks that are multiple of the sequences (e.g., after each block of six or each block of 12 subjects, sequences would be balanced).

This design provides an alternative to the six-sequence, three-period, three-formulation design when there is concern about conducting the design with three periods. It obviously would not be as efficient as the six-sequence, three-period, three-formulation design, and may not be balanced for carry-over effects. Further, there may be no interest in comparing the two test formulations. If this is the case, then sequences three and six could be omitted, but the resulting design would be an incomplete block design, but not balanced.

An appropriate analysis of variance model for this design would be one that accounts for variation among subjects, variation among periods, variation among formulations, and residual variation. If there are multiple subjects per sequence, variation among subjects may be partitioned into variation among sequences and variation among subjects within sequences. As a check on the success of the randomization, sequences may be compared by using the F-ratio of mean square for sequences divided by mean square for subjects within sequences.

TABLE 10.8

Six-by-Two-by-Three BIB Design Schema

	Period 1	Period 2
Sequence 1	Formulation T_1	Formulation R
Sequence 2	Formulation T_2	Formulation R
Sequence 3	Formulation T_1	Formulation T_2
Sequence 4	Formulation R	Formulation T_1
Sequence 5	Formulation R	Formulation T_2
Sequence 6	Formulation T_2	Formulation T_1

10.7.3 Endpoints

Endpoints of interest in the analysis of data collected in a bioequivalence clinical trial are those reflecting bioavailability of the drug in the formulations. These are area under the concentration-by-time curve (AUC_{0-t}), area under the concentration-by-time curve extrapolated to infinity ($AUC_{0-\infty}$), maximum concentration (CMAX), time to reaching maximum concentration (TMAX), terminal elimination rate (β_t), and terminal elimination half-life ($t_{1/2}$).

The first four of these endpoints directly reflect bioavailability; i.e., the rate and extent of absorption. The last two provide information on the elimination phase of the drug in the formulations. Computations of these endpoints for each subject follow in Section 10.7.6.1.

In some bioequivalence trials, there may be other endpoints (functions of the concentration-by-time data) of clinical interest; e.g., the time at which concentrations reach a level that correlates to effectiveness as well as the time at which concentrations reach a level that would create a concern for safety. This was the case in the clinical development of the first receptor antagonist (Cimetidine) for the treatment of duodenal ulcers. Of course, such interest requires some mechanism for correlating concentrations with clinical response. In the case of Cimetidine, since its clinical effectiveness (healing the ulcer) derives from the suppression of gastric acid, gastric antisecretory studies could be conducted in subjects participating in a bioequivalence trial, or in patients with ulcers in whom blood samples are taken for the purpose of determining concentrations.

10.7.4 Sample Size Determination

In the evolution of FDA guidelines for the pharmaceutical industry for the conduct of bioequivalence trials there appeared statements indicating that usually 24–36 subjects were required in a two-sequence, two-period, two-formulation bioequivalence trial. It is relatively rare that such a trial is conducted with a greater number of subjects than 36. However, bioequivalence trials should be designed similar to other clinical trials. That is, a determination should be made at the protocol development stage as to the number of subjects needed to have a high probability (power) that the question (formulations bioequivalent?) will be answered while controlling the false-positive decision rate at some prespecified level α (usually 0.05). The FDA has provided guidance with respect to the choice of power and δ for bioequivalence trials; i.e., there should be at least 80% power to detect a 20% difference (δ) between the test formulation and the reference formulation.

Westlake [17] notes that the roles of α and β in designing clinical trials where rejection of the null hypothesis leads to a conclusion that the regimens are different (not equal) are reversed in bioequivalence trials where rejection of the null hypothesis leads to a conclusion that the regimens are not different in terms of bioavailability endpoints (are considered bioequivalent). The sample size is approximated by the formula

$$n \geq \frac{2\sigma_e^2(z_{1-\alpha} + z_{1-\beta/2})^2}{\delta^2},$$

(10.13)

where
  α is the false-positive decision risk
  β is the false-negative risk
  $1 - \beta$ is the power
  δ is the magnitude of the difference in formulations (in terms of bioavailability endpoints) beyond which they are considered bioinequivalent
  σ_e^2 is an estimate of intrasubject variability
  $z_{1-\alpha}$ and $z_{1-\beta/2}$ are the $(1 - \alpha)$ and $(1 - \beta/2)$ percentiles from the standardized normal distribution
  n is the total number ($n/2$ in each of the two sequences) of subjects in the trial

Table 10.9 provides estimates of the minimum number of subjects per sequence required for a two-sequence, two-period, two-formulation ($2 \times 2 \times 2$) bioequivalence trial for various levels of power and various levels of δ with a false-positive rate of 5%. A previous study provided estimates of σ_e^2 to be 1.2697 and the overall mean μ to be 4.535 (AUC units). The difference δ is a specified percentage of the estimate of the overall mean. To illustrate the computations, substituting the estimates of σ_e^2 and $\delta = .2(4.535) = 0.907$ gives 34 total subjects for a power of 90% ($z_{1-\beta/2} = 1.645$) and a false-positive risk of 5% ($z_{1-\alpha} = 1.645$).

Table 10.9 shows that as power increases for fixed δ, or as δ decreases for fixed power, sample size increases. For example, for $\delta = 20\%$ (of the overall mean), the number of subjects per sequence increases from 13 to 22 as power increases from 80% to 95%. For a power of 80%, the number of subjects per sequence increases from 13 to 208 as δ decreases from 20% to 5%.

TABLE 10.9

Number of Subjects per Sequence for $2 \times 2 \times 2$ Crossover Design for Various δ and Power, and $\alpha = 0.05$

Power	$\delta = 30\%$	$\delta = 20\%$	$\delta = 10\%$	$\delta = 5\%$
0.80	6	13	52	208
0.90	8	17	68	272
0.95	10	22	88	352

If estimates of the intrasubject variation (σ_e^2) and the overall mean (μ) are unknown, but the coefficient of variation (CV) is known, the sample size formula (10.13) may be rewritten as

$$n \geq \frac{2(CV)^2(z_{1-\alpha} + z_{1-\beta/2})^2}{(\%)^2}, \tag{10.14}$$

where
  CV is the estimate of σ_e/μ
  $(\%)^2$ is the numerical percentage represented by δ

Most bioequivalence trials are conducted by either the innovator company of the original drug product or the generic drug industry. The innovator company conducts bioequivalence trials if they want to market a new formulation of an FDA-approved formulation or if they switch manufacturing sites for the approved formulation. For these purposes, estimates of σ_e^2 and μ as well as estimates of the means of bioavailability endpoints for the approved innovator formulation would be known from previous studies. Such information is also usually available to the generic industry through the Freedom of Information (FOI) Act. Thus, the estimates needed for determination of sample size for most bioequivalence trials may be obtained.

However, if they are unknown, a reasonable strategy would be to perform computations to assess what levels of power and CVs 24–36 subjects would provide. In studying the results one would want to have at least 80% power to detect a 20% difference (in the formulation means of bioavailability endpoints) for a CV that is realistic. Here, input from the drug metabolism expert or pharmacokineticist is needed. A companion to this assessment would be to assess whether the attendant CIs on the ratio of means (μ_T/μ_R) of the test formulation (T) to reference formulation (R) are contained in the (80%; 125%) interval.

Other methods may be used to determine sample size. For example, one could assess the sample size necessary to have the length (L) of a $(1 - 2\alpha)$% CI on the difference between the means of $\text{Log}(AUC_T)$ and $\text{Log}(AUC_R)$ to be less than the length of the bioequivalence decision interval on a Log scale $(2\{\text{Log}(5) - \text{Log}(4)\})$. Here we have

$$n > \frac{4\sigma_e^2 z_{1-\alpha}^2}{L^2}, \tag{10.15}$$

where $z_{1-\alpha}^2$ is the square of the $100(1 - \alpha)$ percentile of the standardized normal distribution, and $L = 2\{\text{Log}(5) - \text{Log}(4)\}$. Here α is usually chosen to be 0.05. The intrasubject variation σ_e^2 would be estimated from a previous study based on analysis of log-transformed AUC.

To be technically correct, the percentiles from the standardized normal distribution appearing in formulae (10.13) through (10.15) should be replaced by percentiles from Student's t-distribution. However, using the standardized normal distribution for sample size determination is easier to work with since the percentiles from Student's t-distribution are dependent on the degrees of freedom, which are functions of the sample size trying to be determined. In practice it is not likely to make a difference for moderate to large samples sizes. For example, for $30°$ of freedom, $t_{.05} = 1.697261$ and $z_{.05} = 1.645$; $t_{.05}$ is only 3.18% larger than $z_{.05}$. Sample sizes determined from the formulae in (10.13) through (10.15) can be adjusted upward by the percentage increase reflected by the ratio of the percentile from Student's t-distribution to the percentile from the standardized normal distribution.

The methodology of Makuch and Simon [21] may also be used as a basis for sample size determination. This methodology is more conservative than those previously discussed in the sense that it leads to larger sample sizes, due to recognizing that the endpoints of CIs are themselves random variables and thus exhibit variation. The methodology was developed for positive-control clinical efficacy trials or active-control equivalence studies (ACES) [22].

Sample sizes may also be determined based on Schuirmann's two one-sided test procedure. For a discussion using this approach as well as other methods, the reader may see Chapter 9 of Chow and Liu's [17] book (and later editions).

10.7.5 Randomization and Blinding

In the review of the designs presented in Section 10.7.2.4, the importance of randomization of subjects to sequences of formulation administration was presented. Few textbooks on clinical trial methodology include a focused treatment of bioequivalence trials. Those that do, as well as textbooks on bioavailability and bioequivalence, fail to mention the importance of blinding investigator site personnel as well as personnel involved in assays of the blood samples for determining drug concentrations. It is important for such personnel as well as subjects to be blinded.

The protocol for bioequivalence trials specifies the times of sample collection. Typically, when the concentration-by-time dataset reaches the biostatistician for statistical analysis, both the scheduled times and the actual times of sample collection are included. The first author has supported bioequivalence trials in the pharmaceutical industry for more than 30 years and has analyzed dozens of such trials. In a few of those trials bioequivalence was concluded when using the scheduled times of sample collection but not when using the actual times of sample collection. Slight departures in the actual times of sample collection from the scheduled times of sample collection, particularly if systematic for one formulation more so than for the other formulation, can lead to fairly large differences in the AUCs of formulations. The point here is that bias could be introduced from knowing the identity of the formulation taken by subjects, simply by recording slight departures from the scheduled times (or actual times). Blinding is an important clinical trial methodology to prevent the introduction of bias as well as avoiding the appearance of bias.

10.7.6 The Statistical Analysis Section

Prior to computing bioavailability endpoints and conducting statistical analyses, the biostatistician and the drug metabolism expert and/or pharmacokineticist should examine the concentration-by-time data for quality and reasonableness. If some concentrations are missing, or are below the quantifiable limit (BQL) of the assay, or appear to be outliers, decisions have to be made about how to handle. BQL concentrations are often considered as 0 (provided this does not create a problem in computing the terminal elimination rate). Missing concentrations are often imputed by linear interpolation. Outliers may be handled by any number of outlier detection procedures [12].

Data examination prior to conducting statistical analyses is an important exercise (see Chapter 9) regardless of the data and its source. The first author was once approached to analyze data from a bioequivalence trial comparing a generic aspirin formulation to Bayer aspirin. In examining the concentration data, it was clear that the Bayer aspirin concentrations were considerably lower than those from previous studies. This led to the correct decision of not analyzing the data. It is unethical and a waste of resources to produce inferences from analyses of data known to be deficient in quality, authenticity, or accuracy.

10.7.6.1 Computation of Endpoints for Each Subject

The endpoints AUC_{0-t}, CMAX, TMAX, β_t, $t_{1/2}$, and $AUC_{0-\infty}$ are computed directly from the concentration-by-time data for each subject:

$$AUC = \frac{\sum_i (t_i - t_{i-1})(c_i + c_{i-1})}{2}, \tag{10.16}$$

$$CMAX = Max(c_0, c_1, \ldots, c_k), \tag{10.17}$$

$$TMAX = t_i \text{ at which CMAX is observed}, \tag{10.18}$$

where
  t_i are the times of blood sample collection
  c_i are the blood or plasma concentrations
  $i = 1, 2, \ldots, k$ (the last sample collected)

The formula for computing AUC is the trapezoid rule. The time t_0 is the time (0) at which the first sample is collected and is considered baseline. It is obtained just before the first formulation is administered to each subject. The concentration c_0 of the drug in the first sample should be 0.

The terminal elimination rate β_t for each subject is estimated by the slope of a straight line fit to the log concentration-by-time data for the last "few" samples. The largest number of samples for which the fit of the straight line is best, as measured by the coefficient of determination (R^2), is used. Since a perfect fit is obtained from the last two samples, the last three samples are chosen initially and the value of R^2 (say R_3^2) noted. Then the last four samples are included and the value of R^2 noted (say R_4^2). If $R_4^2 < R_3^2$ then β_t are estimated from the last three samples. If $R_4^2 \geq R_3^2$ then the last five samples are included and the value of R^2 (say R_5^2) compared to R_4^2. If $R_5^2 < R_4^2$ then β_t is estimated from the last four samples, etc.

The terminal half-life and AUC extrapolated to infinity are estimated by

$$t_{1/2} = \frac{-\ln(2)}{\beta_t}, \tag{10.19}$$

$$\mathrm{AUC}_{0-\infty} = \mathrm{AUC}_{0-t} + \frac{c_k}{\beta_t}, \tag{10.20}$$

where
    $\ln(2)$ is the natural logarithm of 2
    β_t is the terminal half-life
    c_k is the concentration in the last sample collected

10.7.6.2 Statistical Analysis of Concentrations and Bioavailability Endpoints

Descriptive analyses of the concentration-by-time data will be performed. These include graphs of mean concentrations-by-time of sample collection by sequence and period and for each formulation. A plot of mean concentrations-by-time will be generated for each formulation. This plot will also contain the actual concentrations for each subject at each time of sample collection—so that the viewer will have an impression of the intersubject variation in concentrations. Different colors and/or different symbols will be used to distinguish between formulations.

Descriptive of the endpoints AUC_{0-t}, $\mathrm{AUC}_{0-\infty}$, CMAX, TMAX, β_t, and $t_{1/2}$ will be performed. Descriptive analyses include means, standard deviations, and standard errors of each endpoint by sequence and period, by sequence, by period, and by formulation.

Inferential analyses of the endpoints will also be performed. These include the analysis of variance table for the model appropriate for the design (see Section 10.7.2.4), the construction of two-sided CIs and the two one-sided tests. The main purpose of the analysis of variance is to obtain the estimate of intrasubject variability needed for CI construction, performing the two one-sided tests, and to test for differential carryover effects (if appropriate for the design).

CIs and the two one-sided tests are needed to address whether the formulations are bioequivalent.

Both the Westlake symmetric and the usual asymmetric CIs on the true differences in formulation means will be computed and their limits converted to reflect the ratio of the test formulation to the reference formulation. The confidence level will be 90%. If the CIs on the ratio of the test formulation to the reference formulation for AUC_{0-t}, $AUC_{0-\infty}$, and CMAX are wholly embedded within the bioequivalence decision interval (80%; 125%), the test formulation will be considered bioequivalent to the reference formulation.

The two one-sided tests will also be performed on AUC_{0-t}, $AUC_{0-\infty}$, and CMAX, each at the 5% level of significance. If both P-values are less than 0.05, the test formulation will be considered bioequivalent to the reference formulation. It is noted that 90% two-sided CIs and the two one-sided tests are operationally inferentially equivalent.

The other endpoints TMAX, β_t, and $t_{1/2}$ will also be inferentially analyzed as they provide comparative pharmacokinetic information of interest about the two formulations.

Typically, these results do not figure into the decision about bioequivalence of the two formulations.

The analysis of TMAX is usually problematic as its estimate of variability often gives the impression of great precision when it is most likely due to the spacing of the times of sample collection. As indicated in Section 10.6.1, TMAX in conjunction with the partial AUC to the left of TAX may be helpful in concluding bioequivalence in terms of the rate and extent of absorption, as well as comparing the formulations in terms of the ratio of CMAX to TMAX.

10.8 Analysis of Bioequivalence Trials

Statistical analyses of bioequivalence trials proceed according to the presentation in statistical analysis section (Section 10.7.6) of the trial protocol. For greater detail about statistical methods used in the analysis of bioequivalence clinical trials, approaches found in references [12,14,16–18] may be reviewed. The FDA Guidance for Industry: Statistical Approaches to Establishing Bioequivalence [23] is also helpful for biostatisticians supporting bioequivalence clinical trials of compounds regulated by the FDA.

In addition, a concentration dataset from a two-sequence, two-period, two-formulation crossover design of an antibiotic drug appears in Appendix 10.A.1. The dataset is analyzed using methods that address the question of bioequivalence and the results summarized in Section 10.12.2. The computer code (in R) used for the analysis also appears in Appendix 10.A.2.

10.9 Analysis of Ratios

As has been previously mentioned, the FDA decision rule for concluding bioequivalence is on the ratio of the mean of the test formulation (T) to the mean of the reference formulation (R). It is well known that the ratio of means is not the same as the mean of ratios. Peace [24] suggested using within-subject ratios rather than using within-subject differences as the analysis unit in the assessment of bioequivalence, and presented the basis for this choice at the 1986 FDA public hearing on the Agency's method of determining bioequivalence of generic drugs for immediate-release, solid oral dosage forms.

In addition to using the within-subject ratios, he suggested constructing a two-sided 90% (lower bound) CI on the mean of the distribution of ratios using the Bienayme–Tchebycheff (BT) inequality for the sole purpose of determining whether the FDA decision rule for concluding bioequivalence was met. If met, since the confidence level would be at least 90% *regardless* of the distribution of ratios, both the FDA and consumers of generic drugs should have greater comfort that the decision was the correct one. If not met, then bioequivalence would be assessed using conventional methods, or by determining a 90% CI on the true mean of the ratios using resampling methods.

The interval

$$CI_r = (\bar{r} - C_\alpha \sigma_{\bar{r}}; \ \bar{r} + C_\alpha \sigma_{\bar{r}})$$

is a $100(1 - 2\alpha)\%$ CI on the true mean μ_r of the distribution of the ratios, where $\bar{r}$ is the (observed) arithmetic mean of the ratios, $\mu_{\bar{r}} = E(\bar{r}) = \mu_r$ is the (true) mean of the distribution of ratios, and $\sigma_{\bar{r}}$ is standard deviation of the sampling distribution of the ratios. If $\alpha = 0.05$ then the interval would be a 90% CI. But the difficulty is in determining C_α because the distribution of ratios is not usually known. As has been indicated, the interval could be determined by sampling repeatedly from the sample of subject ratios.

Alternatively, the BT inequality

$$\Pr\left[|\bar{r} - \mu_r| \leq K\sigma_{\bar{r}}\right] \geq 1 - \frac{1}{K^2},$$

where k is a positive real number, may be used. This inequality says that the probability that the mean of the sample ratios is within K standard error units of the true mean of the ratios is at least $1 - 1/K^2$, regardless of the distribution of ratios. Unraveling the inequality in terms of absolute value yields an interval of the form given by CI_r. Setting the lower bound on the probability to be 90% yields $K = 3.1623$.

10.10 Pharmacokinetic Models

A pharmacokinetic model is a simplified mathematical model with undetermined parameters that attempts to describe the concentration of the drug in the bloodstream. For an oral formulation of a drug, the drug is absorbed from the gut into the bloodstream (the blood compartment) where it is distributed to the tissue compartment and simultaneously eliminated. If it is assumed that the rates of transfer between compartments are proportional to the amount of drug in the compartments, then a set of ordinary linear differential equations is obtained that can be solved to produce a mathematical model for the concentration $C(t)$ of the drug in the blood compartment of the form

$$C(t) = \frac{k_a D}{V} [A_1 \exp(-\alpha t) + A_2 \exp(-\beta t) + A_3 \exp(-k_a t)],$$

where

$$A_1 = \frac{(\alpha - k_{21})}{(\alpha - \beta)(k_a - \alpha)}$$

$$A_2 = \frac{(k_{21} - \beta)}{(\alpha - \beta)(k_a - \beta)}$$

$$A_3 = \frac{(k_a - k_{21})}{(k_a - \alpha)(k_a - \beta)}$$

D is the amount of drug absorbed
V is the volume of distribution of the blood compartment

$$\alpha\beta = k_e k_{21}, \quad \alpha + \beta = k_e + k_{12} + k_{21},$$

where
k_a is the absorption rate constant from the gut to the blood compartment
k_{12} is the forward transfer rate constant from the blood compartment to the tissue compartment
k_{21} is the backward transfer rate constant from the tissue compartment to the blood compartment
k_e is the elimination rate constant from the blood compartment

The equation expressing $C(t)$ above may be fit to the concentration-by-time data collected in a bioavailability/bioequivalence trial and the parameters estimated. The literature is rich with pharmacokinetic models and methods of fitting. Pharmacokineticists are strong proponents for pharmacokinetic modeling and routinely fit such models to estimate bioavailability parameters on a per subject basis and for the entire population of subjects. Such modeling is not necessary for the purpose of assessing bioequivalence of pharmaceutical formulations [17]. For readers who wish to learn about pharmacokinetic modeling, the book by Shargel et al. [25] may be seen.

10.11 Support of Bioequivalence Trials in the Pharmaceutical Industry

Biostatistical support to bioequivalence clinical trials varies across the pharmaceutical industry, ranging from little input to full support by the biostatistician. Some companies, through collaboration between the pharmacokineticist, drug metabolism expert, and biostatistician, have developed software programs that provide analysis results nicely formatted in the study report. In other companies, the biostatistician may provide input at the protocol design stage, at the study implementation stage, during the conduct of the trial, and post trial completion.

Biostatistical input at the protocol design stage includes choice of the most appropriate experimental design, sample size determination, and providing the statistical analysis section of the protocol. Biostatistical responsibilities at trial implementation include generating the randomization schedule and coding memorandum.

Questions regarding logistics often occur during the conduct of the trial. For example, the investigational site conducting the trial may be able to process only one-half the subjects during 1 month (say) and the remainder during the following month, and want to know whether that will have any impact on study conclusions. It is possible to assess any impact at the analysis stage by introducing month as a block and investigating direct formulation effect-by-block interaction. This situation would essentially reflect two identical trials at the same facility, each with one-half the planned sample size. In bioequivalence trials some subjects do not complete all periods of the study design, and the investigational site wants to know whether dropouts need to be replaced. The first author once supported a bioequivalence trial where the length of the washout interval between periods of the experimental design was determined per subject while the trial was ongoing. Here, an assay was used that could rapidly assess concentration of drug in samples taken on a daily basis.

Post-trial-completion responsibilities include data examination, statistical analysis of the data collected, and providing written descriptions of analysis methods, results, and interpretations to the final study report. Data review prior to conducting statistical analyses is an important exercise in any clinical trial. Often decisions have to be made about how to handle trace concentrations (those below the quantifiable limit of the assay), missing concentrations, or concentrations that are atypical or outliers. Of course, the biostatistician should ensure that assumptions underlying the validity of the analysis methods used hold for the data, and that the methods are appropriate for the trial design. During FDA review of the SNDA containing the bioequivalence study reports, the biostatistician may interact with FDA reviewers.

10.12 Examples

10.12.1 Parallel Bioequivalence Clinical Trial of Six Formulations with Sample Size Reestimation

10.12.1.1 Background

A two-sequence, two-period, crossover bioequivalence trial of a new oral formulation (F1) versus the FDA-approved standard (S) formulation of a drug was conducted in 16 subjects. One subject failed to complete the second period. Although an adequate washout period was included, analysis of AUC and CMAX from both periods suggested the presence of a carryover effect (or treatment-by-period interaction). Therefore, the comparison of F1 to S was based on analyses of the AUC and CMAX endpoints from the first period. Not unexpectedly, due to loss of power ($N = 8$ subjects rather than 14 or 15), bioequivalence was not confirmed.

By the time we began to design a new bioequivalence trial, four other formulations (F2, F3, F4, F5) were available. So the new trial was to include the standard S and all five "new" formulations.

10.12.1.2 Six-by-Six Latin Square Design versus Six-Group Parallel Design

Initially, we considered using a **six-by-six Latin square** as the design, with each subject receiving each of the six formulations. We estimated sample size based upon the first period data from the earlier two-sequence, two-period crossover study. We concluded that we needed 20 subjects in each formulation group in order to have 80% power to detect a 20% difference in AUC for each pairwise comparison of a new formulation to the standard with a Type I error rate of 5%—if run as a six **formulation group parallel** study. This gave a total of 120 (between subjects) observations, 20 per group. We were therefore satisfied that running a six-by-six crossover trial with four subjects per sequence (for a total of 24 subjects and 144 observations) would provide at least 80% power to detect a 20% difference in AUC between the formulations in each pairwise comparison.

However, we estimated **costs** of conducting the crossover study versus conducting the parallel study. Obviously, based upon the costs of concentration assays, the crossover study was more expensive. The crossover was also expected to be more expensive in terms of volunteer stipends, since we expected that we would have to pay volunteers "pretty big bucks" to ensure that they participated in all six periods. In addition, facility rental costs for the crossover study (6 weekends) would be more expensive than for the parallel study (5 weekends).

So, the final study design was a parallel blood level trial of six formulation groups of 20 subjects per group.

10.12.1.3 Sample Size Reestimation

As the variance estimate for sample size estimation derived from the first period data from the referenced two-sequence, two-period crossover trial with eight subjects per sequence, we decided to include a sample size reestimation plan. Twenty-four subjects were entered on each of the 5 consecutive weekends. Our data management department developed a computer program that "kicked out" in blinded fashion the variance estimate based upon the analysis model after the data (AUC) were available from the subjects entered on each weekend (before the next weekend). After the second weekend (48 subjects, 8 per group) the variance estimate used for sample size estimation was greater than the variance estimate based upon the 48 subjects. We thus concluded that our sample size estimate of 120 was adequate.

It is noted that the sample size reestimation plan introduced no bias, as under normal theory, the estimators of variance and mean are independent, so that knowledge of the variance estimate as data accumulated gave us no information about mean differences between formulations, neither did the sample size reestimation plan invoke a Type I error penalty.

This trial was conducted in 1978 when the first author worked at Burroughs–Wellcome Pharmaceutical Company in Research Triangle Park, North Carolina 27709. The trial recruited healthy volunteers, primarily students from local universities. We rented rooms at the local Governor's Inn where participants reported for entry, dosing, and blood sample collection. The trial was conducted long before there was much in the literature about sample size reestimation or adaptive designs in general.

10.12.2 Crossover Bioequivalence Trial

10.12.2.1 Background and Endpoint Computations

A clinical bioequivalence trial comparing a test formulation (T) to the reference formulation (R) of an oral antibiotic drug was conducted. The trial followed a two-sequence, two-period, two-formulation crossover design with a total of 30 subjects. The concentration-by-time data for each subject are included in Tables 10.A.1 and 10.A.2. Plots of mean concentrations-by-time for each formulation appear in Figure 10.3. The distributions of the concentrations about the means at each time of sample collection are illustrated in Figure 10.4.

The six bioavailability endpoints were computed with code developed using the R software. The R code is included in Appendix 10.A.2. R is an open-source software (available free at http://www.r-project.org). The computations are detailed line by line for easy understanding by readers. The computations follow the descriptions given in Section 10.7.6.

Table 10.A.3 summarizes the endpoints AUC_{0-t}, CMAX, TMAX, B_t, half-life, and $AUC_{0-\infty}$ for each subject, period, sequence, and formulation. Figure 10.5 graphically illustrates AUC_{0-t} for the 30 subjects for the two formulations (similar figure can be produced for other endpoints).

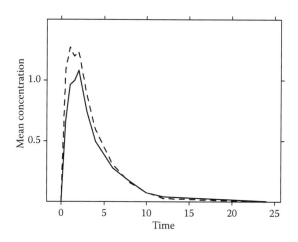

FIGURE 10.3
Mean concentration-by-time curves: solid line is test formulation T and dashed line is the
reference formulation R.

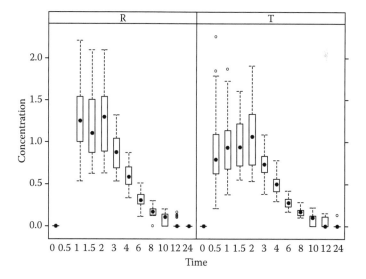

FIGURE 10.4
Boxplot to illustrate the distribution of concentrations at each time of sample collection for the
test (T) and reference (R) formulations.

In addition, descriptive statistics n, mean, and standard deviation for all
endpoints are summarized in Table 10.10 by sequence, period, formulation,
sequence, and period, respectively. In parallel to Table 10.3, Table 10.11
displays the means and the associated marginal means by period and
sequence for the six endpoints.

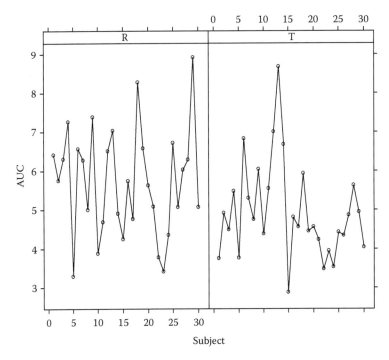

FIGURE 10.5
Plot of AUC_{0-t} for each subject for the two formulations.

10.12.2.2 Test for Differential Carryover Effect

As is indicated in Section 10.7.2.4.2.1, using Model 9 requires one to test whether the difference in carryover effects is 0 prior to conducting analyses addressing bioequivalence in terms of direct effects (see Tables 10.3 and 10.4). The statistical test can be performed using SAS or R. The SAS code and R code appear below:

```
---- SAS Code ---
proc glm;
class subject sequence period formulation;
model AUC = sequence subject(sequence) period formulation/ss3;
lsmeans sequence formulation /pdiff stderr;
estimate 'formulation' formu 1 -1;
test h = sequence e = subject(sequence);
run;


--- R Code ---
cat("Test Carryover(sequence) effect using
SUBJECT(SEQUENCE) as an error term \n")
summary(aov(AUC~period•formulation+Error(subject),
data=Data)).
```

TABLE 10.10

Summary Table of Number of Observations, Mean, and Standard Deviation (STD) for the Six Bioavailability Endpoints

	n	AUC_{0-t} Mean	STD	CMAX Mean	STD	TMAX Mean	STD	Beta Mean	STD	Half-Life Mean	STD	$AUC_{0-\infty}$ Mean	STD
Sequence													
1	32	5.52	1.34	1.42	0.43	1.50	0.64	−0.26	0.10	3.93	5.28	5.54	1.38
2	28	5.11	1.34	1.24	0.39	1.70	0.60	−0.27	0.08	2.99	1.67	5.11	1.34
Period													
1	30	5.15	1.18	1.32	0.41	1.48	0.59	−0.28	0.09	2.97	1.86	5.15	1.18
2	30	5.51	1.50	1.36	0.43	1.70	0.64	−0.25	0.09	4.01	5.37	5.53	1.53
Formulation													
R	30	5.71	1.38	1.48	0.41	1.53	0.69	−0.29	0.09	2.75	1.38	5.71	1.38
T	30	4.94	1.22	1.19	0.38	1.65	0.54	−0.24	0.09	4.24	5.46	4.99	1.27
Sequence/period													
1, 1	16	5.71	1.23	1.53	0.40	1.34	0.65	−0.30	0.10	2.74	1.63	5.71	1.23
2, 1	14	4.50	0.69	1.07	0.27	1.64	0.50	−0.26	0.08	3.24	2.12	4.50	0.69
1, 2	16	5.33	1.46	1.30	0.44	1.66	0.60	−0.22	0.09	5.11	7.21	5.36	1.53
2, 2	14	5.72	1.57	1.42	0.43	1.75	0.70	−0.28	0.08	2.75	1.07	5.72	1.57

TABLE 10.11

Endpoint Means Reflecting Crossover Design

	Sequence	Period 1	Period 2	Margin
AUC_{0-t}	1	5.71	4.50	5.52
	2	5.33	5.72	5.11
	Margin	5.10	5.53	5.32
CMAX	1	1.53	1.07	1.42
	2	1.30	1.42	1.24
	Margin	1.30	1.36	1.33
TMAX	1	1.34	1.64	1.50
	2	1.66	1.75	1.70
	Margin	1.49	1.70	1.60
Beta	1	−0.30	−0.26	−0.26
	2	−0.22	−0.28	−0.27
	Margin	−0.28	−0.25	−0.26
Half-life	1	2.74	3.24	3.93
	2	5.11	2.75	2.99
	Margin	2.99	3.93	3.46
$AUC_{0-\infty}$	1	5.71	4.50	5.54
	2	5.36	5.72	5.11
	Margin	5.10	5.54	5.32

Since bioequivalence is based primarily on AUC and CMAX, differential carryover effect was tested for the AUC and CMAX endpoints only. The associated *P*-values from the F-test are 0.329 and 0.167 for AUC and CMAX, respectively. Therefore, it is concluded that there is no strong evidence of a differential carryover effect and decisions about bioequivalence may be based on comparative analysis of the direct formulation effects. It is interesting to note that the F-test for differential direct effects is strongly statistically significant ($P < 0.0001$ for all endpoints). Thus the formulations are statistically different, but whether the difference is large enough to conclude bioinequivalence will be determined in the following analyses of bioequivalence.

The normality assumption was tested using QQ-plots and the Shapiro–Wilk test for both raw AUC (not modeled) and the residuals from the fitting $2 \times 2 \times 2$ crossover model (9). The QQ-plots indicate that neither deviates significantly from the normal distribution (Figure 10.6). The *P*-values from the Shapiro–Wilk test are 0.095 and 0.951 for the raw AUC values and the model residuals, respectively—which further substantiates the normality assumption. In view of this, AUC was analyzed rather than Log(AUC) to more directly connect with the BT inequality based and resampling-based CI results that follow.

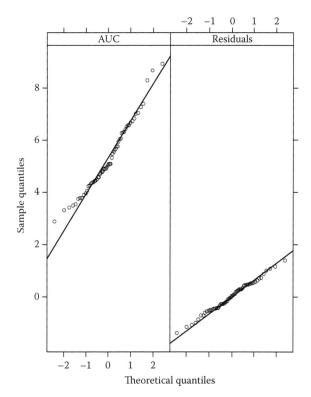

FIGURE 10.6
QQ-plot for AUC (left panel named as "AUC") and residuals after fitting model (9) (right panel named "Residuals").

10.12.2.3 Inferential Analysis of Bioequivalence: Confidence Interval Approaches

The statistical test of equality of direct formulation effects to assess bioequivalence has been criticized in pharmaceutical research [3,17,26] and it is now well known that CI provide a more appropriate inferential framework for assessing bioequivalence. The implementation of the most commonly used CIs to assess the bioequivalence follows.

10.12.2.3.1 The Classical Asymmetric Confidence Interval

The classical (or shortest) asymmetric CI is based on the least squares means for the test and reference formulations and the t statistic:

$$T = \frac{(\overline{Y}_T - \overline{Y}_R) - (\mu_T - \mu_R)}{\hat{\sigma}_e \sqrt{\frac{1}{n_R} + \frac{1}{n_T}}}$$

which follows a central t-distribution with $n_A + n_B - 2$ degrees of freedom where $\hat{\sigma}_e$ is the pooled (intrasubject) variance based upon within-subject formulation differences from both sequences. Based on this distribution, the classical $100(1 - 2\alpha)\%$ CI on $\mu_T - \mu_R$ can be constructed as follows:

$$CI_1 = (L_1, U_1) = \left((\bar{Y}_T - \bar{Y}_R) - (t_\alpha, df)\hat{\sigma}_e \sqrt{\frac{1}{n_R} + \frac{1}{n_T}}, \ (\bar{Y}_T - \bar{Y}_R) + (t_\alpha, df)\hat{\sigma}_e \sqrt{\frac{1}{n_R} + \frac{1}{n_T}} \right)$$

where $df = n_R + n_T - 2$. Since this CI is on the difference in means, the bioequivalence decision interval $(0.80, 1.25)$ on the ratio of μ_T/μ_R is converted to an interval on the difference $\mu_T - \mu_R$; i.e., the decision interval on the difference is $DecisionCI_1 = (\theta_L, \theta_U) = (-0.2\mu_A, \ 0.25\mu_A)$. If CI_1 is completely contained in $DecisionCI_1$ we conclude that the test formulation is bioequivalent to the reference formulation.

Alternatively, the CI_1 on $\mu_T - \mu_R$ may be converted to an interval CI_2 on the ratio of μ_T/μ_R by adding the reference mean to both L_1 and U_1 and dividing the result by the reference mean $\bar{Y}_R$ (since $\bar{Y}_R$ is an unbiased estimator of the true reference mean μ_R); i.e.,

$$CI_2 = \left(\frac{L_1}{\bar{Y}_R} + 1, \frac{U_1}{\bar{Y}_R} + 1 \right) \times 100\%.$$

If CI_2 is completely contained in the decision interval $DecisionCI_2 = (80\%, 125\%)$ then formulation T is considered bioequivalent to the reference formulation R.

For the AUC endpoint, $\bar{Y}_R = 5.713$ and the $DecisionCI_1 = (-0.2 * 5.713, 0.25 * 5.713) = (-1.143, 1.428)$. Since $CI_1 = (-1.148, -0.389)$ is not entirely (the left endpoint misses by 0.005) contained in $(-1.143, 1.428)$ and $CI_2 = (79.908, 93.188)$ is not entirely (the left endpoint misses by 0.092%) contained in $(80\%, 125\%)$, it is concluded that the test formulation T is bioinequivalent to the reference formulation R.

10.12.2.3.2 Westlake's Symmetric Confidence Interval

This classical CI_1 on $\mu_T - \mu_R$ is symmetric about $\bar{Y}_T - \bar{Y}_R$, but not 0, and its conversion to the interval CI_2 on the ratio μ_T/μ_R is symmetric about $\bar{Y}_T/\bar{Y}_R$, but not about unity. Westlake [3] suggested adjusting the CI_1 to be symmetric about 0 and the CI_2 to be symmetric about 1. This is accomplished by finding k_1 and k_2 such that

$$\int_{k_2}^{k_1} T \, dt = 1 - \alpha \quad \text{and} \quad (k_1 + k_2) \times \hat{\sigma}_e \sqrt{\frac{1}{n_R} + \frac{1}{n_T}} = 2(\bar{Y}_T - \bar{Y}_R).$$

The R program in Appendix 10.A.2 solves these two equations for k_1 and k_2. For the AUC endpoint, $k_1 = 8.590$ and $k_2 = -1.697$ which lead to the Westlake CI = $(-1.147, 1.147)$. Since the Westlake CI is not completely within the *Decision*CI$_1$ it is concluded that the test formulation T is not bioequivalent to the reference formulation R.

10.12.2.3.3 Bienayme–Tchebycheff Inequality Confidence Interval

The derivation of this CI is based on the famous BT inequality

$$\Pr(\bar{r} - k\sigma_{\bar{r}} < \mu_r < \bar{r} + k\sigma_{\bar{r}}) > 1 - \frac{1}{k^2},$$

where r is the ratio of AUC for the test formulation T to AUC for reference formulation R for each subject, and is discussed in Section 10.10. $\bar{r}$ and $\sigma_{\bar{r}}$ are the mean and standard deviation of sampling distribution of the ratios. Therefore, to have a lower bound of 90% for the probability $1 - 1/k^2$, $k = 3.162$. For the AUC, $\bar{r} = 0.888$ and $\sigma_{\bar{r}} = 0.036$. Therefore, the CI based on the BT inequality is (0.773, 1.003), which is not entirely contained in the (0.80, 1.25) bioequivalence decision interval. Therefore, bioinequivalence of the formulations is not concluded by this method.

It should be realized that the BT-based CI holds regardless of the true distribution of ratios. If the distribution of the ratios were known, it might be that k determined from that distribution would produce an interval that is contained in the decision interval. Alternatively, resampling methods may be applied to the sample ratios to determine a 90% confidence on the true mean of the ratios.

10.12.2.3.4 Bootstrap- or Resampling-Based Confidence Intervals

We implemented the bootstrapping approach by resampling the n individual subject ratios $(r_1, r_2, \cdots, r_n)$ with replacement for 50,000 runs (samples). The distribution is given in Figure 10.7. The 90% CI (from the 5th to the 95th percentile of the sampling distribution) on the mean of the ratios is (83.0%; 94.8%).

We also performed bootstrapping in another way by resampling the AUCs and computed the ratio of the means of $\overline{Y}_T/\overline{Y}_R$ for each bootstrap sample. The resulting distribution is illustrated in Figure 10.8. The 90% CI on the ratio of means is (80.7%, 92.8%).

It can be noted from Figures 10.7 and 10.8 and the associated CIs that the ratio of means is always smaller than the mean of ratios (which can be proven mathematically). Interestingly, both bootstrap CIs are completely within the decision interval (80%; 125%) and therefore lead to concluding that the test formulation is bioequivalent to the reference formulation (even though clearly they are statistically different). This conclusion is different from those reached from the classical, asymmetric CI and the

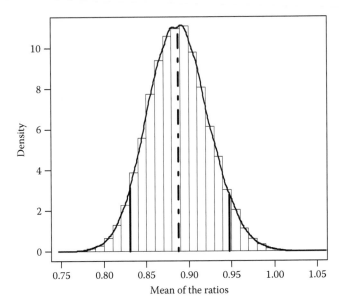

FIGURE 10.7
Bootstrap distribution of the mean of individual ratios. The dashed vertical line in the middle is the observed mean ratio $\bar{r} = 88.8\%$ and the two solid vertical lines are for the 90% CI = (83.0%; 94.8%).

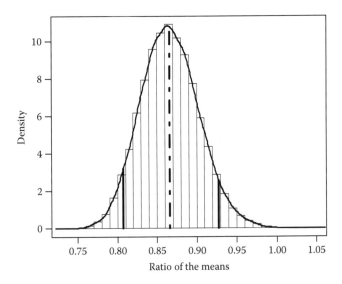

FIGURE 10.8
Bootstrap distribution of the ratio of means. The dashed vertical line in the middle is the observed mean ratio $\bar{r} = 86.5\%$ and the two solid vertical lines are for the 90% CI = (80.7%; 92.8%).

Westlake symmetric CI. The difference between the inferences casts a question about the distributional assumptions underlying the parametric-based CIs (even though the assumption of normality was not violated; see Figure 10.6) and should be investigated further. Since the dataset appears in Appendix 10.A.1, this investigation is a good classroom exercise for students.

10.12.2.4 Inferential Analysis of Bioequivalence: Bayesian Approaches

The Bayesian approach is different from the above frequentist CI methods. The latter assumes that the parameter of interest (such as the direct formulation effect) is *fixed* but unknown and a CI is derived based on the sampling distribution. The Bayesian approach assumes that the unknown direct formulation effect is *a random variable* with some distribution. There are several Bayesian CIs for concluding bioequivalence. We illustrate the one proposed by Rodda and Davis [27] for the bioequivalence trial dataset. This method requires computing the probability that the difference of $\mu_T - \mu_R$ will be within the bioequivalence limits. The detailed derivation may be found in [12,27]. The fundamental conclusion is that the marginal posterior distribution of $\mu_T - \mu_R$ given the observed data is a noncentral t-distribution with $n_T + n_R - 2$ degrees of freedom and noncentrality parameter $\overline{Y}_T - \overline{Y}_R$. Therefore, the posterior probability of $\mu_T - \mu_R$ being within the bioequivalence decision interval *DecisionCI*$_1$ is computed as

$$p_{R.D.} = P(\theta_L < \mu_T - \mu_R < \theta_U) = pt(t_U) - pt(t_L),$$

where pt is the cumulative probability function for central t-distribution with $n_T + n_R - 2$ degrees of freedom and

$$t_L = \frac{\theta_L - (\overline{Y}_T - \overline{Y}_R)}{\hat{\sigma}_e \sqrt{\frac{1}{n_T} + \frac{1}{n_R}}}$$

and

$$t_U = \frac{\theta_U - (\overline{Y}_T - \overline{Y}_R)}{\hat{\sigma}_e \sqrt{\frac{1}{n_T} + \frac{1}{n_R}}}.$$

We then conclude that the test formulation T is bioequivalent to the reference formulation R if $p_{R.D.}$ is $\geq 90\%$. For the AUC endpoint in the example, $t_L = -1.678$ and $t_U = 8.571$, and the degrees of freedom $n_T + n_R - 2 = 14 + 16 - 2 = 28$. The posterior probability is computed to be 80.1%, which is smaller than 90%. We again conclude that the test formulation T is bioinequivalent to the reference formulation R.

10.12.2.5 *Inferential Analysis of Bioequivalence: Two One-Sided Tests*

Another method for assessing bioequivalence is the two one-sided test procedure originally proposed by Schuirmann [6,28]. The null (bioinequivalence) and alternative (bioequivalence) hypotheses are formulated (see Section 10.7.1) as

$$H_{01}: \mu_T - \mu_R \leq \theta_L \quad \text{versus} \quad H_{a1}: \mu_T - \mu_R > \theta_L$$

and

$$H_{02}: \mu_T - \mu_R \geq \theta_U \quad \text{versus} \quad H_{a2}: \mu_T - \mu_R < \theta_U.$$

The method requires conducting two one-sided tests each at the prespecified significance level, $\alpha = 5\%$, and conclude bioequivalence between the test and reference formulations if and only if the two null hypotheses H_{01} and H_{02} are rejected. Similar to Section 10.12.2.3.1, we can reject the two null hypotheses and conclude bioequivalence of the test formulation T to reference formulation R if

$$T_L = \frac{(\overline{Y}_T - \overline{Y}_R) - \theta_L}{\hat{\sigma}_e \sqrt{\frac{1}{n_R} + \frac{1}{n_T}}} > t(0.05, n_R + n_T - 2)$$

and

$$T_U = \frac{(\overline{Y}_T - \overline{Y}_R) - \theta_U}{\hat{\sigma}_e \sqrt{\frac{1}{n_R} + \frac{1}{n_T}}} < -t(0.05, n_R + n_T - 2)$$

For AUC from the bioequivalence trial example $\theta_U = -\theta_L = 1.143$, and therefore the two one-sided hypotheses may be specified as

$$H_{01}: \mu_T - \mu_R \leq -1.143 \quad \text{versus} \quad H_{a1}: \mu_T - \mu_R > -1.143$$

and

$$H_{02}: \mu_T - \mu_R \geq 1.143 \quad \text{versus} \quad H_{a2}: \mu_T - \mu_R < 1.143$$

The values of the test statistics are $T_L = 1.678$ and $T_U = -9.852$. For $\alpha = 10\%$, $t(1 - \alpha/2, 28) = 1.701$. Since $T_L = 1.678 < t(1 - \alpha/2, 28) = 1.701$, we reject H_{01} and conclude that the test formulation T is bioinequivalent to the reference formulation R.

This decision regarding bioequivalence may also be based on the two one-sided P-values; i.e., reject H_{01} and H_{02} and conclude bioequivalence if max $(P_L, P_U) < 0.05$, where P_L and P_U are the one-sided P-values from testing H_{01} and H_{02}, respectively. For AUC from the trial example, the associated

P-values are $P_L = \Pr(T > T_L) = 0.052$ and $P_U = \Pr(T < T_U) < 0.00001$. Since $\max(P_L, P_U) = 0.052 > 0.05$, we conclude that the test formulation T is bio-inequivalent to the reference formulation R.

10.13 Concluding Remarks

Few textbooks on clinical trial methodology include bioequivalence trials. Bioequivalence trials are clinical trials to which clinical trial methodology applies. It is important for students in a course in clinical trial methodology to become acquainted with such trials, in terms of their design, objective, conduct, analysis methodology, and interpretation. This chapter provides an overview of these characteristics for the assessment of bioequivalence in terms of average bioavailability. The methods presented are based on means of bioavailability endpoints and do not take into account the variability of the formulations. Two formulations may differ in variability yet still be bioequivalent in terms of means.

There are two other concepts of bioequivalence: population bioequivalence and individual bioequivalence. Population bioequivalence is assessed using a mixture of both the mean and variance of bioavailability endpoints. Crucial to the concept of population bioequivalence of two formulations of a drug is that patients not yet prescribed either formulation may be effectively and safely treated with either formulation.

Individual bioequivalence implies the notion of switchability from the reference formulation to the (approved) test formulation and vice versa in individual patients. To demonstrate that two formulations exhibit individual bioequivalence requires using a mixture of means and variances of the formulations as well as subject-by-formulation interaction. The textbook by Chow and Liu [12 and later editions] may be seen for a review of methods for assessing population and individual bioequivalence.

Appendix 10.A Bioequivalence Dataset

TABLE 10.A.1

Time–Concentration Data for Formulation R

Formulation R			Time										
Subject	Sequence	Period	0	0.5	1	1.5	2	3	4	6	8	10	12	24
1	1	1	0	2.26	1.12	0.87	0.84	0.8	0.5	0.26	0.18	0.16	0.13	0
2	1	1	0	0.99	1.2	1.32	1.33	1	0.68	0.3	0.19	0	0	0
3	1	1	0	1.28	1.76	1.61	1.61	0.76	0.53	0.32	0.15	0.14	0	0
4	1	1	0	1.79	1.97	1.61	1.54	0.96	0.63	0.38	0.2	0.18	0	0
5	1	1	0	0.45	0.6	0.78	0.68	0.67	0.45	0.15	0.12	0	0	0
6	1	1	0	1	1.25	1.49	1.6	1.04	0.74	0.39	0.17	0.11	0	0
7	1	1	0	0.63	1.26	1.18	0.97	0.7	0.62	0.37	0.24	0.16	0.12	0
8	1	1	0	0.63	0.53	0.65	0.85	1.13	0.82	0.35	0.21	0	0	0
9	1	1	0	1.21	1.67	1.04	1.58	1.32	0.87	0.51	0.18	0.12	0	0
10	1	1	0	1.37	1.24	1.11	1.05	0.53	0.33	0.11	0	0	0	0
11	1	1	0	0.94	1.19	1.08	1.33	0.79	0.53	0.25	0	0	0	0
12	1	1	0	0.91	1.79	1.83	1.66	1	0.63	0.33	0.2	0	0	0
13	1	1	0	1.21	2.21	1.63	1.49	1	0.7	0.34	0.2	0.13	0	0
14	1	1	0	0.76	1.28	1.29	1.28	0.69	0.49	0.28	0.15	0	0	0
15	1	1	0	0.77	1.33	0.9	0.92	0.53	0.39	0.25	0.12	0.11	0	0
16	1	1	0	0.99	1.39	0.86	0.86	1.04	0.67	0.36	0.19	0.17	0	0
17	2	2	0	0.57	0.82	0.64	0.63	1.11	0.64	0.34	0.16	0.11	0	0
18	2	2	0	1.12	1.54	2.05	1.41	1.13	0.78	0.44	0.29	0.17	0.11	0
19	2	2	0	1.23	1.47	1.51	1.63	1	0.58	0.37	0.22	0.1	0	0
20	2	2	0	0.82	1.13	0.9	1.3	0.69	0.5	0.27	0.16	0.12	0.1	0
21	2	2	0	1.25	1.12	1.28	1.3	0.65	0.49	0.31	0.14	0	0	0
22	2	2	0	0.93	0.95	0.72	0.86	0.58	0.53	0.23	0	0	0	0
23	2	2	0	0.8	0.61	0.62	0.82	0.67	0.36	0.29	0	0	0	0
24	2	2	0	0.5	0.61	0.98	0.89	0.75	0.49	0.27	0.18	0.13	0	0
25	2	2	0	0.99	0.82	0.78	0.93	1.04	0.7	0.38	0.24	0.14	0.16	0
26	2	2	0	1.22	1.46	1.21	1.27	0.66	0.44	0.27	0.16	0	0	0
27	2	2	0	1.6	1.69	1.9	1.62	0.86	0.44	0.22	0.13	0	0	0
28	2	2	0	1.85	1.28	1.1	1.37	1.14	0.77	0.28	0.15	0	0	0
29	2	2	0	1.56	1.84	2.1	2.1	0.92	0.75	0.39	0.3	0.2	0.11	0
30	2	2	0	1.07	1	0.97	1.39	0.9	0.58	0.24	0.13	0	0	0

TABLE 10.A.2

Time–Concentration Data for Formulation T

| | Formulation R | | | Time | | | | | | | | | | | |
Subject	Sequence	Period	0	0.5	1	1.5	2	3	4	6	8	10	12	24
1	1	2	0	0.7	0.52	0.55	0.77	0.6	0.42	0.25	0.17	0.11	0	0
2	1	2	0	0.77	1.08	1.17	1.32	0.79	0.51	0.27	0.16	0	0	0
3	1	2	0	1.15	1.66	0.9	0.58	0.64	0.51	0.27	0.13	0	0	0
4	1	2	0	0.78	1.06	1.11	1.21	1.01	0.63	0.31	0.16	0.1	0	0
5	1	2	0	0.52	0.57	0.55	0.53	0.45	0.3	0.21	0.12	0.11	0.11	0
6	1	2	0	0.7	1.87	1.32	1.33	0.87	0.61	0.38	0.18	0.14	0.1	0
7	1	2	0	0.57	0.49	0.72	0.73	0.68	0.4	0.29	0.28	0.2	0.15	0
8	1	2	0	0.56	0.68	0.61	1.91	0.69	0.46	0.23	0.17	0.11	0	0
9	1	2	0	0.83	1.09	1.23	1.14	0.77	0.5	0.35	0.21	0.14	0.1	0
10	1	2	0	0.95	0.99	1.15	1.34	0.65	0.39	0.2	0.1	0	0	0
11	1	2	0	1.12	1.08	1.16	1.71	0.77	0.6	0.31	0.15	0	0	0
12	1	2	0	0.21	1.73	1.61	1.66	1.09	0.63	0.38	0.21	0	0.11	0
13	1	2	0	0.85	1.45	1.47	1.63	1.01	0.78	0.42	0.26	0.17	0.13	0.13
14	1	2	0	1.03	1.35	1.22	1.14	0.83	0.56	0.33	0.23	0.16	0.13	0
15	1	2	0	0.38	0.74	0.72	0.7	0.38	0.29	0.18	0.13	0	0	0

(continued)

TABLE 10.A.2 (continued)

Time–Concentration Data for Formulation T

Formulation R

Subject	Sequence	Period	0	0.5	1	1.5	2	3	4	6	8	10	12	24
16	1	2	0	0.35	0.73	0.82	0.69	1.01	0.73	0.31	0.19	0.12	0	0
17	2	1	0	0.36	0.56	0.71	0.61	0.63	0.4	0.27	0.17	0.17	0.12	0
18	2	1	0	0.72	1.14	1.5	1.39	0.82	0.57	0.35	0.2	0.22	0	0
19	2	1	0	0.65	0.88	0.91	1.05	0.57	0.45	0.32	0.18	0.1	0	0
20	2	1	0	0.9	1.11	1.06	0.84	0.51	0.35	0.17	0.13	0	0.11	0
21	2	1	0	0.72	0.77	1.03	1.09	0.86	0.44	0.21	0.11	0	0	0
22	2	1	0	0.52	0.47	0.66	0.72	0.66	0.49	0.21	0.15	0	0	0
23	2	1	0	0.26	0.37	0.59	0.97	0.81	0.48	0.26	0.17	0.11	0	0
24	2	1	0	0.62	0.58	0.59	0.61	0.59	0.37	0.27	0.15	0.1	0	0
25	2	1	0	0.54	0.69	0.9	1.05	0.78	0.56	0.28	0.2	0	0	0
26	2	1	0	0.71	1.08	0.91	1	0.68	0.5	0.3	0.11	0	0	0
27	2	1	0	0.75	1.3	1.43	1.47	0.71	0.41	0.22	0.13	0	0	0
28	2	1	0	0.72	0.77	0.88	1.18	0.91	0.54	0.34	0.16	0	0.12	0
29	2	1	0	0.65	1.33	1.41	1.08	0.67	0.42	0.28	0.19	0.1	0	0
30	2	1	0	0.29	0.72	0.97	1	0.76	0.51	0.24	0.15	0	0	0

TABLE 10.A.3

Summary Data for each Subject, Period, Sequence, and Formulation

Sequence	Period	Formulation	Subject	AUC_{0-t}	CMAX	TMAX	Beta	Half-Life	$AUC_{0-\infty}$
1	1	R	1	6.42	2.26	0.50	−0.08	8.52	6.42
1	1	R	2	5.75	1.33	2.00	−0.34	2.05	5.75
1	1	R	3	6.31	1.76	1.00	−0.26	2.71	6.31
1	1	R	4	7.27	1.97	1.00	−0.28	2.48	7.27
1	1	R	5	3.31	0.78	1.50	−0.32	2.16	3.31
1	1	R	6	6.56	1.60	2.00	−0.34	2.04	6.56
1	1	R	7	6.27	1.26	1.00	−0.19	3.66	6.27
1	1	R	8	5.02	1.13	3.00	−0.35	2.00	5.02
1	1	R	9	7.39	1.67	1.00	−0.34	2.03	7.39
1	1	R	10	3.89	1.37	0.50	−0.53	1.31	3.89
1	1	R	11	4.69	1.33	2.00	−0.38	1.81	4.69
1	1	R	12	6.52	1.83	1.50	−0.29	2.42	6.52
1	1	R	13	7.03	2.21	1.00	−0.24	2.88	7.03
1	1	R	14	4.91	1.29	1.50	−0.30	2.30	4.91
1	1	R	15	4.27	1.33	1.00	−0.24	2.91	4.27
1	1	R	16	5.75	1.39	1.00	−0.27	2.59	5.75
2	1	T	17	4.56	0.71	1.50	−0.14	4.83	4.56
2	1	T	18	5.94	1.50	1.50	−0.25	2.79	5.94
2	1	T	19	4.45	1.05	2.00	−0.29	2.38	4.45
2	1	T	20	4.57	1.11	1.00	−0.07	10.17	4.57
2	1	T	21	4.24	1.09	2.00	−0.35	2.00	4.24
2	1	T	22	3.48	0.72	2.00	−0.31	2.24	3.48

(continued)

TABLE 10.A.3 (continued)

Summary Data for each Subject, Period, Sequence, and Formulation

Sequence	Period	Formulation	Subject	AUC_{0-t}	CMAX	TMAX	Beta	Half-Life	$AUC_{0-\infty}$
2	1	T	23	3.95	0.97	2.00	−0.22	3.22	3.95
2	1	T	24	3.54	0.62	0.50	−0.25	2.79	3.54
2	1	T	25	4.43	1.05	2.00	−0.29	2.42	4.43
2	1	T	26	4.35	1.08	1.00	−0.35	1.97	4.35
2	1	T	27	4.87	1.47	2.00	−0.29	2.41	4.87
2	1	T	28	5.63	1.18	2.00	−0.23	3.03	5.63
2	1	T	29	4.95	1.41	1.50	−0.23	2.95	4.95
2	1	T	30	4.05	1.00	2.00	−0.33	2.11	4.05
1	2	T	1	3.75	0.77	2.00	−0.21	3.38	3.75
1	2	T	2	4.92	1.32	2.00	−0.29	2.39	4.92
1	2	T	3	4.50	1.66	1.00	−0.34	2.03	4.50
1	2	T	4	5.48	1.21	2.00	−0.31	2.24	5.48
1	2	T	5	3.77	0.57	1.00	−0.02	31.86	3.77
1	2	T	6	6.38	1.87	1.00	−0.15	4.72	6.83
1	2	T	7	5.31	0.73	2.00	−0.16	4.44	5.31
1	2	T	8	4.76	1.91	2.00	−0.18	3.76	4.76
1	2	T	9	6.05	1.23	1.50	−0.19	3.74	6.05
1	2	T	10	4.39	1.34	2.00	−0.34	2.04	4.39
1	2	T	11	5.55	1.71	2.00	−0.35	2.00	5.55

1	2	T	12	7.01	1.73	1.00	−0.22	3.17	7.01
1	2	T	13	8.68	1.63	2.00	−0.13	5.49	9.12
1	2	T	14	6.68	1.35	1.00	−0.16	4.39	6.68
1	2	T	15	2.88	0.74	1.00	−0.22	3.22	2.88
1	2	T	16	4.81	1.01	3.00	−0.24	2.92	4.81
2	2	R	17	4.78	1.11	3.00	−0.30	2.30	4.78
2	2	R	18	8.28	2.05	1.50	−0.23	2.95	8.28
2	2	R	19	6.58	1.63	2.00	−0.33	2.12	6.58
2	2	R	20	5.64	1.30	2.00	−0.12	5.90	5.64
2	2	R	21	5.09	1.30	2.00	−0.30	2.31	5.09
2	2	R	22	3.78	0.95	1.00	−0.32	2.17	3.78
2	2	R	23	3.42	0.82	2.00	−0.27	2.53	3.42
2	2	R	24	4.36	0.98	1.50	−0.18	3.79	4.36
2	2	R	25	6.72	1.04	3.00	−0.22	3.22	6.72
2	2	R	26	5.08	1.46	1.00	−0.25	2.74	5.08
2	2	R	27	6.03	1.90	1.50	−0.30	2.27	6.03
2	2	R	28	6.30	1.85	0.50	−0.42	1.67	6.30
2	2	R	29	8.92	2.10	1.50	−0.25	2.76	8.92
2	2	R	30	5.07	1.39	2.00	−0.40	1.73	5.07

Appendix 10.B R Code with Detailed Annotations

```
###===================================
## Title: Bioequivalence Analysis Methods for Concentration Dataset
##
## Description:
##      1. R= reference T=Test with format
##                           Period 1          Period 2
##          sequence 1          R                 T
##          sequence 2          T                 R
## ===================================
```

```
#
# 0. get the data with following colns:
#        sequence subject period formulation time conc

#
dat                =read.csv("blood.csv", header=T)
num.subj1          =length(unique(sort(dat[dat$sequence==1,]$subject)))# should=14
num.subj2          =length(unique(sort(dat[dat$sequence==2,]$subject))) # should=16
num.subject        =num.subj1+num.subj2
num.sequence       =2
num.period         =2
num.formulation=2
num.time           =12
```

```
#xxxxxxxxxxxxx
# 1. generate one plot of mean concentration by time of
#    sample collection for each formulation (both on same graph)
#

library(lattice)
# the mean time-concentration curve
xyplot(conc~time, group=formulation, ylim=c(0,1.5), dat,
                  xlab="Time", ylab="Mean Concentration", type="a",lty=2:1,lwd=3)
# the boxplot for distribution
bwplot(conc~as.factor(time)|formulation, dat, las=1,xlab="Time", ylab="Concentration")
```

```
#
# 2. compute AUC by the trapezoid rule, and determine CMAX, TMAX,
#    the terminal elimination rate (beta) and terminal halflife,AUC inf
#    on a per subject, per period basis
#

# 2.1. make.beta is the most heavy logic calculation using the iterative approach
make.beta=function(dt, debug=T){
# terminal elimination beta to find the slope for R2(k+1) <R2(k)
n=length(dt$conc) # get the length of data

# end the loop at tmax
tmax=which.max(dt$conc)

for(k in n:tmax){ # loop over starting from the last time-conc point to tmax
if(debug==T) print(k)
dt1=dt[((k-2):n),] # start with last 3 pts and move on
dt2=dt[((k-3):n),] # start with last 4 pts and move on
if(debug==T) print(dt1)
```

```
# some date have 0s at the end of t-c curve and make the lm crash
# so make this data frame at least 3 data points
if( dim(dt1[dt1$conc>0,])[1]>= 3 ){
if(debug==T) print(dt1)
m1    =lm(log(conc)~time, dt1[(dt1$conc>0),]) # then for conc >0
m2    =lm(log(conc)~time, dt2[(dt2$conc>0),])
betat =m1$coef[[2]]
cat("Check=",summary(m1)$r.squared> summary(m2)$r.squared,
        " and Stopped at", k, "with beta=",betat,sep=" ","\n\n")
if(summary(m1)$r.squared> summary(m2)$r.squared) break
if(debug==T) readline()
         } # end of if-loop

} # end of k-for-loop
cat("final beta=",betat,"\n\n")

# return
betat
} # end of make-beta function

# 2.2. make a function to calculate auc for each subj
make = function(dt){
time=dt$time; conc=dt$conc

# do auc
t.dif  =diff(time) # the t(i)-t(i-1)
c.mean= (conc[-1]+conc[-length(conc)])/2
auc    =sum(t.dif*c.mean)

# Cmax
cmax=max(conc)

# tmax
tmax=dt[which.max(dt$conc),]$time

# terminal elimination beta to find the slope for R2(k+1) <R2(k)
betat =make.beta(dt, debug=F)

# terminal halflife
t5=-log(2)/betat

# AUC infinite
aucinf =auc+ conc[length(conc)]/betat

# return the results.
c(auc,cmax,tmax, betat, t5, aucinf)
}

# 2.3. generate the full table
out3 =NULL
for(p in 1:num.period){
        for(s in 1:num.subject){
                d.tmp=dat[(dat$period==p) & (dat$subject==s),]
                out3 =append(out3, c(d.tmp$sequence[1], d.tmp$period[1],
                        (d.tmp$formulation[1]),d.tmp$subject[1], make(d.tmp)))
                        }
                }
out3            =matrix(out3,byrow=T, ncol=6+4)
```

```
colnames(out3) = c("sequence","period","formulation","subject","AUC",
                   "CMAX","TMAX","beta","halflife","AUCinf")
out3

#
# 3. test whether there is evidence of a 'carryover' effect
#        for AUC and Cmax with log-transformed data
#

# 3.1. make the data frame for AUC and cmax
Data       = data.frame(out3)
Data$lAUC  = log(Data$AUC)
Data$lCmax = log(Data$CMAX)
Data$drug  = "A"
Data[Data$formulation == 2,]$drug = "B"
xyplot(AUC~subject|drug, Data[order(Data$drug, Data$subject),],
                type="o", xlab="Subject", ylab="AUC")

# 3.2. for AUC
cat("The ANOVA for 2X2X2 crossover design \n")
m.auc <- lm(AUC ~ sequence + subject:sequence + period + formulation,data=Data)
show(anova(m.auc))
summary(m.auc)
cat("Test carryover(sequence) using SUBJECT(SEQUENCE) as an error term \n")
summary(aov(AUC ~ period * formulation + Error(subject), data=Data))

# 3.3. for Cmax
cat("The ANOVA for 2X2X2 crossover design \n")
m.Cmax <- lm(Cmax ~ sequence + subject:sequence + period + formulation,data=Data)
show(anova(m.Cmax))
summary(m.Cmax)
cat("Test carryover(sequence) using SUBJECT(SEQUENCE) as an error term \n")
summary(aov(Cmax ~ period * formulation + Error(subject), data=Data))

#
# 4. make CI to test bioequivalence
#

# 4.1. calculate the pooled sample variance:
# period difference for each subject within each sequence
prd1          = Data[Data$period == 1,c("sequence","subject","AUC")]
colnames(prd1) = c("sequence","subject","AUC1")
prd2          = Data[Data$period == 2,c("sequence","subject","AUC")]
colnames(prd2) = c("sequence","subject","AUC2")
diff.2to1     = data.frame(merge(prd1,prd2))
diff.2to1$d   = (diff.2to1$AUC2-diff.2to1$AUC1)/2  # equation 3.3.1.
# mean by sequence
mseq          = aggregate(diff.2to1$d,list(sequence=diff.2to1$sequence),mean)
# create the data frame to make the difference for each formulation and subject
dt1           = merge(diff.2to1, mseq)
# the pooled sample variance estimate
dt1$diff      = dt1$d-dt1$x
sig2.d        = sum(dt1$diff^2)/(num.subj1+num.subj2-2)
sig2.d

#
# 4.2 classical shortest 90% CI
#
mdrug  = aggregate(Data$AUC, list(drug=Data$formulation), mean)
alpha  = 1-0.9
```

```
q.alpha=qt(1-alpha/2, num.subj1+num.subj2-2)
low1    =mdrug[2,2]-mdrug[1,2] - q.alpha*sqrt(sig2.d)*sqrt(1/num.subj1+1/num.subj2)
up1     =mdrug[2,2]-mdrug[1,2] +q.alpha*sqrt(sig2.d)*sqrt(1/num.subj1+1/num.subj2)

ref.low=-0.2*mdrug[1,2]
ref.up = 0.25*mdrug[1,2]
cat("The classical CI=(", round(low1,3),",", round(up1,3),")",sep=" ","\n\n")
cat("Ref CI=(", ref.low,",",ref.up,")", sep="", "\n\n")

low2= (low1/mdrug[1,2]+1)*100
up2 = (up1/mdrug[1,2]+1)*100
cat("The Ratio CI=(", round(low2,3),",", round(up2,3),")",sep  =" ","\n\n")

# 4.3 the Westlake CI
# get the k1+k2
k.12=2*(mdrug[1,2]-mdrug[2,2])/sqrt( sig2.d*(1/num.subj1+ 1/num.subj2)) #4.2.8
k2  =uniroot(function(k2) pt(k.12-k2,num.subj1+num.subj2)-
  pt(k2,num.subj1+num.subj2) -0.95,lower=-10, upper=10, tol=0.0001)$root
k1  = k.12-k2
cat("The Westlake k2=",k2," and k1=",k1,sep="", "\n\n")

low.west =k2*sqrt(sig2.d*(1/num.subj1+1/num.subj2)) -(mdrug[1,2]-mdrug[2,2])
up.west  =k1*sqrt(sig2.d*(1/num.subj1+1/num.subj2)) -(mdrug[1,2]-mdrug[2,2])
cat("The Westlake CI for mu_T-mu_A is (",low.west,",",up.west,")", sep="", "\n\n")

# 4.4 Bienayme-Tchebycheff Inequality to conclude Bioequivalence
# Pr( mean r -k*sig_r<mu_r<mean r+k*sig_r) >= 1-1/k^2

# 4.4.1. get the individual ratio
dA          =Data[Data$formulation==1,c("subject","AUC")]
colnames(dA)=c("subject","AUC.A")
dB          =Data[Data$formulation==2,c("subject","AUC")]
colnames(dB)=c("subject","AUC.B")
dAB         =merge(dA,dB)
r.B2A       =dAB$AUC.B/dAB$AUC.A
r.B2A

# 4.4.2 desire for 90%, so Set 1-1/k2=0.90, k=3.1623
K       =1/sqrt(1-.9)
k
low.Tch=mean(r.B2A)-k*sqrt(var(r.B2A)/num.subject)
low.Tch
up.Tch =mean(r.B2A)+k*sqrt(var(r.B2A)/num.subject)
up.Tch

cat("The Tchebycheff CI for mu_T/mu_A is (",low.Tch,",",up.Tch,")",sep="", "\n\n")

# 5 Bayesian: Rodda and Davis:
q.alpha=qt(.95, num.subj1+num.subj2-2)
mB      =mdrug[2,2]
mA      =mdrug[1,2]
m.B2A   =mB-mA
m.B2A

theta.U=0.2*mA # the reference low and upper
theta.L=-theta.U
theta.U
theta.L
```

```
cat("The Bayesian 90% CI = (",low1,",",up1,")",sep=" ","\n\n")
cat("The reference CI = (",theta.L,",",theta.U,")",sep=" ","\n\n")

tU  = (theta.U-m.B2A)/sqrt(sig2.d*(1/num.subj1+1/num.subj2))
tL  = (theta.L-m.B2A)/sqrt(sig2.d*(1/num.subj1+1/num.subj2))
tU
tL
p.RD=pt(tU, num.subject-2, ncp=m.B2A)-pt(tL, num.subject-2,ncp =m.B2A)
cat("The posterior probability that B and A are bioequivalent =",p.RD,sep= " ","\n\n")
```

References

1. Kopacek KB (2007): The Merck manuals online medical library: Pharmacokinetics: Bioavailability. http://www.merck.com/mmpe/sec20/ch303/ch303c.html

2. Food and Drug Administration (2003): Bioavailability and bioequivalence studies for orally administered drug products—General considerations, FDA, Rockville, MD. http://www.fda.gov/downloads/Drugs/GuidanceCompliance RegulatoryInformation/Guidances/ucm070124.pdf

3. Westlake WJ (1976): Symmetric confidence intervals for bioequivalence trials. *Biometrics*; **32**: 741–744.

4. Anderson S, Hauck WW (1983): A new procedure for testing equivalence in comparative bioavailability and other clinical trials. *Communications in Statistics—Theory and Methods*; **12**: 2663–2692.

5. Hauck WW, Anderson S (1984): A new statistical procedure for testing equivalence in two-group comparative bioavailability trials. *Journal of Pharmacokinetics and Biopharmaceutics*; **12**: 83–91.

6. Schuirmann DJ (1987): A comparison of the two one-sided tests procedure and the power approach for assessing the equivalence of average bioavailability. *Journal of Pharmacokinetics and Biopharmaceutics*; **15**(6): 657–680.

7. Food and Drug Administration (2009): Title 21, Part 320—Bioavailability and bioequivalence requirements: Subpart B—Procedures for determining the bioavailability or bioequivalence of drug products, Sections 320.25, 26, 27. http://ecfr.gpoaccess.gov/cgi/t/text/text-idx?c = ecfr&rgn = div5&view = text&node = 21:5.0.1.1.7&idno = 21

8. Grizzle JE (1965): The two period change-over design and its use in clinical trials. *Biometrics*; **21**: 467–480.

9. Koch GG (1972): The use of non-parametric methods in the statistical analysis of the two period change over design. *Biometrics*; **28**: 577–584.

10. Hills M, Armitage P (1979): The two-period crossover clinical trial. *British Journal of Clinical Pharmacology*; **8**: 7–20.

11. Brown B (1980): The crossover experiment for clinical trials. *Biometrics*; **36**(1): 69–79.

12. Chow SC, Liu JP (1992): *Design and Analysis of Bioavailability and Bioequivalence Studies*, Marcel Dekker, New York.

13. Balaam LN (1968): A two-period design with t^2 experimental units. *Biometrics*; **24**: 61–73.

14. Ratkowsky DA, Evans MA, Richard J (1993): *Cross-Over Experiments: Design, Analysis, and Application*, Marcel Dekker, New York.

15. Ebbutt AF (1984): Three-period crossover designs for two treatments. *Biometrics*; **40**: 219–224.
16. Walker GA (2002): *Common Statistical Methods for Clinical Research with SAS Examples*, 2nd edn., SAS Press, Cary, NC.
17. Westlake WJ (1988): Bioavailability and bioequivalence of pharmaceutical formulations. In: *Biopharmaceutical Statistics for Drug Development*, Peace, KE (ed.), Chap. 7, Marcel Dekker, New York.
18. Jones B, Kenward MG (1989): *Design and Analysis of Cross-Over Trials*, Chapman and Hall, London, U.K.
19. Peace KE (1983): Discussion: A critique of the grizzle, Balaam and white designs. In: *Proceedings of the Biopharmaceutical Section*, The American Statistical Association, Las Vegas, NV, pp. 27–28.
20. Williams EJ (1949): Experimental designs balanced for residual effects of treatment. *Australian Journal of Scientific Research*; **2**: 149–168.
21. Makuch R, Simon R (1978): Size requirements for evaluating a conservative therapy. *Cancer Treatment Reports*; **62**: 1037–1040.
22. Makuch R, Pledger G, Hall DB, Johnson MF, Herson J, Hsu JP (1990): Active control equivalence studies. In: *Statistical Issues in Drug Research and Development*, Peace, KE (ed.), Chap. 4, Marcel Dekker, New York.
23. U.S. Department of Health and Human Services; Food and Drug Administration; Center for Drug Evaluation and Research (2001): Guidance for industry: Statistical approaches to establishing bioequivalence. http://www.fda.gov/cder/guidance/index.htm
24. Peace KE (1986): Estimating the degree of equivalence and non-equivalence: An alternative to bioequivalence testing. In: *Proceedings of Biopharmaceutical Section*, The American Statistical Association, Las Vegas, NV, pp. 63–69.
25. Shargel L, Wu-Pong S, Yu ABC (2004): *Applied Biopharmaceutics & Pharmacokinetics*, McGraw-Hill, Columbus, OH.
26. Metzler CM (1974): Bioavailability: A problem in equivalence. *Biometrics*; **30**: 309–317.
27. Rodda BE, Davis RL (1980): Determining the probability of an important difference in bioavailability. *Clinical Pharmacology and Therapeutics*; **28**: 247–252.
28. Schuirmann DJ (1981): On hypothesis testing to determine if the mean of a normal distribution is contained in a known interval (abstract). *Biometrics*; **37**: 617.

11

Dose and Frequency Determination from Phase II Clinical Trials in Stress Test–Induced Angina

11.1 Introduction

Phase II clinical trials represent the first introduction of new drugs into patients that have the disease under the study. These are relatively small trials, and typically there is no determination of sample size for these trials from the point of view of statistical power (see Section 4.4.6). The purpose of Phase II is to identify the doses and the frequency of dosing that should be used in Phase III clinical trials of efficacy. Phase III clinical trials are therefore viewed as confirmatory, pivotal proof-of-efficacy trials—to confirm that the doses and frequency of dosing determined from Phase II are in fact effective.

Prior to the IND/NDA rewrite in the mid-to-late 1980s, pharmaceutical companies did not do much in the way of determining in any optimal sense dose and frequency of dosing in the Phase II program that should be used in the Phase III program. The FDA regulations at that time permitted a pharmaceutical company to produce only two adequate and well-controlled trials at some dose and frequency of dosing, both of which demonstrated effectiveness of the compound to satisfy U.S. regulatory efficacy requirements. The IND and NDA rewrite of the mid-1980s introduced for the first time the dose comparison or clinical dose–response trial. One impact of the IND/NDA rewrite legislation [1], which became effective June 17, 1987, was to serve notice to the pharmaceutical industry that they had to do a better job at identifying dose regimens for drugs to be marketed. It is widely held that Dr. Bob Temple at the FDA was of the opinion that the doses of drugs on the market prior to the IND/NDA rewrite were generally too high. This position is understandable in the absence of regulation requiring evidence of clinical dose response.

Presented in this chapter is a novel application of using response surface methodology (RSM) [2] for identifying dose and frequency of dosing from a Phase II clinical trial of stress test–induced angina. By identifying dose and frequency of dosing it is meant that a dose-by-frequency region is determined such that in this region onset of angina would be expected to be delayed at least 30% (defined as clinically of interest) above baseline. Prior to the application, an overview of RSM including the full quadratic model is presented.

11.2 Overview of Response Surface Methodology

In applying RSM techniques, one is interested in studying the influence of several factors $x_1, x_2, \ldots, x_r$, say, on a measurable response Y where most often the functional form of Y on the x_i, $i = 1, 2, \ldots r$, is unknown. It is assumed that the relationship between Y and the x_i is given by

$$Y = f(x_1, x_2, \ldots, x_r) + \xi \qquad (11.1)$$

where
  f is some specified function (response surface) of the x_i containing
    unknown parameters β_i
  ξ represents random error (with mean 0) in measuring the response Y

An experiment is conducted over some region of the factor space with Y being measured at points (levels of the factors) in the space and the data collected. The model (1) is then fit to the data by some method; e.g., least-squares techniques, enabling estimates $\hat{\beta}_i$ of the unknown parameters to be obtained. After acceptance of reasonable fit within the experimental region of interest, the fitted surface,

$$\hat{Y} = \hat{f}(x_1, x_2, \ldots, x_r) \qquad (11.2)$$

is explored as a function of the factors using computer search methods or classical optimization techniques. Exploring the surface means that one identifies values of the factors that correspond to the optimum (largest or smallest) value of the fitted surface, or identifies a region of the factor space over which the fitted surface is optimal in some predefined manner. For statistical inference on the β_i, one usually assumes that the distribution of the ξ is normal, or resorts to resampling-based methods.

For only two factors x_1, x_2, the potential factor space would be the first quadrant of the Cartesian plane spanned by x_1, x_2. Practical experimental considerations along with what is known about the relationship between the response Y and the factors x_1, x_2 dictate constraining the potential factor space to some rectangular subset of the Cartesian plane. Then certain experimental designs would further restrict the factor space to the actual region of experimentation for a particular experiment. There are many experimental designs that are used in RSM. To some extent the form of the response surface f is constrained by the experimental design and vice versa. Some designs are factorial in nature—for example, two-factor (2^k) or three-factor designs (3^k), each at k levels. There are also composite designs, particularly central composite ones (a 2^k augmented by $2k+1$ center points) as well as equiradial or uniform precision designs. In the Phase II antianginal clinical drug development example in Section 11.4, an equiradial-hexagonal design is used.

11.3 Full Quadratic Response Surface Model

A functional form f that has found application in a wide variety of areas [3–5] is a second-order polynomial model in two variables; i.e., the full quadratic response surface model $\{f(x_1, x_2) = E(Y)$, from Equation 11.1$\}$ is

$$f(x_1, x_2) = \beta_0 + \beta_1 x_1 + \beta_2 x_2 + \beta_{12} x_1 x_2 + \beta_{11} x_1^2 + \beta_{22} x_2^2. \qquad (11.3)$$

It is convenient to rewrite the model in vector-matrix notation as

$$f(x_1, x_2) = \beta_0 + Xb + X\beta X', \qquad (11.4)$$

where

$$X = (x_1, x_2), \quad b' = (\beta_1, \beta_2),$$

and

$$\beta = \begin{bmatrix} \beta_{11} & 1/2\beta_{12} \\ 1/2\beta_{12} & \beta_{22} \end{bmatrix},$$

where X is the 1×2 row vector of factors (x_1, x_2), b is the 2×1 column vector of the coefficients of x_1, x_2, respectively, β is the 2×2 matrix accounting for the quadratic terms in Equation 11.3, and the prime ($'$) denotes vector transpose. In this form, the stationary point $x_0 = (x_{10}, x_{20})$, the point at which relative minima or maxima may occur, is given by

$$x_0 = \frac{-b'\beta^{-1}}{2}, \qquad (11.5)$$

where the -1 superscript denotes the inverse matrix operation. Substituting x_0 into f in Equation 11.3 yields the candidate for the relative optimum

$$f(x_0) = \beta_0 + x_0 \frac{b}{2}.$$

(11.6)

Alternatively, for an experiment with n observations, Equation 11.1 may be written in vector-matrix notation as

$$Y = X\beta + \xi,$$

(11.7)

where Y is an $n \times 1$ vector of responses, X is an $n \times r$ full-rank design matrix, β is the $r \times 1$ vector of unknown parameters, and ξ is the $n \times 1$ vector of unobserved random measurement errors, usually assumed to be independent and identically normally distributed with mean 0 and unknown variance σ_e^2. It is well known that the least-squares estimate (also the maximum likelihood estimate under the independence and normality assumptions on ξ) of the parameter vector β and its variance/covariance matrix $\hat{\sigma}_{\hat{\beta}}^2$ are given by

$$\hat{\beta} = (X'X)^{-1}X'Y,$$

(11.8)

$$\hat{\sigma}_{\hat{\beta}}^2 = (X'X)^{-1}\hat{\sigma}_e^2,$$

(11.9)

respectively, and where $\hat{\sigma}_e^2$ is obtained as the mean-square error from an analysis of variance of Equation 11.7. The estimates of the model parameters along with their variances/covariances may be used to provide inferences (either via significance testing or confidence intervals) on model parameters under normal theory or using resampling-based methods.

The parameter estimates from Equation 11.8 may be substituted into the structural component of Equation 11.6 to obtain the estimated response surface $E(Y) = X\hat{\beta}$. This surface may be searched directly using computer-intensive search procedures (e.g., Nelder–Mead simplex search procedure [6]) to identify optima, or to identify a region of the design variables factor space over which the surface is optimum in some predefined sense. Fletcher's [7] book *Practical Methods of Optimization*, and Björck's [8] book *Numerical Methods for Least Squares Problems* are useful references for function optimization.

Useful textbooks on response surface designs and methods are those by Myers [9], Myers and Montgomery [10], and Khuri [11]. Further the RSREG procedure of SAS [12] is most useful in performing regression analyses of response data deriving from a response surface designed experiment.

11.4 Phase II Clinical Trial Program in Stress Test–Induced Angina

Angina pectoris is the medical term for discomfort or pain in the chest that occurs when the heart muscle receives insufficient oxygen-rich blood. The discomfort may also occur in the back, shoulders, arms, neck, or jaw, and may feel like indigestion. Angina is a symptom of underlying heart or coronary artery disease (CAD) rather than a disease per se [13]. The first drug (coronary vasodilator) approved for the treatment of angina was nitroglycerin, administered sublingually.

RSM was incorporated into two Phase II clinical trials of a new drug thought to have antianginal efficacy. The aim of the RSM was to estimate dose and frequency of dosing that could be used in developing Phase III, pivotal proof of antianginal efficacy protocols. The primary measure of antianginal efficacy in the Phase II protocols was time to onset of exercise-induced angina. An equiradial-hexagonal design—two equilateral triangles with a common center point—and a full second-order response model were used. Design and analysis aspects of these trials are reviewed.

The **original objective** of the Phase II protocols was to obtain dose comparison information on measures reflecting possible antianginal efficacy when given twice-daily (b.i.d.) regimen and to compare the top b.i.d. regimen with a thrice-daily (t.i.d.) regimen at the same total daily dose. As the protocols were exploratory, Phase II studies, sample sizes were not determined from a power perspective, rather clinically chosen to ensure replication in each treatment group (3) per center (2) per protocol (2). Essential features of the protocols are captured in Sections 11.4.1 through 11.4.3.

11.4.1 Treatment Groups in the Original Protocols

The treatment groups for Protocol 1 were 0 mg b.i.d., 4 mg b.i.d., 6 mg b.i.d., and 4 mg t.i.d. The first three regimens permit comparisons among doses: 0 (placebo), 4 and 6 mg when given b.i.d. The last two regimens permit the comparison of the b.i.d. and t.i.d. regimens at the same total daily dose (12 mg).

The treatment groups for Protocol 2 were 2 mg b.i.d., 8 mg b.i.d., and "6 mg t.i.d." The 2 mg b.i.d. regimen was thought to be a "no effect" dose. The last two regimens permit the comparison of the t.i.d. regimen "6 mg t.i.d": 4, 6, and 6 mg, to the 8 mg b.i.d. regimen, at the same total daily dose.

11.4.2 Efficacy Measures

For each protocol, the measures of efficacy were time to stress test–induced anginal onset (primary); total exercise time; double product (heart rate × systolic pressure), at the onset of angina and at the end of the exercise time; maximal *St* wave depression; time to maximal *St* wave depression; and weekly anginal frequency (with nitroglycerin use recorded). **Time to stress test–induced anginal onset** was considered the **primary efficacy measure**.

11.4.3 Stress Testing and Dosing Considerations

Patients who were candidates for protocol entry underwent a stress test prior to randomization. Those who qualified for entry returned to the clinic a week later for a baseline stress test, randomization, and dispensing of study medication. They then returned to the clinic on day 17 for stress tests at 2, 7, or 12 h after the dose taken on day 17.

After randomization, patients were dosed either b.i.d. or t.i.d. for 16 days, plus 0 or 1 tablet on day 17, dependent on the assigned dose group and timing of stress tests on day 17.

11.4.4 Design

At the initial consultation, it was observed that by replicating the 2 mg b.i.d. group and adding a 4 mg b.i.d. group in Protocol 2, the two protocols could be amalgamated under a single equiradial-hexagonal design. This design is a member of the class of uniform precision designs and is rotatable and orthogonal. It permits exploration of the efficacy measures using response surface methods (RSM) as a function of total daily dose (0–16 mg) and time of stress test after the last dose (2, 7, or 12 h). The design matrix was augmented to assess block (protocol and/or center or investigator) differences.

The design represents two equilateral triangles with a common center point (Figure 11.1). The vertices of the hexagon are the vertices of the two equilateral triangles. The vertices have been transformed or coded

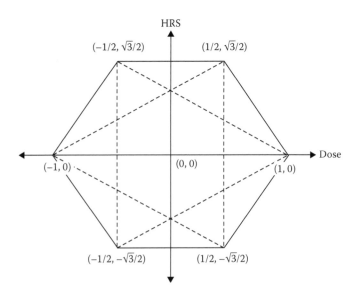

FIGURE 11.1
Equiradial hexagonal design or two equilateral triangles with common center point.

TABLE 11.1

Coded and Uncoded Vertices of Equilateral, Hexagonal Design

	Protocol 1			Protocol 2	
Dosing	Coded Vertices*	Uncoded Vertices	Dosing	Coded Vertices*	Uncoded Vertices
4 t.i.d.	$(1/2, -\sqrt{3}/2)$	(12 mg, 2 h)	2 b.i.d.	$(-1/2, -\sqrt{3}/2)$	(4 mg, 2 h)
6 b.i.d.	$(1/2, +\sqrt{3}/2)$	(12 mg, 12 h)	2 b.i.d.	$(-1/2, +\sqrt{3}/2)$	(4 mg, 12 h)
4 b.i.d.	$(0, 0)$	(8 mg, 7 h)	4 b.i.d.	$(0, 0)$	(8 mg, 7 h)
0 b.i.d.	$(-1, 0)$	(0 mg, 7 h)	6 t.i.d./8 b.i.d.	$(1, 0)$	(16 mg, 7 h)

* Dose is reflected as total daily dose in mg.

(Table 11.1) so that the center point (8 mg, 7 h) becomes (0, 0). The vertex $(-1, 0)$ represents 0 mg (placebo) total daily dose where the stress test is administered 7 h after the last dose (on day 17). The vertex (1, 0) represents 16 mg total daily dose (either 8 mg b.i.d. or "6 mg t.i.d.") where the stress test is administered 7 h after the last dose. The vertex $(-1/2, -\sqrt{3}/2)$ represents 4 mg total daily dose where the stress test is administered 2 h after the last dose. The vertex $(-1/2, \sqrt{3}/2)$ represents 4 mg total daily dose where the stress test is administered 12 h after the last dose. The vertex $(1/2, -\sqrt{3}/2)$ represents 12 mg total daily dose where the stress test is administered 2 h after the last dose. The vertex $(-1/2, +\sqrt{3}/2)$ represents 12 mg total daily dose where the stress test is administered 12 h after the last dose.

11.4.5 Model

The full quadratic response surface model is given by

$$\text{Response} = \beta_0 x_0 + \beta_1 x_1 + \beta_2 x_2 + B x_{00} + \beta_{12} x_1 x_2 + \beta_{11} x_1^2 + \beta_{22} x_2^2 + \xi, \quad (11.10)$$

or in vector-matrix notation

$$Y = X\beta + \xi, \quad (11.11)$$

where
  Y is the column vector of responses (time to anginal onset or change from baseline in anginal onset)
  x_0 is a column of 1's
  x_{00} is a column vector consisting of indicator constants to account for blocks, protocol (2) and investigational site (2) within protocols
  B is the block effect parameter
  ξ represents the vector of random errors in measuring response

The errors are assumed to be independent and identically normally distribute with mean 0 and unknown but common variance.

The design matrix X and the inverse of $X'X$ are given respectively by

$$X = \begin{bmatrix} x_0 & x_1(\text{does}) & x_2(\text{h}) & x_{00} & x_1 x_2 & x_1^2 & x_2^2 \\ 1 & +1/2 & +\sqrt{3}/2 & +1 & +0.433012 & 1/4 & 3/4 \\ 1 & -1/2 & +\sqrt{3}/2 & -1 & -0.433012 & 1/4 & 3/4 \\ 1 & -1/2 & -\sqrt{3}/2 & -1 & +0.433012 & 1/4 & 3/4 \\ 1 & +1/2 & -\sqrt{3}/2 & +1 & -0.433012 & 1/4 & 3/4 \\ 1 & +1 & 0 & -1 & 0 & 1 & 0 \\ 1 & -1 & 0 & +1 & 0 & 1 & 0 \\ 1 & 0 & 0 & -1 & 0 & 0 & 0 \\ 1 & 0 & 0 & +1 & 0 & 0 & 0 \end{bmatrix}$$

and

$$(X'X)^{-1} = \begin{bmatrix} \beta_0 & \beta_1 & \beta_2 & B & \beta_{12} & \beta_{11} & \beta_{22} \\ 0.5 & 0 & 0 & 0 & 0 & -0.5 & -0.5 \\ 0 & 0.33 & 0 & 0 & 0 & 0 & 0 \\ 0 & 0 & 0.33 & 0 & 0 & 0 & 0 \\ 0 & 0 & 0 & 0.125 & 0 & 0 & 0 \\ 0 & 0 & 0 & 0 & 1.33 & 0 & 0 \\ -0.5 & 0 & 0 & 0 & 0 & 1 & 0.33 \\ -0.5 & 0 & 0 & 0 & 0 & 0.33 & 1 \end{bmatrix}.$$

Estimates of the parameters $\hat{\beta}' = (\hat{\beta}_0, \hat{\beta}_1, \hat{\beta}_2, \hat{B}, \hat{\beta}_{12}, \hat{\beta}_{11}, \hat{\beta}_{22})$ are given by Equation 11.8, where Y is the vector containing the time-to-anginal responses. The variance/covariance matrix of the estimates is given by Equation 11.9, which may be determined from the mean-square error from an analysis of variance reflecting the model. The variance/covariance matrix of the estimates may be used for significance testing and to construct 95% confidence intervals on the parameters.

11.4.6 Statistical Analyses

11.4.6.1 Data and Descriptive Analyses

Time-to-anginal onset data appear in Tables 11.2 and 11.3 for Protocols 1 and 2, respectively. The data are descriptively summarized across protocols by treatment group and time of stress test in Tables 11.4 and 11.5, with Table 11.5 summarizing change from baseline in time-to-anginal onset. Mean plots of change from baseline in time-to-anginal onset appear in Figure 11.2.

11.4.6.2 Response Surface Methods Analyses

RSM analyses were performed using change from baseline in time-to-anginal onset as the response variable in the full quadratic model given in

TABLE 11.2

Protocol 1, Time (Minutes)-to-Anginal Onset Data

Group	PAT	Center	Hour 0	Hour 2	Hour 7	Hour 12
0 mg b.i.d.	1101	1	5.1	5.3	5.8	6.1
	1102		6.1	5.4	6.5	7.1
	1103		5.8	6.2	7.0	6.5
4 mg b.i.d.	1104		6.2	8.5	8.1	7.1
	1105		5.4	8.4	7.7	6.1
	1106		6.2	6.8	6.9	5.9
6 mg b.i.d.	1107		4.8	8.1	7.6	5.2
	1108		5.1	7.6	7.1	6.1
	1109		5.9	8.5	7.2	6.8
4 mg t.i.d.	1110		6.0	6.5	6.1	5.6
	1111		5.2	8.2	7.6	6.3
	1112		6.2	7.6	7.8	6.9
0 mg b.i.d.	1201	2	5.1	6.5	6.2	6.4
	1202		6.1	5.8	6.1	6.9
	1203		4.8	5.6	5.2	6.2
4 mg b.i.d.	1204		5.0	7.6	7.1	6.1
	1205		4.4	8.2	7.6	6.4
	1206		5.4	6.1	5.6	5.7
6 mg b.i.d.	1207		5.6	8.2	7.8	7.1
	1208		4.8	7.8	6.2	5.1
	1209		6.0	7.0	7.1	6.4
4 mg t.i.d.	1210		5.4	6.0	6.2	5.8
	1211		5.1	7.2	6.3	5.8
	1212		5.7	5.6	4.9	5.6

Equations 11.10 and 11.11. The block effect was not statistically significant and was thus removed from the model. Since the same total daily dose was achieved by a b.i.d or t.i.d. regimen, three separate response surface analyses were performed. The aim of these analyses was to identify dose and time after dose for which there existed acceptable clinical efficacy (delay in time-to-anginal onset at least 30% above baseline) for chronic dosing regimens at total daily doses of 0, 4, 8, 12, and 16 mg.

To identify the data contributing to the three response surface (RSM) analyses create tables from Tables 11.2 and 11.3 that contain change from baseline (hour 0) in time-to-anginal onset at hours 2, 7, and 12. Then let these data be collectively referenced by cells as in Tables 11.6 and 11.7, respectively. Note for example that the first row of Table 11.6 corresponds to change from baseline data (at hours 2, 7, and 12) on six patients in the 0 mg b.i.d. group (3 from center 1 and 3 from center 2) from Table 11.2. Similarly, for example, the second row of Table 11.7 corresponds to change from baseline

TABLE 11.3

Protocol 2, Time (Minutes)-to-Anginal Onset Data

Group	PAT	Center	Hour 0	Hour 2	Hour 7	Hour 12
2 mg b.i.d.	2101	1	5.1	6.1	4.8	6.2
	2102		4.8	6.0	5.3	4.7
	2103		5.1	4.8	6.1	5.2
4 mg b.i.d.	2104		4.8	6.1	6.3	5.4
	2105		5.2	7.2	6.9	5.9
	2106		5.4	5.6	5.9	5.0
8 mg b.i.d.	2107		5.2	6.4	7.8	7.1
	2108		6.1	8.2	8.5	7.4
	2109		5.8	7.5	7.4	6.9
6 mg t.i.d.[a]	2110		5.2	7.4	7.1	5.8
	2111		5.3	7.8	8.0	6.1
	2112		5.4	6.5	6.2	5.0
2 mg b.i.d.	2201	2	5.4	6.2	6.4	5.1
	2202		5.1	5.4	4.4	5.8
	2203		6.1	7.4	7.6	6.4
4 mg b.i.d.	2204		4.7	5.1	5.1	5.9
	2205		4.8	6.1	6.4	5.4
	2206		6.2	7.0	7.5	6.1
8 mg b.i.d.	2207		4.1	7.0	8.5	6.1
	2208		5.5	7.2	7.9	6.0
	2209		5.3	6.1	6.1	6.7
6 mg t.i.d.[a]	2210		5.1	6.2	6.1	5.4
	2211		5.4	7.2	7.1	6.1
	2212		5.2	6.4	6.7	6.1

[a] 4, 6, and 6 mg.

TABLE 11.4

Descriptive Summary: Mean ± SD, Time (Minutes)-to-Anginal Onset

Group	Hour 0	Hour 2	Hour 7	Hour 12
0 mg b.i.d.	5.50 ± 0.57	5.80 ± 0.47	6.13 ± 0.61	6.53 ± 0.39
2 mg b.i.d.	5.27 ± 0.45	5.98 ± 0.87	5.77 ± 1.17	5.57 ± 0.67
4 mg b.i.d.[a]	5.31 ± 0.62	6.89 ± 1.13	6.76 ± 0.92	5.92 ± 0.54
6 mg b.i.d.	5.37 ± 0.54	7.87 ± 0.53	7.17 ± 0.55	6.12 ± 0.82
8 mg b.i.d.	5.33 ± 0.69	7.07 ± 0.76	7.70 ± 0.89	6.70 ± 0.55
4 mg t.i.d.	5.60 ± 0.44	6.85 ± 0.99	6.48 ± 1.07	6.00 ± 0.51
6 mg t.i.d.[b]	5.27 ± 0.12	6.92 ± 0.64	6.87 ± 0.70	5.75 ± 0.46

Note: $n = 6$, except 4 mg b.i.d.
[a] $n = 12$.
[b] 4, 6, and 6 mg.

TABLE 11.5

Descriptive Summary: Mean ± SD, Change from Baseline
in Time (Minutes)-to-Anginal Onset

Group	Hour 2	Hour 7	Hour 12	Average
0 mg b.i.d.	0.30 ± 0.75	0.63 ± 0.46	1.03 ± 0.27	0.66 ± 0.41
2 mg b.i.d.	0.72 ± 0.61	0.50 ± 0.85	0.30 ± 0.52	0.51 ± 0.32
4 mg b.i.d.[a]	1.58 ± 1.15	1.45 ± 0.89	0.61 ± 0.68	1.21 ± 0.85
6 mg b.i.d.	2.50 ± 0.79	1.80 ± 0.65	0.75 ± 0.47	1.68 ± 0.48
8 mg b.i.d.	1.73 ± 0.73	2.37 ± 1.20	1.37 ± 0.55	1.82 ± 0.71
4 mg t.i.d.	1.25 ± 1.15	0.88 ± 1.13	0.40 ± 0.56	0.84 ± 0.92
6 mg t.i.d.[b]	1.65 ± 0.61	1.60 ± 0.68	0.48 ± 0.48	1.24 ± 0.54

Note: $n = 6$ per group, except 4 mg b.i.d.
[a] $n = 12$.
[b] 4, 6, and 6 mg.

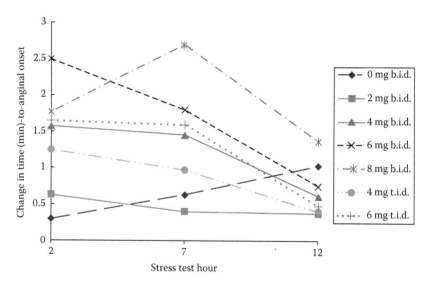

FIGURE 11.2
Change from baseline in time-to-anginal onset.

data (at hours 2, 7, and 12) on six patients in the 4 mg b.i.d. group (3 from
center 1 and 3 from center 2) from Table 11.3.

Now the change from baseline in time-to-anginal onset data contributing to
the three RSM analyses is identified in Table 11.8.

RSM Analysis 1 reflects dose and hour search over 0–16 mg total daily dose
given b.i.d. chronic dosing. RSM Analysis 2 reflects dose and hour search
over 0–16 mg total daily dose given the 12 mg total daily dose was 4 mg t.i.d.
rather than 6 mg b.i.d. The difference between the results in these two

TABLE 11.6

Reference Cells for Analyses of Change from Baseline
in Time-to-Anginal Onset: Protocol 1

Group	Hour 2	Hour 7	Hour 12
0 mg b.i.d.	11	12	13
4 mg b.i.d.	21	22	23
6 mg b.i.d.	31	32	33
4 mg t.i.d.	41	42	43

TABLE 11.7

Reference Cells for Analyses of Change from Baseline
in Time-to-Anginal Onset: Protocol 2

Group	Hour 2	Hour 7	Hour 12
2 mg b.i.d.	11	12	13
4 mg b.i.d.	21	22	23
8 mg b.i.d.	31	32	33
6 mg t.i.d.[a]	41	42	43

[a] 4, 6, and 6 mg.

TABLE 11.8

Reference Cells for Data Used in RSM Analyses

	Protocol 1	Protocol 2
Analysis 1	Cells 12, 22, 31, 33	Cells 11, 13, 22, 32
Analysis 2	Cells 11, 12, 41, 43	Cells 11, 13, 22, 32
Analysis 3	Cells 12, 22, 31, 33	Cells 11, 13, 22, 42

analyses may reflect differences between the 6 mg b.i.d. and 4 mg t.i.d.
regimens or baseline differences among patients in these two groups. RSM
Analysis 3 reflects dose and hour search over 0–16 mg total daily dose given
the 16 mg total daily dose was given as 4, 6, and 6 mg rather than as 8 mg b.i.d.
The difference between the results in Analysis 1 and Analysis 3 may reflect
differences between the 8 mg b.i.d. and 4, 6, and 6 mg regimens or baseline
differences among patients in these groups. Differences between the various
groups at baseline were tested using the pooled t-test and were not statistically
significant ($P > 0.05$).

From the analysis of variance (ANOVA) summaries of the three RSM analyses using PROC RSGEG of SAS in Tables 11.9 through 11.11, respectively,

TABLE 11.9

ANOVA Summary, RSM Analysis 1: 0, 2, 4, 6, and 8 mg b.i.d.

Response mean	1.270833
Root MSE	0.766408
R-square	0.5313
CV	60.3075

Regression	DF	Type I SS	R-Square	F	Prob.
Linear	2	23.286667	0.4424	19.82	<.0001
Quadratic	2	2.015833	0.0383	1.72	0.1922
Cross product	1	2.666667	0.0507	4.54	0.0390
Total regress	5	27.969167	0.5313	9.52	<.0001

Residual	DF	SS	MS	F	Prob.
Lack of fit	1	0.250000	0.250000	0.42	0.5207
Pure error	41	24.420000	0.595610		
Total error	42	24.670000	0.587381		

Parameter	DF	Estimate	SD	T	Prob.
Intercept	1	1.450000	0.221243	6.55	<.0001
X_1	1	0.950000	0.180644	5.26	<.0001
X_2	1	−0.541667	0.156442	−3.46	0.0012
$X_1 * X_1$	1	0.050000	0.312885	0.16	0.8738
$X_1 * X_2$	1	−0.666667	0.312885	−2.13	0.0390
$X_2 * X_2$	1	−0.395833	0.234664	−1.69	0.0991

Factor	DF	SS	MS	F	Prob.
X_1	3	18.926667	6.308889	10.74	<.0001
X_2	3	11.379630	3.793210	6.46	0.0011

common conclusions across the three analyses emerge: (1) the model is not rejected due to lack of fit ($P > 0.07$), with the model from RSM Analysis 3 having the worst fit; (2) the model has predictive capacity; i.e., total regression is statistically significant ($P < 0.0001$); (3) the significance of total regression is explained primarily by the significance of the linear terms ($P < 0.002$) in the model; (4) both dose (X_1: $P < 0.0002$) and time of stress test after last dose (X_2: $P < 0.04$) are statistically significant; and (5) the estimates of the coefficients (slopes) of dose and time of stress test after last dose are intuitively consistent; i.e., the predicted delay in time to anginal onset (P_DTTAO) from the model increases as dose increases (positive slope) and decreases as the time of last stress test after dose increases (negative slope).

The fitted response surfaces from the three RSM analyses appear in Figures 11.3 through 11.5, respectively. These figures depict predicted delay in

TABLE 11.10

ANOVA Summary, RSM Analysis 2: 0, 2, 4, and 8 mg b.i.d. and 4 mg t.i.d. (rather than 6 mg b.i.d.)

Response mean	0.891667
Root MSE	0.777284
R-square	0.4320
CV	87.1720

Regression	DF	Type I SS	R-Square	F	Prob.
Linear	2	12.879138	0.2883	10.66	0.0002
Quadratic	2	6.002451	0.1344	4.97	0.0116
Cross product	1	0.419931	0.0094	0.70	0.4092
Total regress	5	19.301520	0.4320	6.39	0.0002

Residual	DF	SS	MS	F	Prob.
Lack of fit	2	1.211813	0.605907	1.00	0.3758
Pure error	40	4.163333	0.604083		
Total error	42	25.375146	0.604170		

Parameter	DF	Estimate	SD	T	Prob.
Intercept	1	1.173466	0.292047	4.02	0.0002
X_1	1	0.686355	0.174706	3.93	0.0003
X_2	1	−0.314400	0.153174	−2.05	0.0464
$X_1 * X_1$	1	0.323135	0.341151	0.95	0.3490
$X_1 * X_2$	1	−0.225732	0.270759	−0.83	0.4092
$X_2 * X_2$	1	−0.589849	0.266110	−2.22	0.0321

Factor	DF	SS	MS	F	Prob.
X_1	3	10.997076	3.665692	6.07	0.0016
X_2	3	5.718278	1.906093	3.15	0.0346

time-to-anginal onset (P_DTTAO) as a function of dose and time of stress test after last dose. The figures are generally consistent in terms of bracketing a dose by time of stress test after last dose region over which the delay in time-to-anginal onset is predicted is at least 30% above baseline. These results are summarized in Table 11.12.

Across the three RSM analyses, maximal predicted delay in time-to-anginal onset ranged from 2.02 to 3.16 min, representing a delay that ranged from 38% to 59% above baseline. However, the corresponding "troughs" reflected a total daily dose of 16 mg and time of stress test of 2 h after last; suggesting an unrealistic dosing and frequency of dosing regimen of 1.33 mg given 12 times daily. The specified clinically important delay in time-to-anginal onset of 30% is predicted with a total daily dose of 16 mg and frequency of dosing interval that

TABLE 11.11

ANOVA Summary, RSM Analysis 3: 0, 2, 4, and 6 mg b.i.d. and "6 mg t.i.d." (rather than 8 mg b.i.d.)

Response mean	1.175000
Root MSE	0.708975
R-square	0.4817
CV	60.3383

Regression	DF	Type I SS	R-Square	F	Prob.
Linear	2	15.722222	0.3860	15.64	<.0001
Quadratic	2	1.230000	0.0302	1.22	0.3045
Cross product	1	2.666667	0.0655	5.31	0.0263
Total regress	5	19.618889	0.4817	7.81	<.0001

Residual	DF	SS	MS	F	Prob.
Lack of fit	1	1.604444	1.604444	3.37	0.0736
Pure error	41	19.506667	0.475772		
Total error	42	21.111111	0.502646		

Parameter	DF	Estimate	SD	T	Prob.
Intercept	1	1.450000	0.204663	7.08	<.0001
X_1	1	0.694444	0.167107	4.16	0.0002
X_2	1	−0.541667	0.144719	−3.74	0.0005
$X_1 * X_1$	1	−0.333333	0.289438	−1.15	0.2560
$X_1 * X_2$	1	−0.666667	0.289438	−2.30	0.0263
$X_2 * X_2$	1	−0.300000	0.217078	−1.38	0.1743

Factor	DF	SS	MS	F	Prob.
X_1	3	12.013889	4.004630	7.97	0.0003
X_2	3	10.668333	3.556111	7.07	0.0006

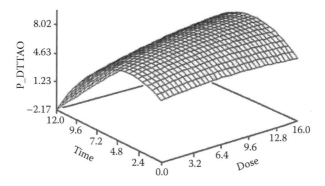

FIGURE 11.3
Plot of fitted response (P_DTTAO) surface: RSM 1.

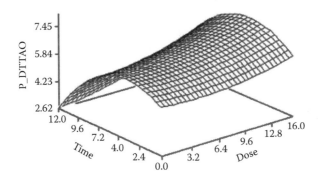

FIGURE 11.4
Plot of fitted response (P_DTTAO) surface: RSM 2.

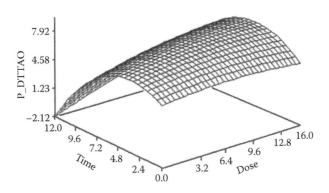

FIGURE 11.5
Plot of fitted response (P_DTTAO) surface: RSM 3.

contains 8 h. Therefore, the results of the RSM analyses suggest a total daily dose of 16 mg given t.i.d. (the 4, 6, and 6 mg regimen) for consideration in Phase III trials. Since the total daily dose was at the end of the dosing interval, it would be advisable for Phase III trials t.i.d dosing regimens to bracket 16 mg per day, or to conduct another Phase II t.i.d. trial that brackets this dose.

The response surface analyses summarized in Tables 11.9 through 11.12 and Figures 11.3 through 11.5 represent analyses of subsets of the data collected. The subsets represent the least amount of all data collected satisfying the requirements of the equiradial-hexagonal design; i.e., representation at all vertices with replication at the center point. For completeness, an

TABLE 11.12

P_DTTAO, Dose and Time of Stress Test RSM Summary

Desired Effect P_DTTAO	Predicted Dose (mg) Increasing	Predicted Time (h) Decreasing
RSM analysis 1		
(2.98 min; 3.16 min)	16	2
(55%; 59%)		
(1.60 min)	8	2–5
(30%)		
(1.60 min)	16	8.5–9.5
(30%)		
RSM analysis 2		
(2.02 min; 2.14 min)	16	3–7
(38%; 40%)		
(1.60 min)	9–14	2–9
(30%)		
RSM analysis 3		
(2.58 min; 2.73 min)	16	2
(48%; 51%)		
(1.60 min)	7.6	2–5
(30%)		
(1.60 min)	16	7–8
(30%)		

RSM Analysis (#4) was performed on all the data (144 observations). The results are summarized in Table 11.13. The results are categorically consistent with those from RSM Analyses 1, 2, and 3.

In this analysis, it is instructive to contrast the degrees of freedom from RSM Analyses 1, 2, and 3 with that of RSM Analysis 4. For RSM Analyses 1, 2, and 3, there are six groups (vertices) each with six observations plus one group (the center point) with 12 observations. Each vertex group contributes 5 df to pure error. The center point group contributes 11 df to pure error. Therefore, the df for pure error from these analyses is 6 * 5 + 11 = 41.

For RSM Analysis 4, there are six groups (0 mg b.i.d. and 2 mg b.i.d. at stress test hours 2, 7, and 12) each with six observations. These contribute 30 df to pure error. There are nine groups (8, 12, and 16 mg total daily dose at stress test hours 2, 7, and 12) each with 12 observations. These contribute 99 df to pure error. Thus df for pure error from RSM Analysis 4 is 129.

TABLE 11.13

ANOVA Summary, RSM Analysis 4: All Data

Response mean	1.147917
Root MSE	0.843294
R-square	0.2601
CV	73.4630

Regression	DF	Type I SS	R-Square	F	Prob.
Linear	2	27.473300	0.2071	19.32	<.0001
Quadratic	2	2.543744	0.0192	1.79	0.1711
Cross product	1	4.484418	0.0338	6.31	0.0132
Total regress	5	34.501462	0.2601	9.70	<.0001

Residual	DF	SS	MS	F	Prob.
Lack of fit	9	9.544580	1.060509	1.54	0.1392
Pure error	129	88.593333	0.686770		
Total error	138	98.137913	0.711144		

Parameter	DF	Estimate	SD	T	Prob.
Intercept	1	1.253513	0.144624	8.67	<.0001
X_1	1	0.492919	0.108691	4.54	<.0001
X_2	1	−0.298874	0.089490	−3.34	0.0011
$X_1 * X_1$	1	−0.022440	0.169301	−0.13	0.8947
$X_1 * X_2$	1	−0.328228	0.130708	−2.51	0.0132
$X_2 * X_2$	1	−0.281250	0.149075	−1.89	0.0613

Factor	DF	SS	MS	F	Prob.
X_1	3	19.499795	6.499932	9.14	<.0001
X_2	3	19.486085	6.495362	9.13	<.0001

11.5 Concluding Remarks

Usually in applying response surface designs and methods to determine dose and frequency of dose in clinical trials, one would use a factorial design [14–16] with specified levels of the dose factor and specified levels of the frequency of dosing factor. The choice of doses would be based on what is known about the dose–response relationship within a safety tolerance range. The choice of frequencies of dosing would typically range from 1 to 4 (providing marketing thinks they could sell a q.i.d drug).

The example presented in this chapter is rather novel. The factor used as dose was total daily dose. Further, although the frequency of dosing was b.i.d. or t.i.d., the frequency of dosing was not explicitly a factor in the RSM approach. Rather, the time after last stress test provided information as to frequency in the sense of a "trough." In bioavailability studies, the trough is the concentration of a drug in the bloodstream just before giving the next dose. In developing dose and frequency of dosing regimens, it is desirable for the trough to be sufficiently high to provide clinical benefit (prior to taking the next dose). Therefore, the response surface was explored over the total daily dose and time after last stress test region to determine a subregion over which the time to anginal onset would be predicted to be delayed at least 30% over baseline (defined as clinically important).

Time-to-anginal onset could also have been analyzed by time-to-event methods. This was not done as the dataset contained no censored observations.

References

1. U.S. Food and Drug Administration: Proposed new drug, antibiotic, and biologic drug product regulations. Code of Federal Regulations Title 21. Retrieved from http://www.fda.gov/oc/gcp/preambles/48fr/48fr.html
2. Peace KE (1989): The use of response surface methodology in the development of anti-anginal drugs. In: *Statistical Issues in Pharmaceutical Drug Development*, Peace, KE (ed.), Marcel Dekker, Inc., New York, pp. 285–303.
3. Madsen JI, Wei S, Haftka RT (2000): Response surface techniques for diffuser shape optimization. *AIAA Journal*; **38**(9): 1512–1518.
4. Wen JG, Zhang YP, Choi SH, Zhang YJ, Kwang-Pill Lee KP (2006): Application of response surface methodologies in capillary electrophoresis. *Microchimica Acta*; **156**(3–4): 327–335.
5. Liu CQ, Chen QG, Tang B, Ruan H, He GQ (2007): Response surface methodology for optimizing the fermentation medium of alpha-galactosidase in solid-state fermentation. *Letters in Applied Microbiology*; **45**(2): 206–212.
6. Nelder JA, Mead R (1965): A simplex method for function minimization. *Computer Journal*; **7**: 308–313.
7. Fletcher R (1987): *Practical Methods of Optimization*, 2nd edn., John Wiley & Sons, New York.
8. Björck A (1996): *Numerical Methods for Least Squares Problems*, SIAM, Philadelphia, PA.
9. Myers RH (1971): *Response Surface Methodology*, Allyn & Bacon, Boston, MA.
10. Myers RH, Montgomery DC (2002): *Response Surface Methodology: Process and Product Optimization Using Designed Experiments*, Wiley Interscience, John Wiley & Sons, New York.
11. Khuri AI (ed.) (2006): *Response Surface Methodology and Related Topics*, World Scientific Publishing, Hackensack, NJ.
12. Statistical Analysis System, Version 9.1 (2009): PROC RSREG; SAS Institute Inc., Cary, NC.
13. http://www.nhlbi.nih.gov/health/dci/Diseases/Angina/Angina_WhatIs.html (retrieved May 26, 2009).

14. Canter D, Frank GJ, Knapp LE, Phelps M, Quade M, Texter M (1994): Quinapril and hydrochlorothiazide combination for control of hypertension: Assessment by factorial design. *Journal of Human Hypertension*; **8**(3): 155–162.
15. Frishman WH, Bryzinski BS, Coulson LR, DeQuattro VL, Vlachakis ND, Mroczek WJ, Dukart G, Goldberg JD, Alemayehu D, Koury K (1994): A multifactorial trial design to assess combination therapy in hypertension: Treatment with bisoprolol and hydrochlorothiazide. *Archives of Internal Medicine*; **154**(13): 1461–1468.
16. Pool JL, Cushman WC, Saini RK, Nwachuku CE, Battikha JP (1997): Use of the factorial design and quadratic response surface models to evaluate the fosinopril and hydrochlorothiazide combination therapy in hypertension. *American Journal of Hypertension*; **10**: 117–123.

12

Confirmation of Clinically Optimal Dosing in the Treatment of Duodenal Ulcers: A Phase III Dose Comparison Trial

12.1 Introduction

Duodenal ulcers are ulcers that occur in the duodenum—the upper portion of the small intestine as it leaves the stomach. A duodenal ulcer is characterized by the presence of a well-demarcated break (ulcer crater) in the mucosa that may extend into the muscularis propria [1].

Cimetidine was the first H_2 receptor antagonist to receive regulatory approval (in the late 1970s) for the treatment of duodenal ulcers. When it was being developed it was widely held that duodenal ulcers were caused by excessive gastric acid production. In fact the prevailing medical opinion was *no acid, no ulcer*. Sir James Black and colleagues at SmithKline and French Laboratories are credited with the discovery of cimetidine. They discovered that histamine released by the H_2-receptor stimulated the production of gastric acid, and that cimetidine by blocking the release of this histamine would suppress both normal- and food-stimulated gastric acid secretion [2]. In a lesser acidic environment, ulcers would be able to heal.

The first cimetidine regimen approved for the treatment of duodenal ulcers in the United Kingdom was 1000 mg per day, given as 200 mg at breakfast, lunch, and dinner, and 400 mg at bed time, for up to 4 weeks. The first regimen approved in the United States for this indication was 1200 mg per day, given as 300 mg q.i.d. for up to 4 weeks. Subsequently, other indications were obtained, and dosing regimens modified; for example, 800 mg per day given as 400 mg b.i.d.

In the mid-1980s, based upon gastric acid suppression data from gastric acid anti-secretory studies at various doses and frequencies of dosing, there was reason to believe that a single nighttime (h.s.) dose of 800 mg of cimetidine (C) for up to 4 weeks would be the clinically optimal way to treat patients with duodenal ulcers. A large, landmark, dose comparison clinical trial [3–6] was undertaken to confirm the effectiveness of 800 mg C h.s. in the treatment of duodenal ulcers for up to 4 weeks. Details of the design and logistics of this trial, biostatistical analysis methods, and results are reviewed in this chapter.

12.2 Background

When the first author was first consulted by the project physician and regulatory affairs expert, the clinical development plan consisted of two randomized, double-blind, placebo-controlled, pivotal proof-of-efficacy trials with single nighttime dosing for 4 weeks:

Trial 1: 800 mg C h.s.   versus   placebo

Trial 2: 1200 mg C h.s.   versus   placebo

Each trial was to enroll 150 patients per treatment group, for a total of 600 patients. One hundred fifty patients per group would provide a power of 95% to detect a 20% difference in 4-week ulcer healing rates between the cimetidine and placebo groups with a one-sided, Type I error [7] of 5%. Investigator and patient costs to conduct both trials were estimated at just over $4.5 M.

   Since conducting these trials would subject half the patients to placebo, the first author recommended amalgamating the two trials into a single trial:

Trial 3: 1200 mg C h.s.   versus   800 mg C h.s.   versus   0 mg C h.s. (placebo)

with 164 patients per treatment group, for a total of 492 patients. One hundred sixty-four patients per treatment group would provide a power of 95% to detect a difference of 20% in 4-week ulcer healing rates between any two of the treatment groups with an experiment-wise Type I error of 5% (1.67% per each one-sided, pair-wise comparison). Not only would this trial require fewer patients and be less expensive to conduct, it would also provide a within-trial comparison between cimetidine doses.

   Further savings could be realized by incorporating into the Trial 3 protocol, a planned interim analysis after half the patients had been entered and completed. At the interim analysis, the efficacy comparisons, 1200 mg C versus placebo, and 800 mg C versus placebo would be tested. If both were statistically significant, then the entire study could be stopped—if efficacy of the doses were the only objective. If comparing the doses of cimetidine was also of clinical importance, then the placebo arm could be stopped and the two cimetidine arms run to full completion to assess dose discrimination. By conducting Trial 3 (instead of the two separate trials) and incorporating the interim analysis, potential savings of 190 patients and approximately \$1.4 M could be realized. Additional savings would be expected due to less time required to conduct the trial [8,9].

The primary objective in conducting a clinical trial of cimetidine in the treatment of duodenal ulcers with a single nighttime dose was to demonstrate that 800 mg C was clinically optimal. We therefore added a 400 mg dose and replaced the 1200 mg dose with a 1600 mg dose (a twofold increase among consecutive doses) in the final trial protocol.

12.3 Objective

Both primary and secondary efficacy objectives were identified in the final protocol. The **primary objective addressed ulcer healing.** The **secondary objective addressed upper gastrointestinal (UGI) pain relief.**

The **primary objective** was to confirm that cimetidine given as a single nighttime dose of 800 mg for up to 4 weeks was clinically optimal in healing duodenal ulcers. Clinically optimal meant that 800 mg C was effective (significantly superior to placebo), that 800 was superior to 400, and that 1600 mg C was not significantly superior to 800 mg C. Symbolically the primary (note p subscript of H) objective derives from three null and alternative hypotheses:

$$H_{p01}: P_{uh800} = P_{uh0}$$
$$H_{pa1}: P_{uh800} > P_{uh0}$$

$$H_{p02}: P_{uh800} = P_{uh400}$$
$$H_{pa2}: P_{uh800} > P_{uh400}$$

$$H_{p03}: P_{uh1600} = P_{uh800}$$
$$H_{pa3}: P_{uh1600} \neq P_{uh800}$$

where P_{uh0}, P_{uh400}, P_{uh800}, and P_{uh1600} represent the 4-week ulcer healing (UH) rates in the placebo, 400, 800, and 1600 mg C treatment groups, respectively, under single nighttime dosing. Specifically, H_{pa1}, H_{pa2}, and H_{p03} comprised the primary study objective.

Symbolically, the **secondary** (note s subscript of H) **objective** derives from the three null and alternative hypotheses:

$$H_{s01}: P_{pr800} = P_{pr0}$$
$$H_{sa1}: P_{pr800} > P_{pr0}$$

$$H_{s02}: P_{pr800} = P_{pr400}$$

$$H_{sa2}: P_{pr800} > P_{pr400}$$

$$H_{s03}: P_{pr1600} = P_{pr800}$$

$$H_{sa3}: P_{pr1600} \neq P_{pr800}$$

where P_{pr0}, P_{pr400}, P_{pr800}, and P_{pr1600} represent the UGI pain relief (PR) rates in the placebo, 400, 800, and 1600 mg C treatment groups, respectively, under single nighttime dosing. Specifically, H_{sa1}, H_{sa2}, and H_{s03} comprised the secondary study objective.

Of the six possible pair-wise comparisons among the four dose groups, only three comprised the study objective.

12.4 Designing and Planning the Investigation

The trial was multicenter, stratified, randomized, double-blind, and placebo-controlled. As there had been reports [10–13] of the influence of smoking on the healing of duodenal ulcers at the time of protocol development, patients were stratified by smoking status within each center prior to randomization to the treatment groups. Smoking strata were light smokers and heavy smokers. Patients who smoked at most nine cigarettes per day comprised the light smoker stratum. Patients who smoked at least 10 cigarettes per day comprised the heavy smoker stratum.

12.4.1 Blinded Treatment Groups

Blinded treatment group medication was packaged using the existing regulatory approved 400 mg C tablet. A 400 mg placebo tablet was formulated identical to the 400 mg C tablet except that it contained 0 mg C. Blinded trial medication for the four treatment groups was packaged in blister packs for 4 weeks of treatment as identified below:

0 mg C Group: Four 400 mg placebo tablets

400 mg C Group: One cimetidine 400 mg tablet + three 400 mg placebo tablets

800 mg C Group: Two cimetidine 400 mg tablets + two 400 mg placebo tablets

1600 mg C Group: Four cimetidine 400 mg tablets.

12.4.2 Sample Size Determination

The trial was designed to recruit and enter enough patients to complete one hundred sixty-four (164) per treatment group, for a total of 656 patients. One hundred sixty-four patients per treatment group would provide a power of 95% to detect a difference of 20% in cumulative 4-week ulcer healing rates between any two of the treatment groups with an experiment-wise Type I error rate of 5% (1.67% per each one-sided, pair-wise comparison). This number was inflated to account for a 15% drop out rate. A cumulative 4-week healing rate of 45% among placebo-treated patients [14: references < 1985] in previous trials was used in the sample size determination.

12.4.3 Entry Requirements and Assessment Schedule

Patients were required at entry to have an endoscopically confirmed duodenal ulcer of size at least 0.3 cm and either daytime or nighttime UGI pain. At the preliminary examination or baseline visit, patients provided a history (including prior use of medications, particularly antiulcer ones or antacids), underwent a physical examination, had vital signs measured, provided blood and urine samples for clinical laboratory assessments, in addition to having UGI pain assessed and undergoing endoscopy. Patients were also instructed how to use a daily diary to record the severity of daytime or nighttime UGI pain, as well as to record any adverse experience or concomitant medication use. Diaries and trial medication were dispensed and the patients instructed to return at weeks 1, 2, and 4 of the treatment period for follow-up endoscopy, UGI pain assessment, and assessment of other clinical parameters. Antacids were provided to patients for relief of severe pain during only the first 6 days/nights of therapy, and were limited to four tablets per day of low acid-neutralizing capacity. Table 12.1 summarizes clinical assessments made throughout the trial.

Follow-up endoscopic evaluation was carried out following strict time windows (Table 12.1) at week 1 (Days 7–8), week 2 (Days 13–15) and week 4

TABLE 12.1

Clinical Evaluation Schedule

Clinical Parameter	Preliminary Examination	Week 1 (Days 7–8)	Week 2 (Days 13–15)	Week 4 (Days 26–30)
History	Y			
Physical exam	Y			
Vital signs	Y	Y	Y	Y
Adv. events		Y	Y	Y
Con. meds	Y	Y	Y	Y
Endoscopy	Y	Y	Y	Y
Pain assessment	Y	Y	Y	Y
Clin. labs.	Y	Y		Y

(Days 26–30). Patients whose ulcers were healed at any follow-up endoscopy were considered trial completers and received no further treatment or endoscopic assessment.

12.4.4 Primary and Secondary Endpoints

The **primary efficacy data** was ulcer healing at week 1, 2, or 4. Ulcer healing was defined as complete *re-epithelization of the ulcer crater* (normal or hyperemic mucosa), *documented by endoscopy*. The **primary efficacy endpoint** was cumulative ulcer healing at week 4.

Secondary efficacy data were the severity ratings of daytime and nighttime UGI pain recorded by the patient on the daily diary card. The severity of daytime pain was recorded just prior to going to sleep at night. The severity of nighttime pain was recorded upon arising in the morning. At each follow-up visit, the physician would review the diary card and record the most severe rating of daytime and nighttime pain since the previous clinic visit. Daytime and nighttime UGI pain were rated separately according to the following scale:

0 = None = I had no pain

1 = Mild = I had some pain, but it did not bother me much

2 = Moderate = I had pain that was annoying, but it did not interrupt my activities

3 = Severe = I had pain which was so bad I could not do my usual activities

For nighttime pain, activities reflected sleep. The **secondary efficacy endpoint** was whether the patient was free of daytime or nighttime pain at weeks 1, 2, or 4.

12.5 Conducting the Investigation

When the trial was conducted, there was great pressure to complete it as quickly as possible. This was due in part to ranitidine's rapid gains into the antiulcer market, of which cimetidine had exclusivity for several years. Approximately 60 centers were recruited. The centers were rigorously and frequently monitored for conformity to protocol and federal regulations, in an attempt to minimize violations to protocol and collection of questionable if not unusable data. Roughly half of the sites were monitored by in-house clinical monitoring personnel (clinical research associates = CRA). The remaining sites were monitored by an outside Contract Research Organization (CRO).

A fairly heavy advertisement campaign was initiated to recruit possible trial participants. Advertisements ran on television and radio and appeared in the print media. In addition, circulars were posted in public areas such as supermarket and laundromat bulletin boards. The ads were targeted to adults who had been having UGI or ulcer-like pain, but who were otherwise healthy.

Weekly meetings were held during the conduct of the trial to monitor progress and deal with any issues. A proactive approach to clinical data management was taken. Data collection forms (DCFs) were expressed by each clinic to the data management group (or picked up by the CRA), where they were rapidly reviewed for completeness, legibility, entered into the computerized trial database, verified, and quality assured. The goal was to provide a quality-assured database for statistical analysis in as short a time as possible after each patient completed the protocol.

At the time the duodenal ulcer trial was conducted, 800 mg C tablets were not commercially available. The commercially available 400 mg C tablet was used. Therefore a blood level trial that demonstrated bioequivalence [15] between a new 800 mg C tablet formulation (to be marketed) and two 400 mg C commercially available tablets had to be conducted with results available by the completion of the duodenal ulcer trial. Results from these two trials as well as that from specified drug interaction studies provided the primary data to support filing a supplemental new drug application (SNDA) to the FDA for the approval of cimetidine as a single 800 mg tablet taken at bedtime for the treatment of duodenal ulcers.

12.6 Statistical Analyses

12.6.1 Statistical Analysis Methods

12.6.1.1 Methods

Descriptive and inferential methods were used in presentations and analysis of the trial data using procedures (PROCS) in the statistical analysis system (SAS) software. Both tables and graphs reflecting the number of patients, the mean (percent for dichotomous data) and standard deviation by treatment group, and time of assessment were developed.

Inferential analyses, significance tests, and confidence intervals derived from an analysis of variance model containing fixed effects of center, strata, and treatment group, with contrasts specified for the pair-wise comparisons of interest. *P*-values for the pair-wise comparisons comprising the primary trial objective were used for statistical inference. Confidence intervals were used as the basis of inference for secondary trial objectives and for the three pair-wise comparisons that were not a part of the trial objective.

Since there were many centers and relatively few patients per treatment group per strata per center, 12 blocks reflecting smoking status (two levels)-by-baseline ulcer size (six levels) were defined a priori (Table 12.2). An analysis of variance model containing the fixed effects of blocks and treatment was also used to assess the effect of treatment adjusted for blocks.

Generalizability (poolability) of treatment effects was assessed by running an analysis of variance model with block, treatment group and block-by-treatment interaction. In these analyses, the sole interest was the *P*-value for the interaction term. The blocking factor was smoking status-by-baseline ulcer size as defined in Table 12.2. A separate analysis that included the factors like smoking status, baseline ulcer size, their interaction, and the interaction of each of these with treatment was also performed.

TABLE 12.2

Smoking Status by Ulcer Size Blocks

Smoking Status	Ulcer Size (cm)
Light	[0.3]
Light	(0.3; 0.4]
Light	(0.4; 0.5]
Light	(0.5; 1.0)
Light	[1.0]
Light	(1.0; 3.0]
Heavy	[0.3]
Heavy	(0.3; 0.4]
Heavy	(0.4; 0.5]
Heavy	(0.5; 1.0)
Heavy	[1.0]
Heavy	(1.0; 3.0]

Bivariate plots of the proportion of patients with ulcers remaining unhealed and the proportion of patients with UGI pain (daytime or nighttime) by time of endoscopic evaluation and treatment group were developed. These plots illustrate the rate of ulcer healing and pain relief across the times of endoscopic evaluation.

12.6.1.2 Interim Analysis

Prior to finalizing the protocol, we considered including an interim analysis plan. Incorporating such a plan could result in completing approximately half the planned number of patients. More importantly, it could reduce the time from starting the trial to filing the SNDA. The idea was accepted initially, but later rejected by upper management; so the final protocol did not include an interim analysis plan.

However after the trial started, there was a push to conduct an interim analysis. A plan was developed to conduct an interim (mid-study) analysis after half the patients had entered. The plan was filed by in-house regulatory affairs personnel with the FDA. Essential features of the plan ensured preservation of the Type I error and safeguarded blindedness among investigators, patients, and in-house personnel.

We hired an external consulting group that generated dummy investigator, patient, and treatment group identification. The group also computed the *P*-values associated with the three pair-wise comparisons comprising the study objectives and reported them to FDA biometrics and in-house personnel. The trial was not stopped and ran to completion, eventually enrolling 768 patients. The final results, based upon more than twice the number of patients in the interim analysis, were similar to those of the interim analysis in terms of estimates of treatment effects.

12.6.2 Interim Analysis Results

12.6.2.1 Numbers of Patients and Baseline Characteristics

Table 12.3 summarizes the number of patients available for the mid-study, interim analysis. Three hundred and thirty-seven (337) were randomized, of which 315 [4,5] were considered evaluatable [16] for efficacy for at least one follow-up visit. The fact that 17 more patients were assigned to the 1600 mg C group illustrates that a slight imbalance across treatment groups can occur in randomized trials consisting of many centers.

Table 12.4 contains descriptive results of data available at baseline for mid-study analysis patients by cimetidine treatment group. The treatment

TABLE 12.3

Number of Patients by Treatment Group (Mid-Study Analysis)

	Total	0 mg	400 mg	800 mg	1600 mg
# Randomized	337	76	83	85	93
# Evaluatable					
Week 1	304	67	80	73	84
Week 2	235	46	63	60	66
Week 4	174	41	47	47	39
≥1 week	315	71	82	75	87

TABLE 12.4

Baseline Characteristics (Mid-Study Analysis)

Characteristic	Statistic	0 mg	400 mg	800 mg	1600 mg
Age (yr)	Mean	42	40	44	42
Height (in.)	Mean	67	67	67	67
Weight (lb)	Mean	169	160	163	160
Sex	Male (N)	50	62	51	55
	Female (N)	26	21	34	38
Race	Caucasian (N)	44	50	58	61
	Black (N)	24	21	18	24
	Other (N)	8	12	9	8
Day pain	Mean	2.89	3.13	2.91	2.92
Night pain	Mean	2.68	2.84	2.80	3.05
Ulcer size (cm)	Mean	0.76	0.71	0.85	0.75
Smoking status	Heavy (N)	40	45	45	48
	Light (N)	36	38	40	45

groups appear balanced in terms of demographic characteristics, UGI pain and ulcer size,
although the 800 mg C group had patients with
the largest ulcers.

12.6.2.2 Distribution of Patients according to Ulcer Size

Table 12.5 provides the distribution of patients at
baseline according to ulcer size. Ten percent (10%)
of patients had ulcers of size 0.30 cm, 12.5% had
ulcers of size greater than 0.30 but at most 0.40 cm,
17.8% had ulcers of size greater than 0.40 cm but
at most 0.50 cm, 27.2% had ulcers of size between
0.50 and 1.00 cm, 17.8% had ulcers 1.00 cm in size,
and 14.7% had ulcers of size greater than 1.00 cm
but at most 3.00 cm.

Table 12.6 provides the distribution of patients
in the placebo group by baseline ulcer size whose
ulcers had healed by 4 weeks. Seventy-one percent (71%) of placebo patients with ulcers of size
0.30 cm healed; 78% of placebo patients with
ulcers of size greater than 0.30 but at most
0.40 cm healed; 45% of placebo patients with
ulcers of size greater than 0.40 cm but at most
0.50 cm healed; 41% of placebo patients with
ulcers between 0.50 and 1.00 cm in size healed; 30% of placebo patients
with ulcers 1.00 cm in size healed; and 25% of placebo patients with ulcers
of size greater than 1.00 cm but at most 3.00 cm healed. Table 12.5 reflects a
strong negative correlation (or trend) between baseline ulcer size and ulcer
healing by 4 weeks; that is, the smaller the ulcer, the greater the ulcer healing
by 4 weeks.

TABLE 12.5

Distribution by Ulcer Size

Ulcer Size (cm)	% Patients
[0.30]	10.0
(0.30; 0.40]	12.5
(0.40; 0.50]	17.8
(0.50; 1.00)	27.2
[1.00]	17.8
(1.00; 3.00]	14.7

TABLE 12.6

Cumulative 4-Week Ulcer
Healing Rates: Placebo
Patients

Ulcer Size (cm)	% Healed
[0.30]	71
(0.30; 0.40]	78
(0.40; 0.50]	45
(0.50; 1.00)	41
[1.00]	30
(1.00; 3.00]	25

12.6.2.3 Influence of Smoking Status and Ulcer Size on Ulcer Healing

Figure 12.1 provides a summary of the cumulative proportion of patients
across all treatment groups with healed duodenal ulcers by week of endoscopy and smoking status. Figure 12.1 reflects a strong negative correlation
between smoking status and ulcer healing; that is, light smokers have a higher
percentage of healed ulcers than do heavy smokers at all weeks of endoscopy.

Figure 12.2 provides a summary of the cumulative proportion of patients
across all treatment groups with healed duodenal ulcers by week of endoscopy and baseline ulcer size. Figure 12.2 reflects a strong negative correlation
between ulcer size and ulcer healing; that is, patients with smaller ulcers have

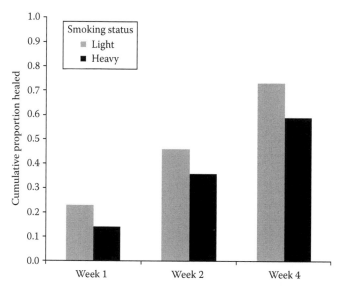

FIGURE 12.1

Cumulative proportion healed: light versus heavy smokers, combined treatment groups.

a higher percentage of healed ulcers than do patients with larger ulcers at all weeks of endoscopy. Note that the categories of ulcer size in Figure 12.2 are those that were defined a priori. The negative correlation between ulcer size and healing is sharpened when collapsing the six ulcer size categories into three (Figure 12.3).

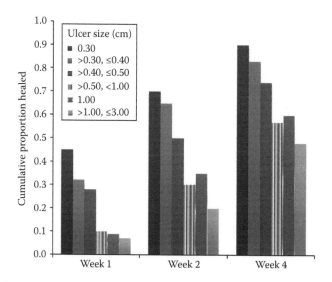

FIGURE 12.2

Cumulative proportion healed by ulcer size, combined treatment groups.

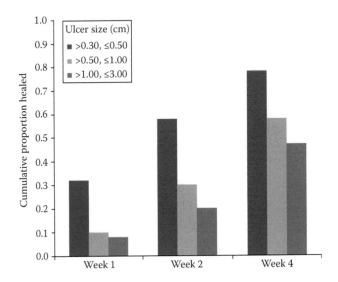

FIGURE 12.3
Cumulative proportion healed by ulcer size, combined treatment groups.

12.6.2.4 Cumulative Ulcer Healing

The cumulative duodenal ulcer healing rates are summarized [4,5] in Figure 12.4 by week of endoscopy and treatment group. The healing rates were 19%, 18%, 16%, and 21% at week 1; 29%, 37%, 38%, and 49% at week 2;

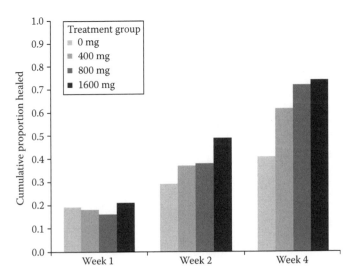

FIGURE 12.4
Cumulative proportions of patients with healed ulcers, by week and treatment group.

and 41%, 62%, 72%, and 74% at week 3; for the placebo, 400, 800 and 1600 mg C groups respectively. At week 4, 800 mg C was effective ($P = 0.0002$) compared to placebo, 800 was marginally superior to 400 ($P = 0.1283$), and 1600 mg C provided no clinically significant greater benefit {$\delta = 0.0156$: 90% CI on ratio of 1600/800 mg C $= (0.86–1.18)$} than did 800 mg C. Even though 800 mg C healed 10% more ulcers than did 400 mg C, the *P*-value for this comparison did not achieve statistical significance. Therefore, the mid-study analysis did not demonstrate that 800 mg C was clinically optimal as formulated in the trial objective.

12.6.2.5 Generalizability Assessment

Table 12.7 provides a summary of the assessment of generalizability (poolability) of treatment effect across smoking status, baseline ulcer size, and smoking status-by-baseline ulcer size. All of the *P*-values are large and therefore provide no evidence of lack of generalizability of treatment effects across these subpopulations.

12.6.2.6 Complete UGI Pain Relief and Ulcer Healing

To illustrate changes in duodenal ulcer healing and complete relief of UGI pain jointly, bivariate plots (Figures 12.5 and 12.6) were generated. To develop these plots, the means (proportions) of each endpoint were computed by treatment or dose group and each endoscopy evaluation. The means, corresponding to each endoscopy evaluation and dose group identification, along with the ranges (0, 1) of each endpoint, were output to a data file. The data file was accessed by a graphical software package and a plot generated of the mean pairs by dose group. In generating the plots, the horizontal axis reflects the range of one endpoint and the vertical axis reflects the range of the other endpoint. In plotting the pairs of means for each dose group, the endoscopy evaluation corresponding to each pair appears as a floating index on the graph of each dose group.

TABLE 12.7

Assessment of Generalizability: Smoking Status by Ulcer Size Subpopulations

Source	F-Value	P-Value
Smoke × size	1.11	0.3559
Smoke × dose	0.40	0.7518
Size × dose	1.12	0.3359
Smoke × size × dose	0.78	0.7038

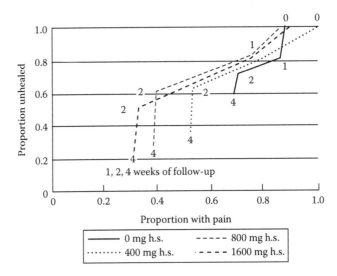

FIGURE 12.5
Proportions of patients with daytime pain and unhealed ulcers, by treatment group (mid-study analysis).

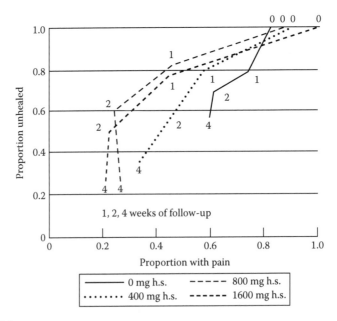

FIGURE 12.6
Proportions of patients with nighttime pain and unhealed ulcers, by treatment group (mid-study analysis).

In Figures 12.5 and 12.6, the horizontal axis reflects the proportion of patients with UGI pain, and the vertical axis reflects the proportion of patients with unhealed ulcers rather than proportions of patients without UGI pain and with healed ulcers. The (1, 1) point therefore reflects where the patients are at baseline, and the (0, 0) point reflects the ideal therapeutic goal of a treatment or dose by the final visit. For a broader discussion of bivariate plots, Peace and Tsai [17] may be seen.

Figure 12.5 is the bivariate plot of daytime UGI pain and lack of ulcer healing. Figure 12.6 is the bivariate plot of nighttime UGI pain and lack of ulcer healing. The fact that all dose groups do not begin at the (1, 1) point is due to the fact that some patients had daytime UGI pain but not nighttime UGI pain and vice versa. Focusing on week 4 results, Figures 12.5 and 12.6 reflect a beautiful picture of dose response, both univariately and bivariately.

12.6.3 Final Analysis Results

At the final study analysis, 168, 182, 165, and 188 patients [6] were efficacy evaluatable, in the placebo, 400, 800, and 1600 mg C groups, respectively. The cumulative duodenal ulcer healing rates are summarized in Figure 12.7 by week of endoscopy and treatment group. The healing rates were: 17%, 16%, 15%, and 21% at week 1; 30%, 40%, 42%, and 48% at week 2; and 41%, 62%, 73%, and 77%; for the placebo, 400, 800, and 1600 mg C groups

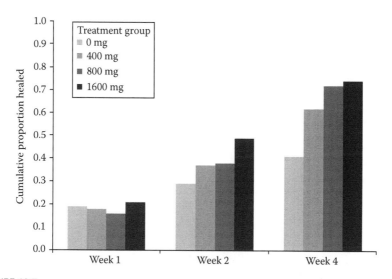

FIGURE 12.7
Cumulative proportions of patients with healed ulcers by week and treatment group (final study results).

respectively. At week 4, 800 mg C was effective $(P < 10^{-8})$ compared to placebo; 800 was superior to 400 $(P = 0.023)$; and 1600 mg C provided no clinically significant greater benefit $\{\delta = 0.04$: 90% CI on ratio of 1600/800 mg C = $(0.96–1.17)\}$ than did 800 mg C. Therefore, the study demonstrated that 800 mg C was clinically optimal.

12.7 Other Considerations

12.7.1 Bioequivalence Trial of Two 400 mg Tablets and One 800 mg Tablet

At the time the duodenal ulcer trial was conducted, 800 mg C tablets were not commercially available. The commercially available 400 mg C tablet was used. Therefore a blood level trial that demonstrated bioequivalence [15] between a new 800 mg C tablet formulation (to be marketed) and two 400 mg C commercially available tablets had to be conducted with results available by the completion of the duodenal ulcer trial.

12.7.2 Cimetidine-by-Drug Interaction Trials

Since cimetidine was widely prescribed (the prescription leader at the time), a change in dosage regimen, particularly a larger dose, required other trials involving the new 800 mg C regimen. We conducted specific drug–drug interaction trials exploring whether 800 mg C altered the circulating levels of other widely prescribed drugs. The drugs selected were theophylline [18–20], lidocaine [21], and warfarin [22].

12.7.3 Study in the Elderly

At the time the duodenal ulcer trial was conducted, the FDA IND/NDA rewrite was in progress, which among other specifics stipulated that pharmaceutical companies should conduct studies in the elderly to explore whether doses of drugs posed a drug dose-by-age interaction. In addition, conducting clinical efficacy trials in the elderly was gaining sway. We actually developed a protocol for a small clinical trial comparing the 800 mg C to placebo in elderly (age $\geq$ 65 years) patients with duodenal ulcers. The trial was to enroll 100 patients balanced across the 800 mg C and placebo groups.

However, prior to starting the trial, the first author subset the final database for the trial described in this chapter and found it contained 101 elderly patients of which 19 were in the placebo group and 23 in the 800 mg C group. Randomization in the large trial did not guarantee balance across treatment groups in this subset of elderly patients. Therefore the treatment groups were compared statistically in terms of baseline characteristics and found to be comparable. Sixteen (16) of 23 (75.6%) elderly patients treated with 800 mg C experienced ulcer healing, as compared to six of 19 (32%) in the placebo group $\{\delta = 0.38\%; 95\%\ \text{CI} = (10.3\text{–}75.6\%)\}$. Since there was evidence in the original trial database that 800 mg C was effective in the elderly, the first author recommended against conducting a separate clinical efficacy trial in the elderly.

Results from the duodenal ulcer trial, the bioequivalence trial, and the cimetidine-by-drug interaction trials provided the primary data to support filing an SNDA to the FDA for the approval of cimetidine as a single 800 mg tablet taken at bedtime for the treatment of duodenal ulcers.

12.8 Innovative Aspects of the Clinical Trial Program

There are several aspects of this program that were rather innovative.

12.8.1 Interim Analyses to Drop Placebo Arms

Interim analysis plans that would allow dropping of the placebo arm after establishing efficacy of the doses, while allowing the dose arms to run to completion for dose discrimination, were developed.

12.8.2 Third-Party Blinding during Interim Analyses

Interim analysis plans that safeguarded company personnel from knowing the identity of investigators, of patients, and treatment groups were developed. These included the following plans: (a) using an outside data management group who generated an analysis data set in which dummy treatment group labels, investigator id and patient id, while preserving the original randomization appeared; and (b) having the outside data management group provide the blinded data set to the company statistician and to the FDA plus the file containing the IDs directly to the FDA.

12.8.3 Trial Objectives as Only Three of Six Pair-Wise Comparisons

The study objective was formulated as only three of six pair-wise comparisons among the four dose groups while preserving the overall experiment-wise Type I error across these three comparisons. The other three comparisons could be investigated, preferably using confidence intervals, but they should not invoke a Type I error penalty on the study objective.

12.8.4 Giving Up Information on Center Differences

Instead of using centers as a blocking factor in the primary analyses, the 12 classifications of smoking status-by-baseline ulcer size was used as the blocking factor due to small numbers of patients per treatment group per center and due to the prognostic importance of smoking status and baseline ulcer size.

12.8.5 Assessment of Type of Monitoring by Treatment Group

An assessment of differences in treatment effect between sites monitored by in-house personnel and those monitored by the CRO was conducted. There was no treatment-by-type of monitoring interaction, although the healing rates were generally lower among CRO monitored sites.

12.8.6 Association between Ulcer Healing and Smoking Status and Ulcer Size

The duodenal ulcer trial definitively established for the first time, negative correlations between ulcer healing and smoking and ulcer healing and baseline ulcer size. Effectiveness estimates of ulcer healing were adjusted for smoking status and baseline ulcer size.

12.8.7 Utilization of Bivariate Graphical Methods

The duodenal ulcer trial was the first to utilize bivariate plots to profile ulcer healing and UGI pain relief jointly. The plots illustrated strong dose–response in terms of ulcer healing and UGI pain relief separately and jointly.

12.8.8 Establishing Effectiveness Based on a Subset Analysis

Efficacy of the 800 mg C dose was established in the elderly based on a subset analysis. The trial entered a large enough elderly population to demonstrate that 800 mg C was effective in elderly. That is a plus for conducting a trial larger than necessary to establish the effectiveness of each dose.

12.8.9 Maximum Use of Patients Screened with UGI Pain

The focus of this chapter has been to review features of the landmark, dose-comparison trial of once nightly cimetidine in the treatment of duodenal ulcer. This trial was one of three clinical trials comprising a major clinical trial program. Each center conducted three protocols: the one discussed in duodenal ulcer, but also one in gastric ulcer and one in dyspepsia.

Patients were recruited on the basis of having experienced ulcer-like symptoms including UGI pain. Those who satisfied general entry criteria and who gave consent were endoscoped. If duodenal ulcer (DU) was confirmed, they entered the DU trial. If gastric ulcer (GU) was confirmed, they entered a GU trial, and if there was no DU or GU, they entered a dyspepsia trial. This latter protocol provided a rather stringent definition of dyspepsia: ulcer like symptoms including UGI pain not explained by the presence of DU or GU. This concurrent protocol method maximized the utility of the advertisement effort to get to the clinic, patients who were experiencing ulcer-like symptoms.

12.9 Concluding Remarks

Since the development of cimetidine and other H_2-receptor antagonists, ranitidine (Glaxo), famotidine (Merck), and Nizatidine (Lilly), more is known about the causes of ulcers in the duodenum and stomach. It is now widely held that duodenal and gastric ulcers are caused by chronic use of NSAIDS, nonsteroidal, anti-inflammatory drugs (that decrease endogenous prostaglandin production), and by interference with the protective gastric mucosal layer from *Helicobacter pylori* infection [1]. Current treatment consists of a combination of an antibiotic, a H_2-receptor antagonist (or a proton pump inhibitor), and a bismuth containing compound, with the primary aim of eradicating *H. Pylori* infection.

References

1. Thomson ABR, Leung YPY, Devlin SM, Meddings J (2009): Duodenal ulcers. eMedicine: emedicine.medscape.com/article/173727-overview (accessed May 6, 2009).
2. Nayak PR, Ketteringham JM (1986): *Tagamet: Repairing Ulcers without Surgery* (in breakthroughs), Rawson Associates, New York, pp. 102–129.

3. Dickson B, Dixon W, Peace KE, Putterman K, Young MD (1985): Cimetidine single-dose active duodenal ulcer protocol design. *Post Graduate Medicine*; **78**(8): 23–26.

4. Peace KE, Dickson B, Dixon W, Putterman K, Young MD (1985): A single nocturnal dose of cimetidine in active duodenal ulcer: Statistical considerations in the design, analysis and interpretation of a clinical trial. *Post Graduate Medicine*; **78**(8): 27–33.

5. Venezuela J, Dickson B, Dixon W, Peace KE, Putterman K, Young MD (1985): Efficacy of a single nocturnal dose of cimetidine in active duodenal ulcer: Result of a United States multicenter trial. *Post Graduate Medicine*; **78**(8): 34–41.

6. Young MD, Frank WO, Dickson BD, Peace K, Braverman A, Mounce W (1989): Determining the optimal dosage regimen for H_2-receptor antagonist therapy—A dose validation approach. *Alimentary Pharmacology & Therapeutics*; **3**(1): 47–57.

7. Peace KE (1991): One-sided or two-sided p-values: Which most appropriately address the question of drug efficacy? *Journal of Biopharmaceutical Statistics*; **1**(1): 133–138.

8. Peace KE (1990): TMO: The trial management organization—A new system for reducing the time for clinical trials. *Drug Information Journal*; **24**: 257–264.

9. Peace KE (1991): Shortening the time for clinical drug development. *Regulatory Affairs Professionals Journal*; **3**: 3–22.

10. Korman MG, Shaw RG, Hansky J, Schmidt GT, Stern AI (1981): Influence of smoking on healing rate of duodenal ulcer in response to cimetidine or high-dose antacid. *Gastroenterology*; **80**: 1451–1453.

11. Korman MG, Hansky J, Eaves ER, Schmidt GT (1983): Influence of cigarette smoking on healing and relapse in duodenal ulcer disease. *Gastroenterology*; **85**: 871–874.

12. Lam SK, Koo J (1983): Accurate prediction of duodenal ulcer healing rate by discriminant analysis. *Gastroenterology*; **85**: 403–412.

13. Barakat MH, Menon KN, Badawi AR (1984): Cigarette smoking and duodenal ulcer healing. *Digestion*; **29**: 85–90.

14. de Craen AJ, Moerman DE, Heisterkamp SH, Tytgat GN, Tijssen JG, Kleijnen J (1999): Placebo effect in the treatment of duodenal ulcer. *British Journal of Clinical Pharmacology*; **48**(6): 853–860.

15. Randolph WC, Peace KE, Seaman JJ, Dickson B, Putterman K (1986): Bioequivalence of a new 800 mg cimetidine tablet with commercially available 400 mg tablets. *Current Therapeutic Research*; **39**(5): 767–772.

16. Peace KE (1984): Evaluable or evaluatable? *Biometrics*; **40**(4): 1180–1181

17. Peace KE, Tsai K-T (2009): Bivariate or composite plots of endpoints. *Journal of Biopharmaceutical Statistics*; **19**: 324–331.

18. Seaman J, Randolph W, Peace KE, Frank WO, Dickson B, Putterman K, Young MD (1985): Effects of two cimetidine dosage regimens on serum theophylline levels. *Post Graduate Medicine*; **78**(8): 47–53.

19. Randolph WC, Seaman JJ, Dickson B, Peace KE, Frank WO, Young MD (1986): The effect of age on theophylline steady-state serum levels and clearance in normal subjects. *British Journal of Clinical Pharmacology*; **22**(5): 603–660.

20. Randolph WC, Peace KE, Frank WD, Seaman JJ (1986): Age-related differences in theophylline clearance at steady state. *Journal of the American Society for Clinical Pharmacology and Therapeutics*; **39**(2): 222–223.

21. Frank WO, Seaman JJ, Peace KE, Myerson RM, Humphries TJ (1983): Lidocaine-cimetidine Interaction. *Annals of Internal Medicine*; **99**(3): 414–415.
22. Sax MJ, Randolph W, Peace KE, Chretian S, Frank WO, Gray DR, McCree L, Braverman AB, Wyle F, Jackson BJ, Beg M (1987): Effect of cimetidine 800 mg h.s. and 300 mg q.i.d. on the pharmaceutics of warfarin in patients receiving maintenance warfarin therapy. *Clinical Pharmacy*; **6**(6): 492–495.

13

Pivotal Proof-of-Efficacy Clinical Trials in the Prevention of NANSAID-Induced Gastric Ulceration

13.1 Introduction

One of the positions the first author had in the pharmaceutical industry provided me the opportunity to run a large-scale clinical research program of the synthetic prostaglandin (PGE_2) analogue, misoprostol. The program consisted of two identical protocols. Clinical and statistical evidence from the program formed the primary basis for FDA approval of misoprostol (Cytotec) in the prevention of gastric ulceration induced by nonaspirin, nonsteroidal, anti-inflammatory drugs (NANSAIDs) in osteoarthritic (OA) patients requiring NANSAIDs in the management of their OA symptoms. A rationale for the program is presented in Section 13.2. The protocols are reviewed in Section 13.3. Monitoring and data management considerations are presented in Section 13.4. Meeting with the U.S. Regulatory Agency is addressed in Section 13.5. Discussion and concluding remarks appear in Section 13.6.

13.2 Rationale

Gastric ulceration induced by the chronic administration of NANSAIDs represents potentially a major health problem. Factors to consider are [1–5] (1) the socioeconomic impact, (2) pathophysiological aspects, (3) clinical management dilemmas, (4) the effect of NANSAIDs on the gastroduodenal mucosa of arthritic patients, and (5) the mucosal protective potential of misoprostol against injury by NANSAIDs. Concerning this last point, two studies [6,7] indicated that misoprostol might prevent gastric mucosal injury due to NANSAID use as assessed by endoscopy. They did not prove that misoprostol was effective in the prevention or treatment of NANSAID-induced symptoms: bleeding, ulceration, or perforation, nor could they be adduced as evidence supporting prostaglandin therapy for peptic ulcer disease. However, since misoprostol was known to increase mucous production and to have gastric anti-secretory properties through increasing the production of bicarbonate, the data clearly pointed to the need for controlled clinical trials of misoprostol in OA patients requiring NANSAIDs.

13.3 The Protocols

The clinical research program consisted of two identical protocols in OA patients requiring any of three NANSAIDs in the management of their OA symptoms. Patients were recruited primarily from the practices of rheumatologists.

After an endoscopy at baseline to document the absence of gastric ulceration, patients who qualified for the studies were randomized in balanced, double-blind fashion to a placebo group, a misoprostol 100 mcg q.i.d. group, or a misoprostol 200 mcg q.i.d. group. All patients were to return for follow-up endoscopy and other clinical evaluations after 4, 8, and 12 weeks of study medication administration. All endoscopies were performed by board-certified gastroenterologists.

13.3.1 Objectives

The primary objective of each trial was to demonstrate the effectiveness of misoprostol in the prevention of NANSAID-induced gastric ulcers in OA patients. That is, the primary objective of each trial is reflected by the alternative hypothesis H_a:

$$H_0: \mu_0 = \mu_{100} = \mu_{200}$$

$$H_a: \mu_0 \leq \mu_{100} \leq \mu_{200}$$

with strict inequality ($<$) holding for at least one $\leq$.

The secondary objective was to assess the effect of misoprostol on UGI symptom relief.

13.3.2 Inclusion Criteria

Inclusion criteria were the following: (1) legal age of consent or older; (2) males, or females of non-childbearing potential (postmenopausal or surgically sterilized), or practicing an acceptable method of birth control; (3) patients taking either ibuprofen, piroxicam, or naproxen as NANSAID therapy for osteoarthritis; (4) patients with abdominal pain; (5) patients who did not have gastric ulcers on endoscopy at baseline and required at least 3 months of NANSAID therapy for the arthritic condition; and (6) informed consent.

13.3.3 Efficacy Endpoints

The **primary efficacy data** was the development of gastric ulcers, as confirmed by endoscopy at weeks 4, 8, or 12. The **primary efficacy endpoint** was the proportion of patients with ulcers by 12 weeks.

Secondary efficacy data were the following: (1) UGI pain relief as derived from pain ratings recorded by the patient in a daily diary and (2) relief of other UGI symptoms. UGI pain was rated by the patient and recorded in a sponsor-provided diary at each follow-up visit according to the scales:

UGI Day Pain Rating Scale:

0 = None = I had no abdominal pain

1 = Mild = I had some abdominal pain but it did not interrupt my normal activities

2 = Moderate = I had some abdominal pain sufficient to interrupt my normal activities

3 = Severe = I had severe disabling abdominal pain

UGI Night Pain Rating Scale:

0 = None = I had no abdominal pain

1 = Mild = I had some abdominal pain but I was able to go back to sleep

2 = Moderate = I had abdominal pain sufficient to keep me awake for long periods

3 = Severe = I had severe abdominal pain that kept me awake most of the night

The **secondary efficacy endpoint** was the proportion of the patients without daytime or nighttime pain.

In addition, data reflecting OA symptoms were collected for the purpose of demonstrating that adding misoprostol to the NANSAID regimens did not compromise the OA effect of the NANSAIDS.

13.3.4 Sample Size Determination

Per protocol sample size determination revealed 450 evaluatable patients, 150 in each treatment group, would be needed to address the primary objective. The numbers were determined on the basis of a one-sided [8] Type I error rate of 5% and a 95% power to detect a 15% difference in ulcer development rates between a misoprostol treated group and the placebo group, given an expected ulcer development rate of 25% in the placebo group.

13.3.5 Statistical Methods

The Mantel–Haenszel [9] or Fisher's exact test (FET) was (to be) used for statistical analyses of the efficacy endpoints. No plans were provided in the protocol for any formal, statistical, or interim analyses of the efficacy endpoints. Accumulating safety data, however, was to be carefully and frequently monitored.

13.4 Monitoring and Data Management

Successful clinical development programs require good clinical trial management. At a minimum, this requires staying current with enrollment, dropout, and completion rates for each clinical trial. This allows taking corrective action early on, if such is needed. Beyond an interest in the progress of clinical trials, there is usually strong interest in knowing safety and efficacy outcomes prior to study completion. These interests are genuine and may represent a concern for patient safety, a need to plan future studies, or a desire to stop the study early to permit earlier filing of the registrational dossier.

All studies should be monitored for safety. Ideally, this should be done on a per patient basis without knowledge of the treatment to which the patient was assigned. Monitoring by treatment group can be done if it is important to make a clinical decision as to whether the study should be stopped for safety reasons. In this case, it is usually sufficient to separate the safety data into treatment groups without revealing group identity [10]. Since the design of a clinical trial of a new drug is almost always based upon efficacy considerations, it is unlikely that monitoring for safety while trial is ongoing will, in itself, compromise (efficacy) objectives. However, it is good practice to indicate in the protocol what procedures will be used to monitor safety.

Most studies of new drugs are designed to provide answers to questions of efficacy. Therefore, monitoring for efficacy while the study is in progress, particularly in an unplanned, ad hoc manner, will almost always be seen to compromise the answers. If it is anticipated that the efficacy data will be looked at prior to study determination, for whatever reason, an appropriate plan for doing so should be included in the protocol. The plan should address Type I error penalty considerations, what steps will be taken to eliminate or minimize bias, and permit early termination.

The early termination procedure of O'Brien and Fleming [11] is usually reasonable. It allows periodic interim analyses of the data while the study is in progress, while preserving most of nominal Type I error for the final analysis upon scheduled study completion, provided there was insufficient evidence to terminate the study after an interim analysis. The paper [12] by the PMA working group addressing the topic of interim analyses provides a good summary of the concerns about, and procedures for, interim analyses.

As previously indicated, we did not plan to perform interim analyses of the two misoprostol trials at the time we developed the protocols. The primary reason was due to the uncertainty associated with our estimate of the placebo ulcer development rate. Although we used 25%, the literature reflected wide variability, and no studies had followed OA patients on the three NANSAIDs required by the protocols for 3 months with monthly endoscopic examination for ulcer development.

We did however monitor the studies closely, and were proactive in computerizing the data. We knew on a weekly basis the status of the studies as to entry, completion, and ulcer development, without splitting the data into the three treatment groups. Table 13.1 summarizes such data at about the half-way point, during the conduct of the studies.

Ignoring study and treatment group and based upon patient information in the computerized database, we noticed that the incidence of ulcer development could range from a best-case crude rate of 8.4% to a worst-case rate of 27.4% (Table 13.2).

TABLE 13.1

Entry/Completion Status at Study Midpoint

Protocol	Patients Entered	Patients Completed
1	275	132
2	253	130
1 and 2	528	262

TABLE 13.2

Ulcer Status of Completed Patients
in Computerized Database

Patients	No Ulcer	Ulcer	Unknown	% Ulcer
215	156	18	41	8.4[a]
215	156	18	41	10.3[b]
215	156	18	41	27.4[c]

[a] Crude or best-case estimate (an underestimate).
[b] Reduced estimate.
[c] Worst-case estimate.

TABLE 13.3

Ulcer Status of Completed Patients
Not in Computerized Data Base

Patients	No Ulcer	Ulcer	Unknown	% Ulcer
43	34	5	4	11.6[a]
43	34	5	4	12.8[b]
43	34	5	4	20.9[c]

[a] Crude or best-case estimate (an underestimate).
[b] Reduced estimate.
[c] Worst-case estimate.

Parenthetically, rates among patients whose case report form data had not yet been computerized were generally comparable to those of patients in the computerized database (Table 13.3).

However, all the ulcers could have been in one of the treatment groups. If this were the case, the incidence within the group could have been three times as high, or anywhere from 25.2% to 82.2%. We therefore felt compelled, on ethical grounds, to meet with the U.S. Food and Drug Administration (FDA) to discuss plans for performing an interim analysis of the trials, with the possibility of stopping them early.

13.5 FDA Meeting

At the FDA meeting, we discussed the data, our procedures for stopping the trials, collecting any remaining data, and statistical analysis methods. Among the information presented is that contained in Tables 13.1 through 13.5.

Table 13.4 reflects data from 215 patients with 18 ulcers being split in a reasonably balanced way across three treatment groups, with numbers of ulcers per group reflecting a reasonable but perhaps conservative dose–response relationship. Table 13.5 reflects comparative analyses of the data in Table 13.4 using confidence intervals and FET—expected to be more conservative than the Mantel–Haenszel test.

It should be stressed that Table 13.4 represents a reasonable distribution of the total number (18) of ulcers under an assumption of dose proportionality. At the time of our meeting with the FDA, the blind had not been broken, nor had we separated the data according to blinded treatment group labels. Since we had not planned to do a formal interim analysis at the protocol development stage, we wanted to make the case that we should perform an interim analysis on ethical grounds, and if dose response was observed, that we may be able to stop the studies early based upon a demonstration of prophylaxis

TABLE 13.4

Ulcer Status of Completed Patients in Database: Possible Grouping Reflecting Dose Proportionality; % = Crude or Best Case

Group	Patients	No Ulcer	Ulcer	Unknown	% Ulcer
A	70	58	0	12	0[a]
B	71	53	6	12	8.5[b]
C	74	45	12	17	16.2[c]
All	215	156	18	41	8.4

[a] Reduced estimate = 0% and worst case = 17.1%.
[b] Reduced estimate = 10.2% and worst case = 25.4%.
[c] Reduced estimate = 21.1% and worst case = 39.2%.

TABLE 13.5

Ulcer Status of Completed Patients in Database: Possible Grouping Reflecting Dose Proportionality – *P*-Values and Confidence Intervals

Comparison	% Difference	Std. Er.	90% C.I.[d]	*P*-Value[e]
(B – A)[a]	8.5	0.033	(3.1 to 13.9)	0.015/0.028
(C – A)[a]	16.2	0.043	(9.2 to 23.2)	0.000/0.000
(B – A)[b]	10.2	0.039	(3.7 to 16.7)	0.014/0.027
(C – A)[b]	21.1	0.054	(12.2 to 30.0)	0.000/0.000
(B – A)[c]	8.3	0.069	(−2.9 to 19.6)	0.162/0.304
(C – A)[c]	13.8	0.064	(3.2 to 24.4)	0.003/0.005

[a] Best case.
[b] Reduced.
[c] Worst case.
[d] Normal approximation.
[e] FET: one-sided/two-sided.

efficacy. We wanted to be convincing that if an interim analysis were performed, it would be in a statistically valid, bona-fide manner.

There were three issues that received discussion at the FDA meeting: (1) When to terminate the trials? (2) To what extent should blinding be maintained during the interim analysis? and (3) At what Type I error level should the interim analysis be conducted?

Three possibilities regarding when to terminate were considered. We could terminate immediately, we could terminate based upon enrollment after 4 additional weeks, or we could continue entry until the interim analysis was completed and then decide on the basis of that analysis. The first two of these possibilities exact no penalty on the Type I error, provided we were prepared to live with the results. The third is consistent with the philosophy for performing interim analyses.

Blinding considerations included to what extent should investigators, patients, and company personnel be blinded as to the results of the interim analysis? The primary concern was to not compromise trial objectives should we fail to terminate the studies on the basis of the interim analysis results.

As to the size of the Type I error for the interim analysis, we could take the O'Brien Fleming approach using 0.005, and if there was insufficient evidence to stop, allow the studies to continue to completion, and conduct the final analysis at the 0.048 level. Another possibility was to use a two stage Pocock [13] procedure that would allocate a Type I error of 0.031 to each stage. Yet another possibility was to conduct the interim analysis at the 0.01 level with the final analysis being conducted at a level determined as per Lan and DeMets [14] if insufficient evidence existed for termination.

The FDA was receptive to us performing an interim analysis subject to us providing them with written plans. Such plans [15] were to address the three issues noted above, as well as any others that would reflect positively on the scientific and statistical validity of the exercise.

13.6 Concluding Remarks

Several facets of the misoprostol treatment and prevention of NANSAID-induced gastric ulceration program merit additional comment. First, the study population consisted of OA patients who required NANSAIDs in the management of their arthritic symptoms. Such patients were being treated for their arthritic condition by a rheumatologist. However, the condition being studied with respect to the effectiveness of misoprostol was gastric ulceration believed to be caused by NANSAID administration. Therefore, for the purpose of the clinical research program, the rheumatologist was not the primary investigator. The gastroenterologist was. At each center, a board-certified gastroenterologist was identified who assessed the degree of ulceration and presence of UGI symptoms.

Second, two identical protocols comprised the program, yet for the purpose of the interim analysis, they were treated as one multicenter protocol. Concerning this point, it is important to realize that since the protocols were identical, and patients were randomized to treatment groups within centers, in actuality, the two protocols were equivalent to just one multicenter study. In addition, the primary reason for performing the interim analysis was due to the ethical dilemma of whether to continue to enroll and treat patients in the studies when more than a quarter of the patients may be developing gastric ulcers—which may lead to perforation and bleeding upon continued administration of NANSAIDs, particularly in an elderly population. To have conducted interim analyses of each trial individually and failed to stop either or both of the trials, because of the lower power from the reduced sample size, would not have been tenable. Since the interim analyses was conducted at about the halfway point of both studies, treating the two trials as one gave us the same statistical power that we had for an individual trial at the time of protocol development. That is, 95% power to detect a 15% difference in ulcer development rates between a misoprostol treated group and the placebo group with a one-sided, Type I error rate of 5%.

Third, would effectively one multicenter trial be sufficient to warrant FDA approval? Concerning this point, the company had conducted several Phase III clinical trials on the use of misoprostol in treating patients with duodenal ulcers (DU); so there was already a large efficacy and safety database on the use of misoprostol in DU patients prior to initiating the clinical trial program in preventing NANSAID-induced ulcers. In fact, the company had submitted a new drug application (NDA) for misoprostol in the treatment of DU, which was recommended for approval by an FDA Gastrointestinal Advisory Committee. The FDA failed to approve the drug for that indication due to the fact that it had not been shown to be significantly superior to the already marketed H_2-receptor antagonists and a concern about the abortifacient capacity of misoprostol. The feeling was that if it could be demonstrated that misoprostol was effective for some indication, for which the H_2-receptor antagonists were not, this would warrant FDA approval. Since the H_2-receptor antagonists had not been shown to be effective in the prevention of NANSAID-induced gastric ulceration and the body of evidence suggested that misoprostol could be, the company decided to develop the drug for this indication.

Fourth, the interim analysis stopping rule was formulated in terms of the single pairwise comparison: misoprostol 200 mcg q.i.d. versus placebo. The other two pairwise comparisons were constructed for interest, but did not impact the statistical decision stopping rule. The reason for this was to try to economize with respect to the overall Type I error by avoiding a multiple comparison issue. The misoprostol 200 mcg dose was seen at the protocol development stage as the target dose. The misoprostol 100 mcg dose was included for dose response purposes. In addition, the dose comparison trial was making its way into the U.S. Federal Food and Drug Regulations in the mid-1980s through the IND/NDA Rewrite. If the misoprostol 200 mcg dose were statistically significantly more effective than placebo (at the 0.01 level), dose response would have been inferred via Williams' methodology [16,17].

Fifth, the interim analysis was based upon FET of the two-by-two table reflecting the misoprostol 200 mcg q.i.d. and placebo groups as rows and the numbers of patients with or without ulcers as columns. That is, the data were lumped across centers for the interim analyses stopping rule. Generally, since randomization was to treatment groups within centers, an analysis such as Mantel–Haenszel, which blocked on centers, would be seen to be more appropriate. The reason for not directly using the Mantel–Haenszel procedure at the interim analysis was that due to small, no, or equal numbers of patients with ulcers (consistent with a large number of investigational centers), the effective sample size was expected to be less than the actual sample size. After stopping the trial, the Mantel–Haenszel procedure was used to address the robustness of the conclusion by collapsing some centers into "pseudo-centers."

Lastly, the interim analysis performed was not included in the protocol. This is not to say that it was unplanned. It was rigorously planned and executed in such a manner as to safeguard blindedness, to preserve the Type I error, and to not compromise trial objectives. The bottom line is that through attentive monitoring, taking a proactive approach to clinical trial and data management, statistical analyses planning and report development, and working proactively with the U.S. FDA, a bona-fide interim analysis was conducted. This led to earlier termination of the clinical trials program, to earlier FDA submission of the NDA for regulatory review, and to earlier regulatory approval and marketing.

References

1. Langman MJS (1987): Nonsteroidal anti-inflammatory drugs: Socioeconomic impact of associated gastropathies. In: *Symposium: Clinical Developments on Misoprostol—Peptic Ulcer Disease and NSAID—Induced Gastropathy*, May 8, Digestive Disease Week, Chicago, IL.
2. Collins AJ (1987): Pathophysiologic aspects of NSAID-induced gastropathies. In: *Symposium: Clinical Developments on Misoprostol—Peptic Ulcer Disease and NSAID—Induced Gastropathy*, May 8, Digestive Disease Week, Chicago, IL.
3. Roth SH (1987): NSAID gastropathy: A rheumatologist's perspective. In: *Symposium: Cytoprotection, NSAIDs, and the Arthritic Patient*, May 29–30, Carlsbad, CA.
4. Lanza FL (1987): The effect of NSAIDs on the gastroduodenal mucosa of arthritic patients and normal volunteers. In: *Symposium: Cytoprotection, NSAIDs, and the Arthritic Patient*, May 29–30, Carlsbad, CA.
5. Cohen MM (1987): Mucosal protection by misoprostol against injury by nonsteroidal anti-inflammatory agents excluding aspirin. In: *Symposium: Clinical Developments on Misoprostol—Peptic Ulcer Disease and NSAID—Induced Gastropathy*, May 8, Digestive Disease Week, Chicago, IL.
6. Lanza FL (1986): A double-blind study of prophylactic effect of misoprostol on lesions of gastric and duodenal mucosa induced by oral administration of tolmetin in healthy subjects. *Digestive Disease Science*; **31**(Suppl): 131S–136S.
7. Aadland E, Fausa O, Vatn M (1986): Misoprostol protection against naproxen-induced gastric damage. In: *Symposium: Advances in Prostaglandins and Gastroenterology; World Congress of Gastroenterology*, September 8, Sao Paulo, Brazil.
8. Peace KE (1989): The alternative hypothesis: One-sided or two-sided? *Journal of Clinical Epidemiology*; **42**: 476.
9. Mantel N, Haenszel W (1959): Statistical aspects of the analysis of data from retrospective studies of disease. *Journal of National Cancer Institute*; **22**: 719–748.

10. Peace KE (1987): Design, monitoring and analysis issues relative to adverse events. *Drug Information Journal*; **21**(1): 21–28.
11. O'Brien P, Fleming T (1979): A multiple testing procedure for clinical trials. *Biometrics*; **35**: 549–556.
12. PMA Biostatistics and Medical Ad Hoc Committee on Interim Analysis (1993): Interim analysis in the pharmaceutical industry. *Controlled Clinical Trials*; **14**: 160–173.
13. Pocock S (1977): Group sequential methods in the design and analysis of clinical trials. *Biometrika*; **64**: 191–199.
14. Lan KKG, DeMets DL (1983): Discrete sequential boundaries for clinical trials. *Biometrika*; **70**: 659–670.
15. Peace KE (1992): *Biopharmaceutical Sequential Statistical Applications*, Marcel Dekker, Inc., New York, pp. 255–270, ISBN 0-8247-8628-9.
16. Williams DA (1971): A test for difference between treatment means when several dose levels are compared with a zero dose control. *Biometrics*; **27**: 103–117.
17. Williams DA (1972): The comparison of several dose levels with a zero dose control. *Biometrics*; **28**: 519–531.

14

Clinical Trials in the Treatment of Alzheimer's Disease Based upon Enrichment Designs

14.1 Introduction

Tacrine or Cognex© is the first drug approved for the treatment of Alzheimer's disease. It was first synthesized in the early 1940s and was discovered by the Australian physician, Dr. Adrian Albert, while trying to advance a new intravenous antiseptic for use by injured battlefield troops in World War II. With the successful production of penicillin by the British, Dr. Albert's efforts ended and little was heard of the drug for the next several decades.

Tacrine once again attracted interest when a physician, Dr. William K. Summers, published an article in *The New England Journal of Medicine* [1] reporting that his studies showed the compound produced marked improvement in cognition and dexterity among Alzheimer's patients. The FDA questioned Dr. Summers' research methods and his conclusions [2]. However, the findings were sufficient to warrant further clinical investigation by Parke-Davis/Warner-Lambert (later acquired by Pfizer) who in-licensed the patent for tacrine from Dr. Summers.

Finding a treatment that improves the quality of life for sufferers of a disease that is marked by progressive mental deterioration is a challenge without equal in pharmaceutical research and development. The disease robs its many elderly victims of their final years. While the disease runs its course—from the early signs of memory loss to the patient's eventual death—family members endure the crippling psychological, emotional, and financial stress of providing long-term care.

The first author was a consultant to Parke-Davis/Warner-Lambert (PD/WL) through his company, Biopharmaceutical Research Consultants, Inc. (BRCI), during the clinical development of tacrine. We provided independent linear model-based analyses [3,4] and nonlinear, mixed-effects models analyses of the primary efficacy endpoints [5–7] from the tacrine clinical trials conducted by PD/WL.

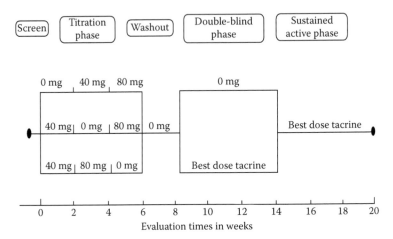

FIGURE 14.1
Enrichment design schema, Protocols 01 and 04.

This chapter reviews aspects of a subset of the clinical trials conducted on tacrine employing an "enrichment design," and analysis methodology conducted on the primary efficacy endpoints requested by the FDA. Analysis methodology presented are the following: Analysis of variance (ANOVA) methods [3,4] for data collected in the titration phase; ANOVA and analysis of covariance (ANCOVA) methods [4] for data collected in the double-blind phase; and methods [5–7] appropriate for data collected in all phases (see Figures 14.1 and 14.2) of the trials such as titration, double-blind, and sustained active, using a pharmacodynamic/pharmacokinetic nonlinear, mixed-effects model.

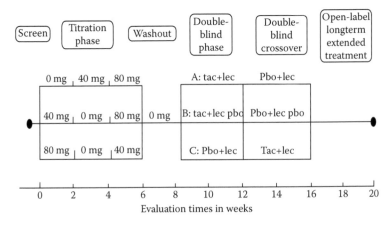

FIGURE 14.2
Enrichment design schema, trial 06.

14.2 Enrichment Design Clinical Trials

Three of the clinical trials: CI-970-01, -04, and -06, employed "enrichment designs" [4–7]. The trials consisted of five phases: a screening phase; a three sequence, three period, crossover titration phase; a washout phase; a double-blind parallel phase; and a sustained active phase, over a 20 week period.

The designs for Protocols 01 (conducted in North America) and 04 (conducted in France) were identical. Following the screening phase, patients who met entry criteria were randomized in double-blind fashion to three possible sequences of treatment with tacrine during the titration phase. Sequence I patients received 0 mg tacrine (placebo) daily for 2 weeks, then 40 mg tacrine daily for 2 weeks, and then 80 mg tacrine daily for 2 weeks. Sequence II patients received 40 mg tacrine daily for 2 weeks, then 0 mg tacrine (placebo) daily for 2 weeks, and then 80 mg tacrine daily for 2 weeks. Sequence III patients received 40 mg tacrine daily for 2 weeks, then 80 mg tacrine daily for 2 weeks, and then 0 mg tacrine (placebo) daily for 2 weeks. The doses reflect total daily dose. Patients were to be dosed every 6 h (q.i.d).

The titration phase reflects the "enrichment" portion of the design. Its purpose was to identify patients (an "enriched population") who responded to tacrine. In determining whether a patient was a responder, the Alzheimer's disease assessment scale (ADAS) total score to each dose of tacrine was compared to the score on placebo. The dose that produced the greater improvement (as compared to placebo) was considered the "best dose," provided that its ADAS score was at least four points smaller than that of placebo or was at least nine points smaller than at baseline. In the case of a tie, the dose having the better clinician's global impression of change (CGIC) was used. If still tied, the smaller dose was used as the best dose.

Following a 2-week washout from the titration phase, patients with a best dose of tacrine were then randomized in double-blind fashion to their best dose of tacrine or to placebo at the beginning of the double-blind, parallel phase and treated for 6 weeks. Thereafter, all patients entered the sustained active phase where they were treated with their best dose of tacrine for an additional 6 weeks (see design schema in Figure 14.1).

Protocol 06 also employed an enrichment design. This protocol differed from Protocols 01 and 04 in the titration phase, in the double-blind phase and in the sustained active phase. By the time Protocol 06 was conducted, there was no longer clinical concern about using 80 mg of tacrine prior to using 40 mg. Therefore sequence III in the titration phase of Protocol 06 was 80 mg tacrine, 0 mg tacrine (placebo), and 40 mg tacrine.

The double-blind phase of Protocol 06 consisted of two consecutive 4-week periods. In the first period, best dose tacrine patients were randomly assigned to three parallel groups: A = tacrine plus lecithin, B = tacrine plus lecithin placebo, or C = lecithin plus tacrine placebo. Patients in group A were crossed over to C in the second period; patients in group B took tacrine placebo plus lecithin placebo in the second period; and patients in group C were crossed over to A in the second period. Note that for blinding purposes both a tacrine placebo and a lecithin placebo are needed.

The sustained active phase (open-label, long-term, extended treatment) of Protocol 06 was 4 weeks in duration as compared to 6 weeks in Protocols 01 and 04. A design schema for Protocol 06 appears in Figure 14.2.

14.3 Objective

The objectives of the trials were to demonstrate that tacrine, at daily doses of 40 or 80 mg per day was effective in treating patients with probable Alzheimer's disease. Symbolically, the objective of each trial is the alternative hypothesis (H_a) of the construct:

$$H_0: D_0 = D_{40,80}$$
$$H_a: D_0 > D_{40,80}$$

where D_0 and $D_{40,80}$ symbolize the efficacy of 0 mg (placebo) and tacrine at 40 or 80 mg during the double-blind, parallel phase of Protocols 01 and 04, and during the double-blind, partial crossover phase of Protocol 06. There were no plans to statistically, inferentially analyze the data collected in the titration and sustained active phases.

As previously indicated, the purpose of the titration phase was to identify a responder population for participation in the subsequent double-blind, placebo-controlled phases. The primary purpose of the sustained active phase was to gather longer-term safety data and to describe longer-term efficacy data in an uncontrolled setting.

14.4 Primary Efficacy Endpoints

The **primary efficacy endpoints** were the cognitive component (**ADAS-C**) of the ADAS [8], measured every 2 weeks and the CGIC [9] measured every 2 weeks with the exception of screening and baseline. The ADAS-C assesses cognitive performance on 11 items: orientation, word recall, word recognition, word finding, naming, language, comprehension, following commands, instruction recall, and constructional and ideational praxis, with a total possible score ranging from 0 to 70 units. CGIC is a subjective rating of clinical change ranging from a score of 1 to a score of 7, with 7 denoting very much worse, 4 denoting no change, and 1 denoting very much improved. A score following treatment that is lower than the baseline score reflects improvement according to the ADAS-C or CGIC scale.

14.5 Sample Size Determination

The enrichment protocols were designed to have enough "best dose" patients in the double-blind parallel phase (Protocols 01, 04) and in the double-blind, partial crossover phase (Protocol 06) to provide an 80% power to detect a 20% difference between the tacrine and placebo groups with a Type I error rate of 5%. The numbers of patients in each protocol were

Protocol	Titration	Double-Blind
01	632	215
04	280	122
06	440	122

14.6 Statistical Methods

Inferential statistical analyses were conducted on the primary efficacy end-points: ADAS-C and CGIC from Protocols 01, 04, and 06. Analysis methodology consisted of fixed effects, linear model methods: (1) analysis of variance (ANOVA) methods [3,4] for data collected in the titration phase, (2) ANOVA and analysis of covariance (ANCOVA) methods [4] for data collected in the double-blind phase, and (3) pharmacodynamic/pharmacokinetic nonlinear, mixed effects model methods [5–7] appropriate for data collected in all phases of the trials such as titration, double-blind, and sustained active. Further, meta-analysis methods were used to combine titration phase results and double-blind phase results, separately, across the protocols.

14.6.1 Linear Model Analyses of Primary Efficacy Measures

Linear models, fixed effect methods were performed on the primary efficacy data collected in the titration phase and in the double-blind phase. These methods were Analysis of Variance (ANOVA) methods [3,4] for titration phase data and ANOVA and analysis of covariance (ANCOVA) methods [4] for double-blind phase data. Meta-analysis methods were used to combine titration phase results and double-blind phase results, separately, across the protocols.

14.6.1.1 Titration Phase

Details of the analysis methodology for analyzing primary efficacy data from the titration phase of Protocols 01 and 04 are presented. Similar methodology based on contrasts for estimating direct and carryover dose effects from the titration phase of Protocol 06 may be similarly developed.

TABLE 14.1

Three-by-Three Crossover Design

		Period	
Sequence	1	2	3
1	D_0	D_1	D_2
2	D_1	D_0	D_2
3	D_1	D_2	D_0

Note: $D_0 = 0$ mg, $D_1 = 40$ mg, $D_2 = 80$ mg.

14.6.1.1.1 ANOVA Model with Carryover Effects

The design for the titration phase of the tacrine enrichment Protocols 01 and 04 appears in Table 14.1 where $D_0 = 0$ mg tacrine (placebo), $D_1 = 40$ mg tacrine, and $D_2 = 80$ mg tacrine. It is noted that no patient received the high dose first. Patients were randomized in double-blind, balanced fashion to the three sequences of dose administration. Patients were dosed daily for 2 weeks within each dosing period. There was no washout between the periods.

The **model for this design with carryover effect** is [3]

$$Y_{ijk} = \mu + S_{ij} + P_k + D_l + C_l + \xi_{ijk} \tag{14.1}$$

where

Y_{ijk} is the response observed on the jth patient in the ith sequence during the kth period

μ is an effect common to all responses

S_{ij} is the effect of the jth patient in the ith sequence

P_k is the fixed effect of the kth period

D_l is the direct fixed effect of the lth dose

C_l is the residual or carryover fixed effect of the lth dose received in one period into the immediately succeeding period

ξ_{ijk} is the within-patient random measurement error inherent in observing Y_{ijk}; $i = 1, 2, 3$; $k = 1, 2, 3$; $l, l' = 0$ (0 mg),1 (40 mg), 2 (80 mg); and $j = 1, 2, \ldots, n$

For statistical inference purposes, the ξ_{ijk} are assumed to be independent and to follow a symmetric distribution with mean 0 and common variance σ_e^2. The S_{ij} may or may not be considered random, but if so, they are assumed to be independent (and independent of the ξ_{ijk}), and their distribution is also assumed to be symmetric with mean 0 and common variance σ_s^2.

To develop statistical tests for direct dose effects and carryover dose effects, appropriate within-patient contrasts are defined [3]. Here a contrast is defined as a linear combination of contrast constants and the raw data from a block of three patients, one per sequence, rather than as a linear

TABLE 14.2

Model (1) Contrast Constants for Direct and Carryover Effects

	Sequence/Period Combination								
Effect	11	12	13	21	22	23	31	32	33
$D_1 - D_0$	$-2/3$	$+1/3$	$+1/3$	$+2/3$	$-1/3$	$-1/3$	0	0	0
$D_2 - D_0$	0	0	0	$+1$	-1	0	-1	$+1$	0
$C_1 - C_0$	$-1/3$	$-1/3$	$+2/3$	$+1/3$	$+1/3$	$-2/3$	0	0	0
$C_2 - C_0$	0	0	0	$+2$	-1	-1	-2	$+1$	$+1$
Data	Y_{1j1}	Y_{1j2}	Y_{1j3}	Y_{2j1}	Y_{2j2}	Y_{2j3}	Y_{3j2}	Y_{3j2}	Y_{3j3}

combination of group means. This is mainly of interest for understanding and for a nonparametric analysis with Wilcoxon signed ranks statistics. The contrast constants and the data from the *j*th patient in each sequence are symbolized and displayed in Table 14.2.

The contrast constants in Table 14.2 are augmented by the symbolized data for ease in formulating the contrasts for estimating direct and carryover dose effects. The estimators of these effects are obtained by averaging the values of each contrast based on a block of three patients over the number of blocks.

Contrasts for estimating $P_2 - P_1 + C_0$ and $P_3 - P_1 + C_0$ may also be developed. Differencing these enables one to test the null hypothesis, H_0: $P_3 - P_2 = 0$, and under the assumption that the carryover effect of placebo or the 0 dose is nil, one can also test the null hypotheses, H_0: $P_2 - P_1 = 0$ and H_0: $P_3 - P_1 = 0$.

Contrasts for estimating the effects $D_2 - D_1$ and $C_2 - C_1$ may be obtained by subtracting row 1 from row 2 and row 3 and row 4, respectively, in Table 14.2. For a balanced design with *n* patients per sequence, the variances of the contrasts estimating the direct and carryover dose effects are given in Table 14.3.

It is noted that the contrast whose constants are given by $(-1/2, -1/2, -1/2, -1/2, -1/2, -1/2, 1, 1, 1)$ for estimating $C_2 - C_0$ on an among-patient basis has variance $\{27\sigma_s^2 + 9\sigma_e^2\}/2n$, where σ_s^2 is the between-patient and σ_e^2 is the within-patient variation. When σ_s^2 is very small, this contrast would be useful because it is more efficient (the relative efficiency may be as large as $12/4.5 = 2.67$) than the within-patient contrast.

TABLE 14.3

Model (1) Variances of Direct Dose and Carryover Effects

$D_1 - D_0$	$D_2 - D_0$	$D_2 - D_1$	$C_1 - C_0$	$C_2 - C_0$	$C_2 - C_1$
$4\sigma_e^2/3n$	$4\sigma_e^2/n$	$10\sigma_e^2/3n$	$4\sigma_e^2/3n$	$12\sigma_e^2/n$	$34\sigma_e^2/3n$

14.6.1.1.2 ANOVA Model without Carryover Effects

The **model without carryover effect** is [3]

$$Y_{ijk} = \mu + S_{ij} + P_k + D_l + \xi_{ijk} \tag{14.2}$$

For this model, contrast constants for the unweighted least squares, within-patient contrasts for estimating direct dose effects, $D_1 - D_0$, $D_2 - D_0$, and $D_2 - D_1$, and period effects, $P_2 - P_1$, $P_3 - P_1$, and $P_3 - P_2$ are given in Table 14.4. For a balanced design with n patients per sequence, the variances of the contrasts estimating the direct dose and period effects are given in Table 14.5.

It is noted that for the usual 3×3 Latin square with n patients per row, each of the contrasts for estimating pair-wise direct dose effects and pair-wise period effects has variance $2\sigma_e^2/3n$. Therefore, the crossover design specified in the enrichment phase of the protocols with explanatory model given in Model (2) has relative efficiency $(2/3)/(4/5) = 5/6$ for estimating the direct effect of either the low dose ($D_1 - D_0$) or the high dose ($D_2 - D_0$), and relative efficiency of only $(2/3)/(6/5) = 5/9$ for estimating the differential dose ($D_2 - D_1$) effect. Consequently, the enrichment design requires a 20% increase in sample size to maintain power against placebo and an 80% increase in sample size to maintain power for differential dose effects.

To analyze data from a clinical trial using the enrichment crossover design (titration phase), one could estimate σ_e^2 as the mean square error from PROC

TABLE 14.4

Model (2) Contrast Constants for Direct Dose and Period Effects

Effect	Sequence/Period Combination								
	11	12	13	21	22	23	31	32	33
$D_1 - D_0$	$-8/15$	$+7/15$	$+1/15$	$+4/15$	$-5/15$	$+1/15$	$+4/15$	$-2/15$	$-2/15$
$D_2 - D_0$	$-2/15$	$-2/15$	$+4/15$	$+1/15$	$-5/15$	$+4/15$	$+1/15$	$+7/15$	$-8/15$
$D_2 - D_1$	$+6/15$	$-9/15$	$+3/15$	$-3/15$	0	$+3/15$	$-3/15$	$+9/15$	$-6/15$
$P_2 - P_1$	$-7/15$	$+8/15$	$-1/15$	$-4/15$	$+5/15$	$-1/15$	$-4/15$	$+2/15$	$+2/15$
$P_3 - P_1$	$-9/15$	$+6/15$	$+3/15$	$-3/15$	0	$+3/15$	$-3/15$	$-6/15$	$+9/15$
$P_3 - P_2$	$-2/15$	$-2/15$	$-4/15$	$+1/15$	$-5/15$	$+4/15$	$+1/15$	$-8/15$	$+7/15$
Data	Y_{1j1}	Y_{1j2}	Y_{1j3}	Y_{2j1}	Y_{2j2}	Y_{2j3}	Y_{3j1}	Y_{3j2}	Y_{3j3}

TABLE 14.5

Model (2) Variances of Direct Dose and Period Effects

$D_1 - D_0$	$D_2 - D_0$	$D_2 - D_1$	$P_2 - P_1$	$P_3 - P_1$	$P_3 - P_2$
$4\sigma_e^2/5n$	$4\sigma_e^2/5n$	$6\sigma_e^2/5n$	$4\sigma_e^2/5n$	$6\sigma_e^2/5n$	$4\sigma_e^2/5n$

GLM of SAS specifying either Model (1) or (2). Then form *t*-statistics using the contrasts and their variances from Tables 14.2 and 14.4. Alternatively, one could apply the Wilcoxon signed rank test to the contrasts based on blocks of three patients.

14.6.1.2 Double-Blind Phase

Correlation analyses were performed to assess the association between ADAS-C and CGIC scores during the double-blind, parallel, placebo treatment phase and potential covariates: age, gender, height, weight, serum creatinine clearance at screening, and ADAS-C score at screening and at double-blind baseline (if collected). If a covariate had significant correlation ($P \leq 0.05$) with either ADAS-C or CGIC in at least one of the three trials, it was included in the common ANCOVA model used to analyze response data from each of the three trials.

Preliminary repeated measures, fixed effects ANCOVA were then performed to assess whether treatment effect was consistent over time. If the treatment-by-time interaction was significant ($P \leq 0.05$), separate ANCOVA were performed at each double-blind phase assessment time. If not significant, ANCOVA were performed using the average of the double-blind treatment scores as response. Least squares means (LSMEANS) from a common ANCOVA model for ADAS-C and CGIC were determined using PROC GLM of SAS.

The preliminary repeated measures ANCOVA model was

$$Y_{jklm} = \mu + C_j + \beta_{jk}X_{jkm} + \Psi_k + T_l + (\Psi * T)_{kl} + \xi_{jklm} \qquad (14.3)$$

where
  Y_{jklm} is the response (ADAS-C or CGIC) on the mth ($m = 1, 2, \ldots, n_{ijk}$) patient at the lth ($l = 1, 2, 3$: every 2 weeks) double-blind time of assessment in the kth ($k = 1, 2$) treatment group of the jth ($j = 1, 2, \ldots, n_i$) investigational center in each protocol (01, 04, 06)
  μ is an effect common to all responses
  C_j is the effect of the jth center in each protocol
  X_{jkm} is a covariate on the mth patient in the kth ($k = 1, 2$) treatment group of the jth ($j = 1, 2, \ldots, n_{kj}$) investigational center in each protocol (01, 04, 06)
  β_{jk} is the covariate parameter corresponding to X_{jkm}
  Ψ_k is the effect of the kth treatment
  $(\Psi * T)_{kl}$ is the interactive effect between the kth treatment group and the lth double-blind time of assessment
  ξ_{jklm} is the random measurement error corresponding to observing Y_{jklm}, where the ξ_{jklm} are assumed to be independent and follow a common symmetric distribution with mean 0 and variance σ_e^2

Following the investigation of the treatment-by-time interaction term of Model (3), the reduced common Model (4) was obtained:

$$Y_{jkm} = \mu + C_j + \beta_{jk} X_{jk} + \Psi_k + \xi_{jkm} \qquad (14.4)$$

where Y_{jkm} is either the average response across times of double-blind assessment (if nonsignificant treatment-by-time interaction) or the response at each double-blind assessment time of the mth patient in the kth ($k = 1$, 2) treatment group of the jth ($j = 1$, 2,..., n_{kj}) investigational center in each protocol (01, 04, 06). Least squares means from Model (4) were used for estimating treatment effects and providing statistical inference. A treatment-by-center interaction term was then added to the model to explore generalizability of treatment effects across centers (see Chapter 8).

Other models were run to explore generalizability of double-blind treatment effects. For example, sequences in the titration phase represented a natural blocking factor for analysis of double-blind phase response data. Thus an extended model that also included ***titration sequence*** and ***double-blind treatment***-by-***titration phase sequence*** was also run. In addition, to try to assess the contribution of each dose to the estimate of treatment effect (recall that both the tacrine group and the placebo group had patients whose best dose was 40 mg tacrine and patients whose best dose was 80 mg tacrine during the titration phase), double-blind data were post-stratified by best dose.

14.6.1.3 Meta-Analyses of Results across Trials

Following Dersimonian–Laird [10], a random effects model was used to facilitate meta-analyses of individual trial results across the protocols. Separate meta-analyses were performed for the titration phase and for the double-blind phase. The Model (5) is

$$d_i = \theta_i + \xi_i = \mu + \delta_i + \xi_i \qquad (14.5)$$

where
$\quad$ d_i is the observed (estimated) comparative treatment effect in the ith trial
$\quad$ θ_i is the true treatment effect for the ith trial
$\quad$ μ is the overall mean treatment effect for the population of treatments
$\quad$ δ_i is the deviation of ith trial's treatment effect from μ
$\quad$ ξ_i is the sampling error
$\quad$ $\mathrm{Var}(\xi_i) = S_i^2$ is the within-trial sampling variance corresponding to d_i

That is, the d_i are regarded as a random sample from a population with mean μ and variance Δ^2 [which includes both within-trial sampling variance, S_i^2, and the between-trial variation, $\mathrm{Var}(\delta_i)$].

The overall comparative treatment effect μ is estimated as

$$\hat{\mu} = \sum_i w_i d_i \tag{14.6}$$

where

$$w_i = \frac{s_i^{-2}}{\sum_i s_i^{-2}}$$

where s_i^{-2} is the reciprocal of the sample variance from the ith trial. It is noted that the variance of $\hat{\mu}$ is the weighted sum of the variances of the d_i (which incorporates within- and between-trial heterogeneity):

$$\text{Var}(\hat{\mu}) = \sum_i w_i^2 \text{Var}(d_i) = \sum_i w_i^2 \{s_i^2 + \text{Var}(\delta_i)\} \tag{14.7}$$

Several estimated effects (the d_i in Equations 14.5 and 14.6) from the titration phase and the double-blind phase of the individual trials were meta-analyzed to provide both point estimates of μ and corresponding large sample 95% confidence intervals. The **effects from the titration phase** were the following: (1) the effectiveness of each dose as compared to placebo $(D_1 - D_0$ and $D_2 - D_0)$ and the differential dose effect $(D_2 - D_1)$; (2) differential carryover effects $\{C_1 - C_0, C_2 - C_0,$ and $C_2 - C_1 -$ Model (1) only$\}$; and (3) differential period effects $\{P_2 - P_1, P_3 - P_1,$ and $P_3 - P_2 -$ Model (2) only$\}$.

The **effects from the double-blind phase** were the least squares means from the common ANCOVA Model (4) for the effectiveness of tacrine as compared to placebo and the effectiveness of each dose of tacrine as compared to placebo. Meta-analyses of these effects were performed at each double-blind assessment time (2, 4, and 6 weeks) as well as the average response across times of double-blind assessment. In addition, these effects stratified by titration sequence and best dose were also meta-analyzed.

It is noted that since the actual data were available on individual patients, meta-analyses could have been performed by using a model that incorporated protocol as an effect in Model (4). Equivalently, Model (4) could be expanded where the center effect accounted for all centers across the three trials (with center sums of squares partitioned into two components: between protocols and between centers within protocols).

14.6.2 Population Pharmacodynamic/Pharmacokinetic, Nonlinear Mixed Effects Model Analyses

Following the first FDA Advisory Committee hearing on the tacrine NDA [11], Dr. Carl Peck, Director of the Center for Drug Evaluation and Research, requested that a population, pharmacodynamic/pharmacokinetic (PD/PK) nonlinear, mixed effects model [5,6] be used to analyze the ADAS-C and CGIC data collected in all phases of the trials such as screening, titration, washout, double-blind, and sustained active. Data available for committee members to review derived primarily from the parallel, double-blind phase of Protocol 01. The consulting services of Biopharmaceutical Research Consultants, Inc (BRCI) were selected to comply with the request with the first author providing the biostatistical input and Professor Nick Holford of the University of Auckland and consultant to BRCI, providing the PD/PK modeling input.

Some of the unanswered questions raised at the first FDA Advisory Committee hearing [11] were based upon the desire to have greater assurance that the efficacy results observed in the double-blind phase of Protocol 01 were in fact due to the direct effect of tacrine rather than reflecting artifacts of the design (enriched population) employed. In addition, there was a desire to better understand how tacrine induced its effectiveness in both a pharmacodynamic and pharmacokinetic sense.

Protocol 01 was initially analyzed [5,6]. Then Protocols 04 and 06 were analyzed as they became available. Separate analyses were performed on data from each protocol and on data combined (01 and 04, then 01, 04, and 06) across protocols [4,7]. In addition, two later protocols, 26 and 61, were also analyzed [7]. These protocols utilized a parallel (non-enriched) design, at higher doses and are not a part of this chapter.

14.6.2.1 Objectives

The objectives of the PD/PK modeling and analysis effort were to

1. Develop a model to describe the clinical pharmacology of tacrine as a potential modifier of the progression of Alzheimer's disease
2. Fit the model to the data on all patients from screening to the end of their participation in each study to allow for more efficient use of the data

14.6.2.2 Requirements of the Model

The population PD/PK model was a nonlinear regression model that contained both fixed and random (mixed) effects. It incorporated sequences of active or placebo treatments and accounted for carryover effects of both placebo and tacrine. The time courses of placebo and tacrine response and the development of tolerance to placebo and tacrine were described. The model described disease progression without treatment, the placebo effect, and the effect of tacrine as a function of daily dose. Placebo and tacrine effects were modeled by effect site concentration components. Requirements of the model were to

- Describe the time course of the Alzheimer's disease state and account for the effect of different doses of tacrine and placebo
- Incorporate parameters that reflected a potential delay in the onset of response to tacrine and placebo and the waning of response to tacrine or placebo
- Determine the influence of secondary covariates such as age, gender, renal function, and tacrine concentrations on efficacy parameters contained in the model

The population PD/PK model represented a composite of the effect of placebo and tacrine treatment and several structural forms. These forms incorporated pharmacokinetic and pharmacodynamic features of the dosing regimens in the trials under the assumption that the effect of tacrine was mediated by its concentration in an effect site.

14.6.2.3 Model Parameters

The primary structural model parameters were the following:

1. Disease characteristics:
   Baseline disease status—S_0
   Disease progression rate—α
2. Pharmacodynamic (PD) characteristics:
   Tacrine potency—β_T
   Placebo potency—β_P
3. Pharmacokinetic (PK) characteristics:
   Tacrine equilibration half-time—$t_{1/2eq,T}$
   Placebo equilibration half-time—$t_{1/2eq,P}$
   Placebo elimination half-time—$t_{1/2el,P}$
   Placebo tolerance half-time—$t_{1/2tol,P}$

14.6.2.4 Model Formulation

The PD/PK model contained a disease progression component, a pharmacodynamic component and a treatment effect component. The *disease progression component* included a parameter (S_0) representing disease status at baseline and a parameter (α) reflecting the linear progression of Alzheimer's disease. The progression $\{S(t)\}$ of Alzheimer's disease was initially described by the model

$$S(t) = S_0 + \alpha \cdot t$$

where t denotes time.

The *pharmacodynamic component* accounted for the effect of tacrine and the effect of placebo, which could be a linear function

$$PD(C_e) = \beta \cdot C_e$$

or a nonlinear function

$$PD(C_e) = \frac{E_{max} \cdot C_e}{(EC_{50} + C_e)}$$

of the concentration in the effect site (C_e)

where
  β is the potency parameter
  E_{max} is the maximum possible effect
  EC_{50} is the concentration producing 50% of E_{max}

The tacrine *treatment effect component* could be explained in terms of an *effect in the progression rate* parameter, α:

$$S(t) = S_0 + \{PD(C_{eT}) + \alpha\} \cdot t = S_0 + (\beta \cdot C_{eT} + \alpha) \cdot t = S_0 + \beta \cdot C_{eT} \cdot t + \alpha \cdot t$$

or a *shift* in the disease progression curve

$$S(t) = S_0 + PD(C_{eT}) + \alpha \cdot t = S_0 + \beta \cdot C_{eT} + \alpha \cdot t$$

The pharmacodynamic model for the *combined treatment effects of tacrine and placebo* for the shift in disease progression model (Figure 14.3) is therefore

$$S(t) = S_0 + PD(C_{eT}) + PD(C_{eP}) + \alpha \cdot t = S_0 + \beta_P \cdot C_{eP} + \beta_T \cdot C_{eT} + \alpha \cdot t$$

where
  C_{eT} denote the concentration of tacrine
  C_{eP} denotes the "concentration" of placebo in the effect site

Tacrine concentrations in the effect site were modeled as

$$C_{eT}(t) = C_{ss,T}\{1 - \exp(-K_{eq,T} \cdot t)\}$$

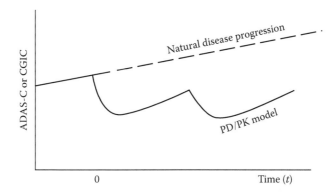

FIGURE 14.3
Schema for PD/PK offset model incorporating disease characteristics and placebo and tacrine effects.

where
$C_{ss,T}$ is the steady-state plasma concentration of tacrine
$K_{eq,T}$ is the equilibration rate constant of tacrine

Placebo "concentration" in the effect site was modeled as

$$C_{eP}(t) = \frac{C_{0,P} \cdot K_{eq,P}}{K_{eq,P} - K_{el,P}} \cdot \left\{ \exp\left(-K_{el,P} \cdot t\right) - \exp\left(-K_{eq,P} \cdot t\right) \right\}$$

where
$C_{0,P}$ is the instantaneous "concentration" of placebo
$K_{eq,P}$ and $K_{el,P}$ are related to the equilibration $t_{1/2eq,P}$ and elimination $t_{1/2el,P}$
half-times of placebo

In addition, other parameters were estimated to test special models [5]. These parameters were tacrine placebo factor (T_{PF}), tacrine tolerance factor half-time ($t_{1/2tol,T}$), tacrine tolerance factor potency ($TOL_{50,T}$), maximum tacrine effect ($E_{max,T}$) and tacrine potency ($EC_{50,T}$).

14.6.2.5 Computational Methods

Parameters in the PD/PK nonlinear mixed effects model were estimated using the NMTRAN/NONMEM [12] software package. The models were specified in NMTRAN (Version II, Level 1.1). Maximum likelihood parameter estimates along with estimates of their variability (the diagonal elements of the estimated variance–covariance matrix) derived from NONMEM (Version IV, Level 1.2). The convergence criterion was three significant digits.

Confidence intervals based upon the parameter estimates were determined by examining the log-likelihood profile. Estimates of the disease status at baseline (S_0), the disease progression rate (α), and tacrine potency (effectiveness), as well as 95% confidence intervals on tacrine potency (β_T) are summarized in Section 14.7.3. Holford and Peace [5–7] present estimation results for other parameters in the model and results from testing other models.

14.7 Results

14.7.1 Titration Phase Data

Descriptive and inferential statistical analyses [3,4] of ADAS-C from the titration phase of Protocol 01 are presented in this section. Analyses results of the titration phase data (ADAS-C and CGIC) from Protocols 04 and 06 are summarized in Section 14.7.1.2.

14.7.1.1 Detailed Titration Phase Results: Protocol 01

In Protocol 01, a total of 632 patients were randomized to the three sequences of dose titration administration. Twenty-four of these had no data past the screening phase. Of the remaining 608 patients, 206 were in sequence I, 203 were in sequence II, and 199 were in sequence III (Table 14.6). One hundred and four of the 608 did not complete all three periods. Thus 504 patients completed all three periods.

To apply the methods (of Sections 14.6.1.1.1 and 14.6.1.1.2), a subset of the data balanced across the three sequences has to be determined. A balanced data subset of 157 patients per sequence was chosen by using patient accession numbers, stopping at the largest subset for which sequences were balanced (Table 14.6). Thus, data on 33 patients who completed all three periods of the titration phase were excluded from the balanced data subset of 471 patients.

Sequences I, II, and III were completed by 185, 157, and 162 patients, respectively. It is to be noted that 28 completed patients from sequence I and five from sequence II could have been randomly excluded to form the balanced dataset of 157 patients per sequence.

Descriptive statistics of the change from baseline in ADAS-C appear in Table 14.6. The symbols N_a and $\overline{Y}_a$, N_c and $\overline{Y}_c$, and N_b and $\overline{Y}_b$ refer to the numbers of patients and means for all (a) patient (608), completed (c) patient (504), and balanced (b) patient (471) datasets, respectively.

14.7.1.1.1 Model with Carryover Effects

To obtain estimates of direct dose and carryover dose effects, one can apply the appropriate contrast constants of Table 14.2 to the cell means of Table 14.6

TABLE 14.6

Descriptive Statistics of ADAS-C, Protocol 01

Sequence	Statistic	Period		
		1	2	3
I		0 mg	40 mg	80 mg
	N_a	206	199	187
	N_c	185	185	185
	N_b	157	157	157
	$\overline{Y}_a$	−0.495	−0.759	−2.112
	$\overline{Y}_c$	−0.632	−0.870	−2.070
	$\overline{Y}_b$	−0.433	−0.701	−2.032
II		40 mg	0 mg	80 mg
	N_a	203	190	157
	N_c	157	157	157
	N_b	157	157	157
	$\overline{Y}_a$	−1.468	−1.337	−2.796
	$\overline{Y}_c$	−1.433	−1.350	−2.796
	$\overline{Y}_b$	−1.433	−1.350	−2.796
III		40 mg	80 mg	0 mg
	N_a	199	188	169
	N_c	162	162	162
	N_b	157	157	157
	$\overline{Y}_a$	−1.814	−2.681	−2.118
	$\overline{Y}_c$	−1.574	−2.562	−2.167
	$\overline{Y}_b$	−1.624	−2.586	−2.280

rather than averaging (over blocks) the contrast based on blocks of three patients. The estimates produced will be unbiased, regardless of whether sequences are balanced, provided that patients contribute data to all three periods. However, if unbalanced, the variances of the contrasts based on cell means are different. For example, from Table 14.3, the variance of the estimate of $(D_1 - D_0)$ would be $\{2\sigma_e^2/3\}\{1/n_1 + 1/n_2\}$ in the unbalanced case. Further for the Model (2) without carryover effects, the contrast would not have minimum variance.

So the analysis strategy for the titration phase data was to apply the methods developed to the balanced dataset, provide point estimates based on the full dataset, and apply model 2 to the full dataset using pair-wise dose effects contrasts. If the point estimates of effects based on the balanced dataset are close to those from the full dataset, one feels comfortable that the statistical inference from the balanced dataset generalizes to the population studied.

Since there was no washout between periods of dose administration in the titration phase, the Model (1) with carryover effects is reasonable to

TABLE 14.7

ADAS-C Direct Dose Effect Estimates, Std. Errors, and *P*-Values: Protocol 01, Model (1)

Completers		Balanced Dataset			
Effect	Estimate	Estimate	Std. Err.	*t*-Statistic	*P*-Value
$D_1 - D_0$	−0.132	−0.195	0.281	−0.695	0.4783
$D_2 - D_0$	−1.071	−1.045	0.487	−2.145	0.0322
$D_2 - D_1$	−0.939	−0.849	0.444	−1.911	0.0564

consider first. Estimates of the direct dose effects based on completed patients (c) and the largest subset of completed patients with balance (b) across sequences appear in Table 14.7. *P*-values for providing statistical inferences on the direct dose effects based on the contrasts from Table 14.2 and variances from Table 14.3, where σ_e^2 is estimated as the mean square error from Model (1) run on the balanced dataset, also appear in Table 14.7. It is noted that only the effectiveness of 80 mg tacrine as compared to placebo is statistically significant ($P = 0.0322$), and 80 mg tacrine compared to 40 mg tacrine is borderline statistically significant ($P = 0.0564$).

Estimates of the carryover effects, $(C_1 - C_0)$ and $(C_2 - C_0)$, based on the balanced dataset were −0.04031 ($P = 0.8859$) and 0.3376 ($P = 0.6890$), which are not statistically significant. It should be noted that although the estimators of direct dose effects and carryover dose effects are unbiased, they are not orthogonal. Pearson product-moment correlation coefficient estimates for $(D_1 - D_0)$ and $(C_1 - C_0)$, $(D_1 - D_0)$ and $(C_2 - C_0)$, $(D_2 - D_0)$ and $(C_1 - C_0)$, and $(D_2 - D_0)$ and $(C_2 - C_0)$, are 0.5313, 0.5549, −0.0558, and 0.8712, respectively.

14.7.1.1.2 Model without Carryover Effects

Since carryover effects from Model (1) were not statistically significant, Model (2) was utilized. These results are summarized in Table 14.8. *P*-values were based on the contrasts from Table 14.4 and variances from Table 14.5—with σ_e^2 estimated as the mean square error from Model (2) run on the balanced dataset.

TABLE 14.8

ADAS-C Direct Dose Effect Estimates, Std. Errors, and *P*-Values: Protocol 01, Model (2)

Completers		Balanced Dataset			
Effect	Estimate	Estimate	Std. Err.	*t*-Statistic	*P*-Value
$D_1 - D_0$	−0.115	−0.134	0.218	−0.617	0.5375
$D_2 - D_0$	−0.888	−0.881	0.218	−4.068	<0.0001
$D_2 - D_1$	−0.773	−0.747	0.266	−2.802	0.0052

TABLE 14.9

ADAS-C Direct Dose Effect Estimates, Std. Errors, and *P*-Values: Protocol 01, Model (2), All Patients

Effect	Estimate	Std. Err.	*t*-Statistic	*P*-Value
$D_1 - D_0$	−0.132	0.195	−0.683	0.4969
$D_2 - D_0$	−0.886	0.206	−4.287	0.0001
$D_2 - D_1$	−0.754	0.244	−3.091	0.0020

The comparison of 40 mg tacrine to placebo is not statistically significant based on analysis results from either Model (1) ($P = 0.4783$) or Model (2) ($P = 0.5375$). The comparison of 80 mg tacrine to placebo is statistically significant based on analysis results from Model (1) ($P = 0.0322$) and Model (2) ($P < 0.0001$). The comparison of 80 mg tacrine to 40 mg tacrine is statistically significant based on analysis results from Model (2) ($P = 0.0052$), but not from Model (1) ($P = 0.0564$).

Interestingly, the data exhibit a period effect, based on Model (2). The *P*-values for the period effects, $(P_2 - P_1)$ and $(P_3 - P_1)$ are 0.5401 and 0.0080, respectively. Since the contrasts for direct dose effects are unbiased estimators and not confounded with period effects, the existence of period effects does not contaminate inferences on direct dose effects.

As a check on the inference from the balanced dataset to all patients who entered the titration phase and who had data in at least one period, the direct dose effects based on these data were estimated using pair-wise contrasts from Model (2) using the CONTRAST option of GLM in SAS. The results appear in Table 14.9.

The results are consistent with those based upon the analyses of the balanced dataset. The maximum difference between any of the three datasets in terms of the direct dose effects ranges from −0.026 to +0.019 ADAS-C units (Table 14.10).

In addition, the results of the Model-based parametric analyses are consistent with those from a nonparametric approach using the Wilcoxon signed rank test (Table 14.11).

TABLE 14.10

Differences in ADAS-C Direct Dose Effect Estimates for the Three Datasets: All Patients, Completed Patients, and Balanced; Protocol 01, Model (2)

Effect	Estimate		
	All − Completers	Completers − Balanced	All − Balanced
$D_1 - D_0$	−0.017	+0.019	+0.002
$D_2 - D_0$	+0.002	−0.007	−0.005
$D_2 - D_1$	+0.019	−0.026	−0.007

TABLE 14.11

Comparison of Inferences from Models 1 and 2 Parametric Analyses with Those from the Nonparametric Wilcoxon Signed Rank Test; Protocol 01, ADAS-C

	P-Values			
	Parametric		Wilcoxon	
Effect	Model (1)	Model (2)	Model (1)	Model (2)
$D_1 - D_0$	0.478	0.538	0.455	0.397
$D_2 - D_0$	0.032	<0.0001	0.028	<0.0001
$D_2 - D_1$	0.056	0.005	0.089	0.006

14.7.1.2 Titration Phase Results Summary: Protocols 01, 04, and 06

Inferential analysis results of direct dose effects based on ANOVA (Model 1) of the ADAS-C (Table 14.12) and CGIC (Table 14.13) data from the titration phases of Protocols 01, 04, and 06 are summarized for all patients (full population) and for the subset of patients who had a best dose. Meta-analytic results across all three protocols also appear.

14.7.2 Double-Blind Parallel Phase Results Summary: Protocols 01, 04, and 06

Inferential analysis results based on the ANCOVA of the ADAS-C (Table 14.14) and CGIC (Table 14.15) data from the double-blind, parallel phases of Protocols 01, 04, and 06 are summarized by titration phase sequence

TABLE 14.12

ADAS-C Direct Dose Effect Estimates from Titration Phase of Protocols 01, 04, and 06, Model (1)

		Direct Dose Effects		
Population	Protocol	40 − 0 mg	80 − 0 mg	80 − 40 mg
Full	01	−0.195	−1.145[a]	−0.849[b]
	04	−0.708[b]	−1.288[b]	−0.579
	06	−0.355	−0.818[a]	−0.462
	MA	−0.354	−0.947[a]	−0.593[b]
Best dose	01	−2.731[a]	−4.774[a]	−2.043[a]
	04	−2.638[a]	−3.800[a]	−1.162
	06	−2.511[a]	−2.978[a]	−0.467
	MA	−2.663[a]	−3.834[a]	−1.171[b]

[a] $P \leq 0.05$.
[b] $0.05 < P < 0.10$.

TABLE 14.13

CGIC Direct Dose Effect Estimates from Titration Phase of Protocols 01, 04, and 06, Model (1)

Population	Protocol	Direct Dose Effects		
		40 − 0 mg	80 − 0 mg	80 − 40 mg
Full	01	0.032	−0.019	−0.051
	04	−0.067	−0.113	−0.046
	06	−0.087	−0.061	0.026
	MA	−0.027	−0.055	−0.028
Best dose	01	−0.074	−0.254[b]	−0.180
	04	−0.048	−0.286	−0.238
	06	−0.427[a]	−0.255[b]	0.172
	MA	−0.174	−0.259[a]	−0.085

[a] $P \leq 0.05$.
[b] $0.05 < P < 0.10$.

TABLE 14.14

ADAS-C Effectiveness Contrasts Estimates from Parallel, Double-Blind Phase of Protocols 01, 04, and 06, ANCOVA Model

Population	Protocol	Effectiveness Contrasts		
		Tacrine − 0 mg	40 − 0 mg	80 − 0 mg
Seq 1	01	−1.15	−0.91	−1.58
	04	−0.13	0.66	−0.25
	06	−4.48[a]	−3.31	−5.50[a]
	MA	−1.64	−1.03	−2.30
Seq 2	01	−4.64[a]	−0.70	−6.03[a]
	04	−3.88	0.96	−3.95
	06	−2.61[a]	−2.63[b]	−2.20
	MA	−3.37[a]	−2.00[b]	−3.76[a]
Seq 3	01	−3.11	0.47	−4.58[a]
	04	−1.13	1.20	−1.67
	06	−0.38	−0.95	4.01
	MA	−1.74	0.12	−1.64
Overall	01	−2.60[a]	−0.72	−4.19[a]
	04	−1.37	0.97	−2.32[a]
	06	−1.06	−1.02	−1.09
	MA	−1.86[a]	−0.54	−2.61[a]

[a] $P \leq 0.05$.
[b] $0.05 < P < 0.10$.

TABLE 14.15

CGIC Effectiveness Contrasts Estimates from Parallel, Double-Blind Phase
of Protocols 01, 04, and 06, ANCOVA Model

Population	Protocol	Effectiveness Contrasts		
		Tacrine − 0 mg	40 − 0 mg	80 − 0 mg
Seq 1	01	−0.03	−0.004	−0.09
	04	−0.64[a]	−0.47	−0.82[a]
	06	0.10	0.11	0.11
	MA	−0.13	−0.04	−0.19
Seq 2	01	−0.38[b]	−0.25	−0.43[b]
	04	−0.60	−0.77	−0.58
	06	−0.18	−0.13	−0.46
	MA	−0.35[a]	−0.26	−0.47[a]
Seq 3	01	0.15	0.26	−0.10
	04	−0.40	−0.34	−0.41
	06	−0.24	−0.06	−0.68
	MA	−0.02	0.12	0.20
Overall	01	−0.17[b]	−0.12	−0.21[b]
	04	−0.33[a]	−0.20	−0.40[a]
	06	−0.09	0.03	−0.20
	MA	−0.17[a]	−0.08	−0.24[a]

[a] $P \leq 0.05$.
[b] $0.05 < P < 0.10$.

and across sequences (overall). Meta-analytic (MA) results across all three
protocols also appear.

14.7.3 Data from All Phases, PD/PK Results Summary: Protocols 01, 04, and 06

Estimates of the disease status at baseline (S_0), the disease progression rate
(α), and tacrine potency (effectiveness), as well as 95% confidence intervals
on tacrine potency (β_T), based upon the nonlinear mixed effects modeling of
ADAS-C and CGIC data from the screening phase through the sustained
active phase of Protocols 01, 04, and 06 are summarized in Table 14.16.
   Data from only the titration phase were used in the ANOVA Model (1)
analyses. Data from only the parallel double-blind phase were used in the
ANCOVA Model analyses. All data from the screening phase, the titration
phase, the washout phase, the parallel double-blind phase, and the sustained
active phases were used in the PD/PK Model analyses. To tie the results from
these three separate methodological analyses together, estimates of the effectiveness of tacrine in terms of ADAS-C and CGIC appear in Table 14.17.

TABLE 14.16

Estimates of Baseline Disease Status, Disease Progression Rate, and Potency (β_T) of Tacrine: All Phases of Protocols 01, 04, and 06

	Protocols			Combined	
Parameter	01	04	06	01 + 04	01 + 04 + 06
ADAS-C					
S_0	28.6	31.3	27.3	28.7	28.5
α	4.34	9.38	0.09	6.17	4.49
β_T	-2.52^a	-5.37^a	-2.26^a	-2.99^a	-2.64^a
95% CI on β_T					
Lower	-3.85	<-8.00	-5.36	-4.44	-3.82
Upper	-1.55	-1.77	-1.04	-1.99	-1.81
CGIC					
S_0	4^b	4^b	4^b	4^b	4^b
α	0.342	0.207	0.058	0.402	0.265
β_T	-0.318^a	-0.413^a	-0.239^a	-0.387^a	-0.359^a
95% CI on β_T					
Lower	-0.60	-0.80	-1.38	-0.98	-1.07
Upper	-0.05	-0.10	-0.013	-0.17	-0.17

[a] $P < 0.05$.
[b] Baseline set at no change score (4).

TABLE 14.17

Summary of the Effectiveness of Tacrine: Titration, Double-Blind, and All Phases of Protocols 01, 04, and 06

	All Patients in Titration[a]	All (Best Dose) Patients in Double Blind[b]	All Patients in All Phases[c]
ADAS-C			
Estimate	-0.95	-2.61	-2.64
95% CI	$(-1.46; -0.43)$	$(-4.54; -0.68)$	$(-3.82; -1.81)$
CGIC			
Estimate	-0.06	-0.24	-0.36
95% CI	$(-0.16; +0.05)$	$(-0.39; -0.09)$	$(-1.07; -0.17)$

[a] ANOVA Model (1).
[b] ANCOVA Model.
[c] PD/PK Model.

14.8 Concluding Remarks

Design and statistical analysis features of three enrichment clinical trials in the development of tacrine in the treatment of patients with probable Alzheimer's disease are presented in this chapter. The trials consisted of five phases: a screening phase; a 3-sequence, crossover titration phase; a washout phase; a double-blind parallel phase; and a sustained active phase. The purpose of the titration phase was to identify a responder (enriched) subpopulation who would subsequently be randomized to treatment with tacrine or placebo in the parallel double-blind phase. No statistical analyses of data from the titration phase or from the sustained active phase were planned at the design stage. Inferences on the effectiveness of tacrine were to be based only on analyses of data from the parallel double-blind phase.

Statistical methods appropriate for analyses of the primary efficacy data from the titration phase only, from the parallel double-blind phase only, and from all phases were developed and applied. Primary efficacy data were the cognitive component of the ADAS-C and the CGIC. Statistical analysis methods for titration phase data were based on ANOVA models with and without carryover effects. Statistical analysis methods for parallel double-blind phase data were based on ANCOVA models. Statistical analysis methods for data from the screening phase through the sustained active phase utilized a pharmacodynamic/pharmacokinetic (PD/PK) nonlinear mixed effects model. Meta-analytic methods were used to combine tacrine effectiveness estimates from the titration phase and from the parallel double-blind phase across the three enrichment trials.

Analyses of ADAS-C and CGIC from the three trials provide evidence that tacrine is effective in treating patients with probable Alzheimer's disease, particularly in terms of improving cognition (as measured by ADAS-C). This is true based upon all patients who entered the titration phase (ANOVA model methods), the "enriched" patients who then entered the double-blind phase (ANCOVA model methods), and all patients from screening through the sustained active phase (PD/PK model methods).

During the titration phase, the tacrine effect was −0.95 ADAS-C units, with a 95% confidence interval (CI) ranging from −1.46 to −0.43. During the double-blind phase, the tacrine effect was −2.61 ADAS-C units, with a 95% CI ranging from −4.54 to −0.68. Over all phases, the tacrine effect was −2.64 ADAS-C units, with a 95% CI ranging from −3.82 to −1.81.

There was also statistical evidence to support the effectiveness of tacrine in terms of clinical improvement (as reflected by analyses of CGIC). During the double-blind phase, the tacrine effect was −0.24 CGIC units, with a 95% CI ranging from −0.39 to −0.09. Over all phases, the tacrine effect was −0.36 CGIC units, with a 95% CI ranging from −1.07 to −0.17.

Much criticism, unwarranted in the first author's opinion, has been leveled that the FDA is not thorough enough in the NDA review process. The tacrine

NDA serves as a counter example. The NDA submission came at a time when there was a lot of public pressure on the FDA to approve some experimental drugs for desperate patients suffering from incurable diseases such as Alzheimer's. The FDA sought the advice of the CNS Advisory Committee in March 1991 [11]. Even though there was some evidence that tacrine was effective at this time, without taking a formal vote, the committee agreed by consensus that tacrine should not be approved. Although recommendations of such advisory committees are not binding, the FDA rarely overrules such guidance.

The FDA CNS Advisory Committee met again in July 1991 [13], at which time the methodology and results of PD/PK nonlinear, mixed effects model were presented. Again, the committee recommended that tacrine not be approved. They did however urge the company to conduct more studies using higher doses over an extended treatment time, and recommended that the drug be made available to a larger number of patients. In December 1991, FDA granted a Treatment IND (Investigational New Drug) to Parke-Davis/Warner-Lambert that led to the enrollment of several thousand patients.

In March 1993 [14], 2 years after the committee's first rejection, they recommended approval of tacrine (Cognex®). The agency granted marketing rights for the drug the following September. Although the additional studies were costly and served to confirm the efficacy findings of the initial 01 trial, they contributed greatly to the safety information and conditions for use. Cognex was on the market 3 years before the next drug for the treatment of Alzheimer's disease was approved.

Much of the criticism about how the FDA does its job comes from those who have little or no understanding of the drug research and clinical development, and regulatory review and approval processes. Often the relationship between the FDA and pharmaceutical industry personnel is considered adversarial, due in part to the extremely high stakes involved. But a component is due to their roles and responsibilities being at opposite ends of the spectrum reflecting the strength of evidence to support claims contained in the regulatory dossier (NDA, SNDA, etc.).

The pharmaceutical company making the submission to the FDA obviously believes that the strength of evidence is sufficient for approval—else the submission would not be made, and is therefore a proponent of the drug. Becoming a proponent is achieved only after company personnel and expert consultants thoroughly review and analyze the safety and efficacy information collected in the clinical development program and conclude that the compound is efficacious and its potential benefits outweigh its potential risks. The FDA is charged with protecting the public's health in the sense of not allowing inefficacious or unsafe drugs to be marketed and therefore has to take an opposing view—operating during the review process as an opponent of approvability. Only if the submission passes the most comprehensive and stringent review does the FDA feel justified in approving the submission.

Regardless of the due diligence exhibited by the pharmaceutical company in conducting the clinical development program, gathering, reviewing, and analyzing the data generated on the safety and efficacy of a compound, and by the FDA in its review of the submission, recent history makes it clear that neither the FDA nor the U.S. pharmaceutical industry is entirely successful in attaining its goals. This is not unexpected, regardless of how well the pharmaceutical industry and the FDA meet their legal and ethical responsibilities.

First, no drug is approved on the basis of "zero" risk. Drugs are approved on the basis of the benefit in the patient population studied, substantially outweighing the risk in that population. It is impossible to prove definitively that a drug has no risk. The history of FDA regulation recognizes this. Whereas the 1962 Kefauver–Harris Amendment to the Pure Food, Drug and Cosmetics Act requires that efficacy claims be proven, there is no statutory requirement for proof of safety. Second, there are nonzero decision risks associated with claims of efficacy and safety and with the approval process. The FDA following its efficacy review will decide that the drug is efficacious or that it is not.

If the FDA concludes that the drug is not efficacious, then it will not be marketed. This is the correct decision if the drug is truly not efficacious. It is the incorrect decision if the drug is truly efficacious—and not being able to market the drug means a huge loss of research and development dollars to the pharmaceutical company. If the FDA concludes that the drug is efficacious, then it may be marketed if the FDA also concludes that the benefits of the drug outweigh its risks. This is the correct decision if the drug is in fact efficacious and its benefits outweigh its risks. It is the incorrect decision if the drug is truly not efficacious or if its benefits do not outweigh its risks.

Both the pharmaceutical industry and the FDA control the magnitude of this type of decision error, by requiring that it be no more than 5%, and in almost all cases that it be much less than 5%. It is a fact that the smaller the regulatory or consumer's risk, the larger the population studied prior to approval has to be. To require that it be closer to zero than it already is would lead to a situation where few if any companies could afford the investment dollars or time to bring new drugs to the market.

References

1. Summers WK, Majovski LV, Marsh GM, Tachiki K, Kling A (1986): Oral tetra-hydroaminoacridine in long-term treatment of senile dementia, Alzheimer type. *New England Journal of Medicine*; **315**(20): 1241–1245.
2. Small GW, Spar JE, Plotkin DA (1987): Oral tetrahydroaminoacridine in the treatment of senile dementia, Alzheimer's type [Letter]. *New England Journal of Medicine*; **316**(25): 1603–1605, June 18.

3. Peace KE, Koch GG (1993): Statistical methods for a three-period crossover design in which high dose cannot be used first. *Journal of Biopharmaceutical Statistics*; **3**(1): 103–116.

4. Peace KE (1993): Linear models analysis of primary efficacy data in the study of Tacrine in Alzheimer's disease. In: *Annual DIA Meeting on Statistical Issues in Clinical Development*, Hilton Head, SC, March.

5. Holford NHG, Peace KE (1992): Methodologic aspects of a population pharmacodynamic model for cognitive effects in Alzheimer's patients treated with Tacrine. *Proceedings of the National Academy of Science*; **89**(23): 11466–11470, December.

6. Holford NHG, Peace KE (1992): Results and validation of a population pharmacodynamic model for cognitive effects in Alzheimer's patients treated with Tacrine. *Proceedings of the National Academy of Science*; **89**(23): 11471–11475, December.

7. Holford NHG, Peace KE (1994): The effect of Tacrine and lecithin in Alzheimer's disease: A population pharmacodynamic analysis of five clinical trials. *European Journal of Clinical Pharmacology*; **47**(1): 17–23.

8. Rosen WG, Mohs RC, Davis KL (1984): A new rating scale for Alzheimer's disease. *American Journal of Psychiatry*; **141**(11): 1356–1364.

9. Schneider LS, Olin JT, Doody RS, Clark CM, Morris JC, Reisberg B, Schmitt FA, Grundman M, Thomas RG, Ferris SH (1997): Validity and reliability of the Alzheimer's cooperative study—Clinical global impression of change: The Alzheimer's disease cooperative study. *Alzheimer Disease and Associated Disorders*; **11**(Suppl 2): S22–S32.

10. Dersimonian R, Laird N (1986): Meta-analysis in clinical trials. *Controlled Clinical Trials*; 7: 177–188.

11. Department of Health and Human Services, Public Health Service, Food and Drug Administration (1991): *Peripheral and Central Nervous System Drugs Advisory Committee*, March 15, 1991, Transcript: Miller Reporting Company, Washington, DC.

12. Beal SL, Sheiner LB (1980): The NONMEM system. *Statistician*; **34**: 118–119.

13. Department of Health and Human Services, Public Health Service, Food and Drug Administration (1991): *Peripheral and Central Nervous System Drugs Advisory Committee*, July 15, 1991, Transcript: Miller Reporting Company, Washington, DC.

14. Department of Health and Human Services, Public Health Service, Food and Drug Administration (1993): *Peripheral and Central Nervous System Drugs Advisory Committee*, March 18, 1993, Transcript: Miller Reporting Company, Washington, DC.

15

A Clinical Trial to Establish Reduction of CHD Risk

15.1 Introduction

Gemfibrozil (Lopid®) was developed by Parke-Davis, the pharmaceutical research division of Warner-Lambert, and approved by the FDA in 1981 for the treatment of adults with high triglyceride levels—those who were considered at risk of developing pancreatitis (inflammation of the pancreas) and who do not respond to a strict diet. Based upon data collected in the Helsinki Heart Study Primary Prevention (HHSPP) trial, Lopid was the first drug approved for the broader indication of reducing the risk of coronary heart disease (CHD) while increasing high-density lipoproteins (HDL)-cholesterol (the "good" component of total cholesterol) and lowering low-density lipoproteins (LDL)-cholesterol (the "bad" component of total cholesterol).

The HHSPP trial was a landmark clinical trial in dyslipidemic, middle-aged Finnish males, who were otherwise healthy and without a history of myocardial infarction (MI) [1]. Subjects who satisfied eligibility criteria were randomized in a balanced fashion to either Gemfibrozil or Placebo and followed in double-blind manner for 5 years. Subjects who exhibited symptoms or signs of possible CHD were eligible to participate in an ancillary treatment protocol [2,3].

Following completion of the 5-year double-blind study phase, all subjects living at that time, including those who dropped out during the double-blind phase, were given the option of taking Gemfibrozil or no drug, and participate in open-label follow-up for up to 5 years [4,5]. This chapter presents an overview of the HHSPP trial and an analysis of data on major events occurring during the double-blind and open-label phases that attempts to adjust for differential exposure to study medication.

15.2 Objective

The objective of the HHSPP trial was to demonstrate that Gemfibrozil by reducing serum total cholesterol and LDL-cholesterol and increasing HDL-cholesterol would reduce the risk of CHD as compared to Placebo in asymptomatic, dyslipidemic, middle-aged men at high risk of developing CHD, and to evaluate the long-term safety of Gemfibrozil [6].

Data from the 5-year double-blind phase of the HHSPP was to be used to address the efficacy objective. Data from the double-blind phase and data from the open-label phase were to be used to address the long-term safety objective.

Symbolically, the efficacy objective is the alternative hypothesis (H_a) of the construct

$$H_0: \lambda_G = \lambda_P \quad \text{versus} \quad H_0: \lambda_G < \lambda_P,$$

where λ_G denotes the hazard (or risk) of developing CHD among Gemfibrozil-treated subjects and λ_P denotes the hazard (or risk) of developing CHD among Placebo-treated subjects, and where CHD is reflected by the numbers of cardiac endpoints among subjects in the double-blind phase of the HHSPP.

The long-term safety objective may be symbolized similarly where the hazards would reflect the risk of experiencing events related to safety during the double-blind and open-label phases of the HHSPP trial.

15.3 Designing and Planning the Investigation

The double-blind phase of the HHSPP trial was conducted from November 1980 through March 1987. Conduct of the HHSPP trial was overseen by the International Advisory Council (IAC). The IAC consisted of experts in cardiology, metabolic disease, clinical toxicology, epidemiologists, biostatisticians, and physicians from the participating institutions and Parke-Davis/Warner-Lambert pharmaceutical research division. IAC reviewed and approved the protocol and met twice yearly [6].

Subcommittees of IAC were formed for various activities. The Executive Committee managed day-to-day activities of the trial through its operational staff at the Helsinki Heart Council central office in Helsinki. The Ethics Committee, consisting of Finnish members of the IAC, was responsible for ethical and safety aspects and had decision-making authority as to whether the trial should be stopped [6].

Participants in the HHSPP trial were employed by the Finnish Postal and Rail Services and five private industrial companies. Participants were seen at

37 clinics and 77 subclinics that employed approximately 90 nurses under the direction of the central office in Helsinki [6–8].

15.3.1 Blinded Treatment Groups

Subjects who were randomized to the Gemfibrozil group received capsules containing 300 mg of Gemfibrozil. Subjects randomized to the Placebo group received matching 300 mg capsules containing 0 mg of Gemfibrozil. Subjects took two, 300 mg capsules twice daily (bid), for a total of four capsules and 1200 mg of double-blind study medication per day [8]. The double-blind treatment groups were

Gemfibrozil (G): 600 mg of Gemfibrozil bid
Placebo (P): 0 mg of Gemfibrozil bid

A cholesterol-lowering diet was also prescribed for all trial participants.

15.3.2 Sample Size Determination

For sample size determination, it is helpful to rewrite the null (H_0) and alternative (H_a) hypotheses of Section 15.2 as H_0: $\lambda_G/\lambda_P = 1$ versus H_a: $\lambda_G/\lambda_P = 1 - \delta$, where $\delta < 0$. The HHSPP trial was designed with a power of 90% to detect a reduction of 33% (δ) in the Gemfibrozil group as compared to the Placebo group in terms of cardiac endpoints over the 5-year double-blind phase assuming a two-sided Type I error rate of 5% [6]. The Placebo cardiovascular event rate was obtained from Finnish statistics and estimated to be 15/1000. A reduction of 33% reflected an expected cardiovascular event rate of 10/1000 in the Gemfibrozil group. Inflating the calculated sample size by an anticipated 20% dropout rate yielded a total sample size of approximately 4000; 2000 per treatment group.

15.3.3 Entry Requirements

To be eligible to enter the HHSPP, subjects had to be symptom-free dyslipidemic Finnish males, 40–55 years of age, without a history of MI or other major illnesses. Dyslipidemia was defined as non-HDL-cholesterol ≥ 200 mg per deciliter on two separate occasions 2–3 months apart prior to entry [1,6–8].

Subjects who satisfied the dyslipidemia criterion were then provided cholesterol-lowering dietary counseling. Those that were free of CHD and other major illnesses were accepted for study participation.

15.3.4 Primary Efficacy and Safety Endpoints

Primary efficacy endpoints were cardiovascular endpoints (CE) defined as any definite fatal or nonfatal (MI), sudden cardiac death, or unwitnessed cardiac death. Other major endpoints, related primarily to safety, were all-cause mortality (ACM) and diagnosis of cancer (CA). All-cause mortality was categorized as cardiac related (CR) or noncardiac related (NCR). Noncardiac related death was further classified according to cancer (CAD) or noncancer (NCRNCA). It is noted that ACM contains deaths that were cardiac related (a subset of CE).

15.4 Conducting the Investigation

The double-blind phase of the HHSPP trial was conducted from November 1980 through March 1987. Conduct of the HHSPP trial was overseen by the International Advisory Council (IAC). The IAC consisted of experts in cardiology, metabolic diseases, clinical toxicology, epidemiologists, biostatisticians, and physicians from the participating institutions and Parke-Davis/Warner-Lambert pharmaceutical research division. IAC reviewed and approved the protocol and met twice yearly [6].

Subcommittees of IAC were formed for various activities. The Executive Committee managed day-to-day activities of the trial through the operational staff of its Helsinki Heart Council central office in Helsinki. The Ethics Committee, consisting of Finnish members of the IAC, was responsible for ethical and safety aspects of the trial. An independent Ad Hoc Committee, consisting of four scientists not involved in the HHSPP trial, was formed as an independent decision-making group. The Ad Hoc Committee provided advice to the Ethics Committee as to whether the trial should be terminated early. The Ethics Committee had final decision-making authority as to whether the trial should be stopped [6].

Upon satisfying entry criteria and providing informed consent subjects were randomized in balanced fashion to either Gemfibrozil or Placebo at the baseline visit. They were provided a 3-month supply of 300 mg capsules and instructed to return to the clinic for follow-up per protocol assessments every 3 months thereafter [7]. Subjects returned any unused medication at each follow-up visit for compliance assessment [9]—at which time they were given another 3-month supply of study medication.

All clinics followed the common protocol and used identical data collection forms for data recording. All clinics were monitored frequently for strict adherence to protocol and consistency of data recording [6].

Following completion of the 5-year double-blind study phase, all subjects living at that time, including those who dropped out during the double-blind phase, were given the option of taking Gemfibrozil or no drug, and participate in open-label follow-up for up to 5 more years [4,5]. Subjects who chose to take Gemfibrozil were provided a 3-month supply of 300 mg capsules and instructed to take two capsules twice daily. All subjects who participated in the open-label (OL) follow-up phase, whether taking Gemfibrozil or not, were instructed to return to the clinic for follow-up assessments every 3 months [7].

15.5 Data Management

Data were collected and recorded at each clinic visit on case report forms (CRFs) designed for the trial. The CRFs were shipped to the clinical data management department at Parke-Davis in Ann Arbor, Michigan for entry into the computerized database. The data was doubly entered and verified. The database was quality assured per standard operating procedures prior to releasing to the biometrics department for statistical analyses [6]. Over one-half million CRF pages were entered [8].

The clinical study report for the HHSPP was developed by the medical writing department. The clinical data management department, the biometrics department, and the medical writing department were in the Division of Technical Operations in the Parke-Davis Pharmaceutical Research Division.

15.6 Statistical Analyses

15.6.1 Methods for Double-Blind Phase

The efficacy objective of the HHSPP trial reflects two components: (1) demonstrate that Gemfibrozil reduces CHD risk as compared to Placebo; and (2) demonstrate that Gemfibrozil lowers serum total cholesterol and LDL-cholesterol and raises HDL-cholesterol as compared to Placebo.

To address the first component, the Gemfibrozil group could be compared to the Placebo group in terms of CHD events using a number of time-to-event statistical methods, such as the Mantel–Haenszel [10] statistic or Gehan's modification [11] to the Wilcoxon statistic. Analysis of variance, analysis of covariance, regression, and correlation methods could be used to compare the Gemfibrozil and Placebo groups in terms of changes in serum total cholesterol, LDL-cholesterol, and HDL-cholesterol concentrations.

However, this strategy would address each component separately. The efficacy objective requires addressing the first component *while* simultaneously addressing the second component. Therefore the Cox proportional hazards model [12] was used to address the first component while simultaneously addressing the second component through the use of serum total cholesterol, LDL-cholesterol, and HDL-cholesterol concentrations as time-dependent covariates [13–16].

This analysis approach enables one to assess whether the reduction in risk (Gemfibrozil compared to Placebo) in terms of cardiac endpoints is correlated with changes in serum total cholesterol, LDL-cholesterol, and HDL-cholesterol concentrations. Negative estimates of the parameters associated with serum total cholesterol and LDL-cholesterol concentrations and a positive estimate of the parameter associated with HDL-cholesterol concentrations. Statistical significance of the parameter estimates and of risk reduction in CE may be construed as evidence confirming the efficacy objective.

An interim analysis was performed [6] after all subjects had completed 3 years of the double-blind phase. Two-thirds of subjects had completed 4 years at this time.

Statistical analyses were performed using programs written in SAS or BMDP. The programs were validated for accuracy by programmers and biostatisticians prior to data analyses.

15.6.2 Methods for Double-Blind and Open-Label Phases

Statistical methods and analysis results of major events in the double-blind and open-label phases have been reported elsewhere [4,5,17]. The statistical methods presented in this section were developed by the first author [3,17–20] when he was a consultant to the Pharmaceutical Research Division of Parke-Davis.

15.6.2.1 Classification Groups

There were two randomized treatment groups at the beginning and end of the double-blind treatment phase. Since subjects could elect to participate in the open-label phase by choosing Gemfibrozil (G) or no drug (N), there were four study groups at the beginning of the open-label phase: PN, PG, GN, GG, where

PN = those subjects on Placebo during double-blind and chose to take no drug during open-label

PG = those subjects on Placebo during double-blind and chose to take Gemfibrozil during open-label

GN = those subjects who were on Gemfibrozil during double-blind and chose to take no drug during open-label

GG = those subjects who were on Gemfibrozil during double-blind and chose to take Gemfibrozil during open-label respectively

15.6.2.2 Data on Major Events

Data from the double-blind phase and 3 years into the open-label phase, on the major events cardiac endpoints (CE), all-cause mortality (ACM), and cancer diagnosis (CA) were analyzed. All-cause mortality was categorized as cardiac related (CR) or noncardiac related (NCR). Noncardiac related death was further broken down according to cancer (CAD) versus noncardiac, noncancer (NCRNCA).

These data are summarized according to the four open-label groups in Tables 15.1 through 15.7. The data from the double-blind phase for these major events also appear in these tables.

15.6.2.2.1 Cardiac Endpoints

Table 15.1 shows that during the double-blind phase, 84/2035 (4.13%) Placebo subjects and 56/2046 (2.74%) Gemfibrozil subjects experienced cardiac endpoints. This means that Gemfibrozil-treated subjects experienced a 33.7% reduction {(2.74% − 4.13%)/4.13%} in the risk of cardiac endpoints.

Table 15.1 also shows that during the open-phase, 19/686 (2.77%) subjects randomized to Placebo but who took no drug in the open-label phase (PN); 28/1242 (2.25%) subjects randomized to Placebo but who took Gemfibrozil in the open-label phase (PG); 24/780 (3.08%) subjects randomized to Gemfibrozil but who took no drug in the open-label phase (GN); and 30/1181 (2.54%) subjects randomized to Gemfibrozil and who took Gemfibrozil (GG) in the open-label phase experienced cardiac endpoints.

Further, among subjects who took Placebo during the double-blind phase, those who took Gemfibrozil during the open-label phase experienced a reduction of 18.8 (81.2 − 100)% in cardiac endpoints during the open-label phase compared to those who took no drug during the open-label phase. Similarly, among subjects who took Gemfibrozil during the double-blind phase, those who took Gemfibrozil during the open-label phase experienced a reduction of 17.5 (82.5 − 100)% in cardiac endpoints during the open-label phase compared to those who took no drug during the open-label phase.

Finally, among subjects who switched (GN or PG) at the beginning of the open-label phase, those who switched off Gemfibrozil (GN) experienced

TABLE 15.1

HHSPP DB and OL 8-Year Follow-Up: Cardiac Endpoints

	Double blind (DB) phase			
Statistic	P		G	
E/N	84/2035		56/2046	
%	4.13		2.74	
Ratio		G/P		
%		66.3		
	Open label (OL) phase			
Statistic	PN	PG	GN	GG
E/N	19/686	28/1242	24/780	30/1181
%	2.77	2.25	3.08	2.54
Ratio	PG/PN		GG/GN	
%	81.2		82.5	
Difference	Switch		No switch	
G − P (%)	+0.83		−0.23	

a slight increase of 0.83 (3.08 − 2.25)% in cardiac events during the open-label phase as compared to those who switched onto Gemfibrozil (PG). In contrast, among subjects who did not switch (GG or PN; here PN is regarding as not switching) at the beginning of the open-label phase, those who continued to take Gemfibrozil (GG) experienced a slight decrease of 0.23 (2.54−2.77)% in cardiac events during the open-label phase as compared to those who continued to take no drug (PN).

15.6.2.2.2 All-Cause Mortality

Table 15.2 shows that during the double-blind phase, 43/2035 (2.11%) Placebo subjects and 44/2046 (2.15%) Gemfibrozil subjects died from all causes. This means that Gemfibrozil-treated subjects experienced a 1.9% increase {(2.15% − 2.11%)/2.11%} in the risk of death from all causes.

Table 15.2 also shows that during the open-phase, 20/709 (2.82%) subjects randomized to Placebo but who took no drug in the open-label phase (PN); 20/1283 (1.56%) subjects randomized to Placebo but who took Gemfibrozil in the open-label phase (PG); 27/795 (3.40%) subjects randomized to Gemfibrozil but who took no drug in the open-label phase (GN); and 30/1207 (2.49%) subjects randomized to Gemfibrozil and who took Gemfibrozil (GG) in the open-label phase died from all causes.

Further, among subjects who took Placebo during the double-blind phase, those who took Gemfibrozil during the open-label phase experienced a reduction of 44.7 (55.3 − 100)% in deaths during the open-label phase compared to those who took no drug during the open-label phase. Similarly, among subjects who took Gemfibrozil during the double-blind phase, those who took Gemfibrozil during the open-label phase experienced a reduction

TABLE 15.2

HHSPP DB and OL 8-Year Follow-Up: All-Cause Mortality

Statistic	Double blind (DB) phase			
	P		G	
E/N	43/2035		44/2046	
%	2.11		2.15	
Ratio		G/P		
%		101.9		
	Open label (OL) phase			
Statistic	PN	PG	GN	GG
E/N	20/709	20/1283	27/795	30/1207
%	2.82	1.56	3.4	2.49
Ratio		PG/PN		GG/GN
%		55.3		73.2
Difference		Switch		No switch
G − P (%)		+1.84		−0.33

of 26.8 (73.2 – 100)% in deaths during the open-label phase compared to those who took no drug during the open-label phase.

Finally, among subjects who switched (GN or PG) at the beginning of the open-label phase, those who switched off Gemfibrozil (GN) experienced an increase of 1.84 (3.40 – 1.56)% in deaths during the open-label phase as compared to those who switched onto Gemfibrozil (PG). In contrast, among subjects who did not switch (GG or PN) at the beginning of the open-label phase, those who continued to take Gemfibrozil (GG) experienced a decrease of 0.33 (2.49 – 2.82)% in deaths during the open-label phase as compared to those who continued to take no drug (PN).

It is noted that the denominators of mortality rates during the open-label phase are consistent across Tables 15.2 through 15.6 summarizing mortality. The denominators of cardiac endpoints during the open-label phase in Table 15.1 differ from their counterparts in the tables summarizing mortality. The reason for this is that subjects who experienced a cardiac event during the double-blind phase and who did not die were not at risk of a cardiac event during the open-label phase (consistent with the protocol entry/exclusion criteria at the beginning of the double-blind phase); but they were at risk of dying during the open-label phase. A similar explanation holds for the inconsistency of denominators in the open-phase for cancer diagnosis and their counterparts in the tables summarizing mortality.

15.6.2.2.3 Cardiac Deaths

Table 15.3 shows that during the double-blind phase, 19/2035 (0.93%) Placebo subjects and 14/2046 (0.68%) Gemfibrozil subjects experienced

TABLE 15.3

HHSPP DB and OL 8-Year Follow-Up: Cardiac Deaths

Statistic	Double blind (DB) phase			
	P		G	
E/N	19/2035		14/2046	
%	0.93		0.68	
Ratio		G/P		
%		73.1		
	Open label (OL) phase			
Statistic	PN	PG	GN	GG
E/N	7/709	12/1283	10/795	12/1207
%	0.99	0.94	1.26	0.99
Ratio	PG/PN		GG/GN	
%	94.7		79.0	
Difference	Switch		No switch	
G – P (%)	+0.32		+0.003	

cardiac deaths. This means that Gemfibrozil-treated subjects experienced a 26.7% decrease {(0.68% − 0.93%)/0.93%} in the risk of cardiac death.

Table 15.3 also shows that during the open-phase, 7/709 (0.99%) subjects randomized to Placebo but who took no drug in the open-label phase (PN); 12/1283 (0.94%) subjects randomized to Placebo but who took Gemfibrozil in the open-label phase (PG); 10/795 (1.26%) subjects randomized to Gemfibrozil but who took no drug in the open-label phase (GN); and 12/1207 (0.99%) subjects randomized to Gemfibrozil and who took Gemfibrozil (GG) in the open-label phase experienced cardiac deaths.

Further, among subjects who took Placebo during the double-blind phase, those who took Gemfibrozil during the open-label phase experienced a reduction of 5.3 (94.7 − 100)% in cardiac deaths during the open-label phase compared to those who took no drug during the open-label phase. Similarly, among subjects who took Gemfibrozil during the double-blind phase, those who took Gemfibrozil during the open-label phase experienced a reduction of 21 (79.0 − 100)% in cardiac deaths during the open-label phase compared to those who took no drug during the open-label phase.

Finally, among subjects who switched (GN or PG) at the beginning of the open-label phase, those who switched off Gemfibrozil (GN) experienced a slight increase of 0.32 (1.26 − 0.94)% in deaths during the open-label phase as compared to those who switched onto Gemfibrozil (PG). In contrast, among subjects who did not switch (GG or PN) at the beginning of the open-label phase, those who continued to take Gemfibrozil (GG) had the same rate of cardiac deaths (0.99% versus 0.99%) during the open-label phase as compared to those who continued to take no drug (PN).

15.6.2.2.4 Noncardiac Deaths

Table 15.4 shows that during the double-blind phase, 24/2035 (1.18%) Placebo subjects and 30/2046 (1.47%) Gemfibrozil subjects experienced noncardiac related death. This means that Gemfibrozil-treated subjects experienced a 24.6% increase {(1.47% − 1.18%)/1.18%} in the risk of noncardiac related death.

Table 15.4 also shows that during the open-phase, 13/709 (1.83%) subjects randomized to Placebo but who took no drug in the open-label phase (PN); 8/1283 (0.62%) subjects randomized to Placebo but who took Gemfibrozil in the open-label phase (PG); 17/795 (2.14%) subjects randomized to Gemfibrozil but who took no drug in the open-label phase (GN); and 18/1207 (1.49%) subjects randomized to Gemfibrozil and who took Gemfibrozil (GG) in the open-label phase experienced noncardiac related deaths.

Further, among subjects who took Placebo during the double-blind phase, those who took Gemfibrozil during the open-label phase experienced a reduction of 66.1 (33.9 − 100)% in noncardiac related deaths during the open-label phase compared to those who took no drug during the open-label phase. Similarly, among subjects who took Gemfibrozil during the double-blind phase, those who took Gemfibrozil during the open-label phase experienced a reduction of 30.4 (69.6 − 100)% in noncardiac related

TABLE 15.4

HHSPP DB and OL 8-Year Follow-Up: Noncardiac Deaths

	Double blind (DB) phase			
Statistic	P		G	
E/N	24/2035		30/2046	
%	1.18		1.47	
Ratio		G/P		
%		124.6		
	Open label (OL) phase			
Statistic	PN	PG	GN	GG
E/N	13/709	8/1283	17/795	18/1207
%	1.83	0.62	2.14	1.49
Ratio	PG/PN		GG/GN	
%	33.9		69.6	
Difference	Switch		No switch	
G − P (%)	+1.52		−0.34	

deaths during the open-label phase compared to those who took no drug during the open-label phase.

Finally, among subjects who switched (GN or PG) at the beginning of the open-label phase, those who switched off Gemfibrozil (GN) experienced an increase of 1.52 (2.14 − 0.62)% in noncardiac related deaths during the open-label phase as compared to those who switched onto Gemfibrozil (PG). In contrast, among subjects who did not switch (GG or PN) at the beginning of the open-label phase, those who continued to take Gemfibrozil (GG) experienced a decrease of 0.34 (1.49 − 1.83)% in cardiac related deaths during the open-label phase as compared to those who continued to take no drug (PN).

15.6.2.2.5 Noncardiac, Noncancer Deaths

Table 15.5 shows that during the double-blind phase, 13/2035 (0.64%) Placebo subjects and 20/2046 (0.98%) Gemfibrozil subjects experienced noncardiac, noncancer related death. This means that Gemfibrozil-treated subjects experienced a 53.1% increase {(0.98% − 0.64%)/0.64%} in the risk of noncardiac, noncancer related death.

Table 15.5 also shows that during the open-phase, 6/709 (0.85%) subjects randomized to Placebo but who took no drug in the open-label phase (PN); 7/1283 (0.55%) subjects randomized to Placebo but who took Gemfibrozil in the open-label phase (PG); 5/795 (0.63%) subjects randomized to Gemfibrozil but who took no drug in the open-label phase (GN); and 11/1207 (0.91%) subjects randomized to Gemfibrozil and who took Gemfibrozil (GG) in the open-label phase experienced noncardiac, noncancer related deaths.

Further, among subjects who took Placebo during the double-blind phase, those who took Gemfibrozil during the open-label phase experienced

TABLE 15.5

HHSPP DB and OL 8-Year Follow-Up: Noncardiac,
Noncancer Deaths

	Double blind (DB) phase			
Statistic	P		G	
E/N	13/2035		20/2046	
%	0.64		0.98	
Ratio		G/P		
%		153.1		
	Open label (OL) phase			
Statistic	PN	PG	GN	GG
E/N	6/709	7/1283	5/795	11/1207
%	0.85	0.55	0.63	0.91
Ratio		PG/PN	GG/GN	
%		64.5	144.9	
Difference	Switch		No switch	
G − P (%)	+0.08		+0.06	

a reduction of 35.5 (64.5 − 100)% in noncardiac, noncancer related deaths during the open-label phase compared to those who took no drug during the open-label phase. Similarly, among subjects who took Gemfibrozil during the double-blind phase, those who took Gemfibrozil during the open-label phase experienced an increase of 44.9 (144.9 − 100)% in noncardiac, noncancer related deaths during the open-label phase compared to those who took no drug during the open-label phase.

Finally, among subjects who switched (GN or PG) at the beginning of the open-label phase, those who switched off Gemfibrozil (GN) experienced a slight increase of 0.08 (0.63 − 0.55)% in noncardiac, noncancer related deaths during the open-label phase as compared to those who switched onto Gemfibrozil (PG). In contrast, among subjects who did not switch (GG or PN) at the beginning of the open-label phase, those who continued to take Gemfibrozil (GG) experienced a slight increase of 0.06 (0.91 − 0.85)% in noncardiac, noncancer related deaths during the open-label phase as compared to those who continued to take no drug (PN).

15.6.2.2.6 Cancer Deaths

Table 15.6 shows that during the double-blind phase, 11/2035 (0.54%) Placebo subjects and 10/2046 (0.49%) Gemfibrozil subjects died from cancer. This means that Gemfibrozil-treated subjects experienced a 9.3% decrease {(0.49% − 0.54%)/0.54%} in the risk of death from cancer.

Table 15.6 also shows that during the open-phase, 7/709 (0.99%) subjects randomized to Placebo but who took no drug in the open-label phase (PN); 1/1283 (0.08%) subjects randomized to Placebo but who took Gemfibrozil in the open-label phase (PG); 12/795 (1.51%) subjects randomized to

TABLE 15.6

HHSPP DB and OL 8-Year Follow-Up: Cancer Deaths

Statistic	Double blind (DB) phase			
	P		G	
E/N	11/2035		10/2046	
%	0.54		0.49	
Ratio		G/P		
%		90.7		
Statistic	Open label (OL) phase			
	PN	PG	GN	GG
E/N	7/709	1/1283	12/795	7/1207
%	0.99	0.08	1.51	0.58
Ratio		PG/PN		GG/GN
%		8.1		38.4
Difference		Switch		No switch
G − P (%)		+1.43		−0.41

Gemfibrozil but who took no drug in the open-label phase (GN); and 7/1207 (0.58%) subjects randomized to Gemfibrozil and who took Gemfibrozil (GG) in the open-label phase died from cancer.

Further, among subjects who took Placebo during the double-blind phase, those who took Gemfibrozil during the open-label phase experienced a reduction of 91.9 (8.1 − 100)% in cancer deaths during the open-label phase compared to those who took no drug during the open-label phase. Similarly, among subjects who took Gemfibrozil during the double-blind phase, those who took Gemfibrozil during the open-label phase experienced a reduction of 61.6 (38.4 − 100)% in cancer deaths during the open-label phase compared to those who took no drug during the open-label phase.

Finally, among subjects who switched (GN or PG) at the beginning of the open-label phase, those who switched off Gemfibrozil (GN) experienced an increase of 1.43 (1.51 − 0.08)% in cancer deaths during the open-label phase as compared to those who switched onto Gemfibrozil (PG). In contrast, among subjects who did not switch (GG or PN) at the beginning of the open-label phase, those who continued to take Gemfibrozil (GG) experienced a slight decrease of 0.41% (0.58% − 0.99%) in cancer deaths during the open-label phase as compared to those who continued to take no drug (PN).

15.6.2.2.7 Cancer Diagnosis

Table 15.7 shows that during the double-blind phase, 28/2035 (1.38%) Placebo subjects and 25/2046 (1.22%) Gemfibrozil subjects were diagnosed with cancer. This means that Gemfibrozil-treated subjects experienced an 11.6% decrease {(1.22% − 1.38%)/1.38%} in the risk of being diagnosed with cancer.

Table 15.7 also shows that during the open-phase, 10/693 (1.44%) subjects randomized to Placebo but who took no drug in the open-label phase (PN);

TABLE 15.7

HHSPP DB and OL 8-Year Follow-Up: Cancer Diagnosis

	Double blind (DB) phase			
Statistic	P		G	
E/N	28/2035		25/2046	
%	1.38		1.22	
Ratio		G/P		
%		88.4		
	Open label (OL) phase			
Statistic	PN	PG	GN	GG
E/N	10/693	13/1282	8/782	18/1207
%	1.44	1.01	1.02	1.49
Ratio	PG/PN		GG/GN	
%	70.1		146.1	
Difference	Switch		No switch	
G − P (%)	+0.01		+0.05	

13/1282 (1.01%) subjects randomized to Placebo but who took Gemfibrozil in the open-label phase (PG); 8/792 (1.02%) subjects randomized to Gemfibrozil but who took no drug in the open-label phase (GN); and 18/1207 (1.49%) subjects randomized to Gemfibrozil and who took Gemfibrozil (GG) in the open-label phase were diagnosed with cancer.

Further, among subjects who took Placebo during the double-blind phase, those who took Gemfibrozil during the open-label phase experienced a reduction of 29.9 (70.1 − 100)% in cancer diagnosis during the open-label phase compared to those who took no drug during the open-label phase. Similarly, among subjects who took Gemfibrozil during the double-blind phase, those who took Gemfibrozil during the open-label phase experienced an increase of 46.1 (146.1 − 100)% in cancer diagnosis during the open-label phase compared to those who took no drug during the open-label phase.

Finally, among subjects who switched (GN or PG) at the beginning of the open-label phase, those who switched off Gemfibrozil (GN) experienced a slight increase of 0.01 (1.02 − 1.01)% in cancer diagnosis during the open-label phase as compared to those who switched onto Gemfibrozil (PG). In contrast, among subjects who did not switch (GG or PN) at the beginning of the open-label phase, those who continued to take Gemfibrozil (GG) experienced a slight increase of 0.05% (1.49% − 1.44%) in cancer diagnosis during the open-label phase as compared to those who continued to take no drug (PN).

15.6.2.3 Inferential Statistical Methods

One analysis strategy is the so-called intention-to-treat (ITT). (Parenthetically, ITT is not an analysis; rather it defines the population of subjects who were randomized. But the literature is replete with the phrase "intent-to-treat analysis" which has been interpreted as "analyze what you randomize.") Such a strategy permits assessing the degree to which response is correlated with the random assignment to the original double-blind treatment groups. This strategy would not take into account differential exposure to study medication. A subject who was on study medication for only 1 day, and one who was on study medication for several years would both contribute the same information. In fact, since response information on the major events was obtained on all subjects in the HHSPP, including those who withdrew, the usual ITT strategy would treat all subjects as having full exposure (to the intervention to which they were originally randomized) over the entire length of follow-up, and also ignore the fact that many subjects switched off or onto Gemfibrozil at the beginning of the open-label phase.

More than 30% of the subjects who entered the study and were randomized to study medication voluntarily withdrew prior to the scheduled completion of the double-blind phase. In addition, many of these subjects were exposed to study medication for only a short period of time. Furthermore, 64% of the subjects originally randomized to the Placebo group elected to switch to Gemfibrozil, and 40% of the subjects originally randomized to Gemfibrozil, elected to switch off Gemfibrozil (take no drug) at the beginning of the open-label phase.

To account for differential exposure to study medication and the choice made at the beginning of open-label as to take or not take Gemfibrozil during open-label, one strategy would be to introduce a dose metameter or exposure index, which is monotonic in the length of time a subject is in the study and taking study medication, and then correlate major events with the exposure metameter. Penultimately, a regression analysis of major events on the exposure index could be performed for each treatment group separately. The treatment groups could then be compared in terms of the parameters of the regression models; e.g., in terms of slopes or intercepts. This strategy may be particularly illustrative in displaying relationships between major events and exposure within treatment groups.

The regression analysis of major events on exposure index within a Placebo group would address the extent to which major events are correlated with exposure to study and no drug treatment. The regression analysis of major events on the exposure index within a drug-treated group would address the extent to which major events are correlated with exposure to study plus treatment with the drug. Therefore, comparing these two groups in terms of regression, major events/exposure parameters could provide an inference as to the effect of drug adjusted for differential exposure to study medication.

The strategy [3,17] presented in this section is to directly compare treatment groups in terms of major events patterns adjusted for exposure using Cox's proportional hazard model with exposure as a time-dependent covariate. This permits an assessment to be made as to whether there is evidence of an association between the times-to-events distributions and explanatory or regression variables, including exposure as well as other covariables.

The regression variables were (1) the baseline measurements that were previously used [1,8] as fixed covariates in the analysis of major events in double-blind phase of the study: past and present smoking habits, age, systolic blood pressure, HDL, and LDL; (2) the original double-blind random treatment group assignment (T) as a fixed covariate; (3) switching status at the beginning of the open-label phase (S) as a time-dependent covariate; (4) the interaction between random group assignment and switching status (T * S); and (5) exposure (E) to study conditions. More specifically,

$T = +1$ if the subject was randomized to Gemfibrozil

    $= -1$ if the subject was randomized to Placebo

$S = 0$ as long as the subject was in double-blind

    $= +1$ if the subject did not switch at the beginning of open-label

    $= -1$ if the subject switched at the beginning of open-label

$S * T =$ the interaction between S and T

$E =$ time-dependent covariate representing the total time the subject participated in the study under study conditions

Running this model on the major event data using SAS or BMDP provides estimates of the log relative risk (Log RR) of the effect of each model covariate parameter and the associated standard error and *P*-value. The estimates of Log RR for the effect of each regression parameter are adjusted for the effects of the other regression parameters in the model. The objective of these analyses was to try to provide an inferential basis for drawing conclusions with respect to the original randomized treatment groups (G versus P) by accounting for differential exposure to trial medication. Of particular interest is the comparative inference between the original randomized groups (G versus P) adjusted for the other covariates in the model.

The estimate of relative risk (RR) may be obtained by exponentiating the estimate of Log RR. The estimate of RR from exposure may be obtained by multiplying the estimate of Log RR by mean exposure time prior to exponentiating. Confidence intervals (CIs) may be obtained by exponentiating the limits of the 95% CIs constructed on Log RR.

15.7 Results

15.7.1 Double-Blind Phase

Results from the HHSPP trial [1,8] established that increases in HDL and decreases in LDL—particularly increases in HDL, attributed to Gemfibrozil over the 5-year double-blind study phase—were significantly correlated with a reduction of 33.7% in the risk of CHD.

Further, an increase of 8% in HDL and a decrease of 7% in LDL were predicted to lead to reductions of 23% and 15%, respectively, in CHD, when taken individually. When the changes in HDL and LDL were considered simultaneously, the estimated CHD risk reduction of 28% − 5% greater than from the increase in HDL cholesterol alone, and 13% greater than from the decrease in LDL-cholesterol alone [8].

15.7.2 Double-Blind and Open-Label Phases

The results of analyses for each major event appear in Tables 15.8 through 15.14. A negative parameter estimate indicates descriptively that subjects originally randomized to the Gemfibrozil group are at less risk of experiencing a major event than subjects originally randomized to the Placebo group. It should be kept in mind that the estimates of these risks are adjusted for the switching experience, the interaction between double-blind randomized group assignment and the switching experience, and differential exposure to study conditions.

15.7.2.1 Cardiac Endpoints

Estimates for each model parameter adjusted for baseline covariates and other effects in the model for cardiac endpoints appear in Table 15.8.

TABLE 15.8

HHS DB and OL 8-Year Follow-Up: RR Estimates for Cardiac Endpoints

Parameter	Log RR	RR	Std. Err	P-Value	95% CI
Randomized groups	−0.14	0.87	0.07	0.03	(0.77, 0.99)
Switching effect	0.06	1.07	0.10	0.52	(0.88, 1.29)
Group-by-switching					
Interaction effect	0.28	1.33	0.11	0.009	(1.07, 1.64)
Exposure	−0.001	0.99	0.0001	<0.0001	(0.98, 0.99)

TABLE 15.9

HHS DB and OL 8-Year Follow-Up: RR Estimates for All-Cause Mortality

Parameter	Log RR	RR	Std. Err	P-Value	95% CI
Randomized groups	0.03	1.03	0.07	0.72	(0.89, 1.19)
Switching effect	0.08	1.09	0.10	0.42	(0.89, 1.33)
Group-by-switching					
Interaction effect	0.71	2.03	0.11	<0.0001	(1.63, 2.52)
Exposure	−0.002	0.99	0.0001	<0.0001	(0.998, 0.99)

TABLE 15.10

HHS DB and OL 8-Year Follow-Up: RR Estimates for Cardiac Related Deaths

Parameter	Log RR	RR	Std. Err	P-Value	95% CI
Randomized groups	−0.11	0.90	0.12	0.37	(0.71, 1.14)
Switching effect	0.04	1.04	0.17	0.83	(0.74, 1.46)
Group-by-switching					
Interaction effect	0. 91	2.49	0.19	<0.0001	(1.73, 3.59)
Exposure	−0.002	0.99	0.0001	<0.0001	(0.998, 0.99)

TABLE 15.11

HHS DB and OL 8-Year Follow-Up: RR Estimates for Noncardiac Deaths

Parameter	Log RR	RR	Std. Err	P-Value	95% CI
Randomized groups	0.12	1.13	0.10	0.21	(0.93, 1.37)
Switching effect	0.13	1.14	0.13	0.33	(0.88, 1.46)
Group-by-switching					
Interaction effect	0.58	1.79	0.14	<0.0001	(1.35, 2.36)
Exposure	−0.002	0.99	0.0001	<0.0001	(0.998, 0.99)

15.7.2.2 All-Cause Mortality

Estimates for each model parameter adjusted for baseline covariates and other effects in the model for all-cause mortality appear in Table 15.9.

15.7.2.3 Cardiac Deaths

Estimates for each model parameter adjusted for baseline covariates and other effects in the model for cardiac deaths appear in Table 15.10.

TABLE 15.12

HHS DB and OL 8-Year Follow-Up: RR Estimates for Noncardiac, Noncancer Deaths

Parameter	Log RR	RR	Std. Err	P-Value	95% CI
Randomized groups	0.06	1.06	0.13	0.67	(0.82, 1.37)
Switching effect	0.13	1.14	0.18	0.48	(0.80, 1.62)
Group-by-switching					
Interaction effect	0.91	2.49	0.19	<0.0001	(1.71, 3.65)
Exposure	−0.002	0.99	0.0002	<0.0001	(0.998, 0.99)

TABLE 15.13

HHS DB and OL 8-Year Follow-Up: RR Estimates for Cancer Deaths

Parameter	Log RR	RR	Std. Err	P-Value	95% CI
Randomized groups	0.22	1.24	0.16	0.17	(0.91, 1.69)
Switching effect	0.14	1.16	0.20	0.47	(0.78, 1.70)
Group-by-switching					
Interaction effect	0.17	1.18	0.22	0.45	(0.77, 1.83)
Exposure	−0.002	0.99	0.0002	<0.0001	(0.998, 0.99)

15.7.2.4 Noncardiac Deaths

Estimates for each model parameter adjusted for baseline covariates and other effects in the model for noncardiac deaths appear in Table 15.11.

15.7.2.5 Noncardiac, Noncancer Deaths

Estimates for each model parameter adjusted for baseline covariates and other effects in the model for noncardiac, noncancer deaths appear in Table 15.12.

15.7.2.6 Cancer Deaths

Estimates for each model parameter adjusted for baseline covariates and other effects in the model for cancer deaths appear in Table 15.13.

15.7.2.7 Cancer Diagnosis

Estimates for each model parameter adjusted for baseline covariates and other effects in the model for cancer diagnosis appear in Table 15.14.

Table 15.15 provides a more concise summary of the results with respect to inference on differences between the originally randomized treatment groups. A negative parameter estimate indicates descriptively that subjects

TABLE 15.14

HHS DB and OL 8-Year Follow-Up: RR Estimates for Cancer Diagnosis

Parameter	Log RR	RR	Std. Err	P-Value	95% CI
Randomized groups	−0.05	0.96	0.10	0.66	(0.86, 1.06)
Switching effect	0.20	1.22	0.14	0.17	(1.06, 1.41)
Group-by-switching					
Interaction effect	0.16	1.68	0.16	0.0009	(1.00, 1.37)
Exposure	−0.001	0.99	0.0001	<0.0001	(0.998, 0.99)

TABLE 15.15

HHS DB and OL 8-Year Follow-Up: RR Estimates for Randomized Group
Effect for Major Events

Event	Log RR@	RR	Std. Err	P-Value	95% CI
CE	−0.14	0.87	0.07	0.03	(0.77, 0.99)
ACM	+0.03	1.03	0.07	0.72	(0.89, 1.19)
CR	−0.11	0.90	0.12	0.37	(0.71, 1.14)
NCR	+0.12	1.13	0.10	0.21	(0.93, 1.37)
CAD	+0.22	1.24	0.16	0.17	(0.91, 1.69)
NCRNCA	+0.06	1.06	0.13	0.67	(0.82, 1.37)
CA	−0.04	0.96	0.10	0.66	(0.86, 1.06)

originally randomized to the Gemfibrozil group are at less risk of experiencing a major event than subjects originally randomized to the Placebo group.
It should be kept in mind that the estimates of these risks are adjusted for the
switching experience, the interaction between double-blind randomized
group assignment and the switching experience, and differential exposure
to study conditions.

Among the seven major events, only the estimate of RR of cardiac endpoints is statistically significant—corresponding to a RR reduction of 13%
(87% − 100%; Tables 15.8 and 15.15) for subjects originally randomized to
the Gemfibrozil group as compared to subjects originally randomized to the
Placebo group. The P-values and CIs for the RR of the other six major events
are consistent with chance findings.

15.8 Summary

In many clinical trials, subjects are treated with a fixed daily dose of study
medication for a fixed length of time. The length of time on treatment should
be at least as long as needed to observe a beneficial response to treatment, if
the treatment provides benefit. For some drugs, the benefits are expected to
accrue only from long-term treatment. The primary objectives of Phase III
clinical trials of a drug not yet regulatory approved for a specific indication,
whether for the treatment or prevention of disease, should be "Is the drug
efficacious and safe?" [21] and "How are efficacy and safety of the
drug related to its use?"

Time-to-event data on the major events cardiac endpoints (CE), all-cause
mortality (ACM), and cancer diagnosis (CA), from the double-blind phase
and the 3-year open-label extension of the HHSPP trial were analyzed.
Statistical analyses utilized Cox's proportional hazards model to regress

time to major events on explanatory variables taken at the time of randomization and occurring during study. The explanatory variables were (1) baseline measurements—past and present smoking habits, age, systolic blood pressure, HDL, and LDL; (2) the original double-blind random treatment group assignment; (3) switching status at the beginning of the open-label phase as a time-dependent covariate; (4) the interaction between random group assignment and switching status; and (5) exposure to study conditions as a time-dependent covariate. For a given subject, exposure to study conditions may be thought of as the total time a subject was participating in the study, in double-blind and in open-label, and returning for regular follow-up visits uninterruptedly.

Since due to withdrawal, subjects were exposed to medication and study conditions for different lengths of time, and many subjects originally randomized to Placebo elected to switch to Gemfibrozil and vice versa at the beginning of the open-label phase, it is felt that analyses adjusting for these effects are more appropriate than the usual intent-to-treat analyses that ignore the length of time or the amount of study medication taken by subjects.

The statistical significance of the model parameters from these analyses are summarized in Table 15.16 (S means $P \leq 0.05$; NS means $P > 0.05$).

Although small, exposure effect is significant for all seven major events. From Tables 15.8 through 15.14, it is noted that the estimate of Log RR for the exposure parameter is negative for all major events. An interpretation of this estimate is that risk of experiencing such events decreases as a function of exposure. This interpretation is illustrated in Table 15.17 by the general decrease in the percentages of subjects experiencing major events across quartiles (Q1 = 0–2157 days, Q2 = 2157–2778 days, Q3 = 2778–3219 days, Q4 ≥ 3219 days) of exposure (Exp) time in study.

Further, although the effect of switching is not statistically significant (Table 15.16) for any major event, the interaction between the original randomized groups and switching status is statistically significant for all major events except cancer deaths. An interpretation of this result is that the difference between the group originally randomized to Gemfibrozil and the group originally randomized to Placebo is not the same for subjects who switched versus those who did not switch.

TABLE 15.16

Summary of Statistical Significance of Main Model Parameters

Effect	CE	ACM	CR	NCR	NCRNCA	CAD	CA
DB treatment (T)	S	NS	NS	NS	NS	NS	NS
Switching (S)	NS	NS	NS	NS	NS	NS	NS
Interaction (T * S)	S	S	S	S	S	NS	S
Exposure	S	S	S	S	S	S	S

TABLE 15.17

Quartile Distribution for Major Events (%) by Randomized DB Group

Group	Exp	CE	ACM	CR	NCR	NCRNCA	CAD	CA
P	Q1	14.4	14.4	6.6	7.8	4.3	3.5	5.8
	Q2	6.1	2.2	1.0	1.2	0.8	0.4	2.0
	Q3	3.9	0.4	0.2	0.2	0.2	0.0	2.0
	Q4	1.9	0.0	0.0	0.0	0.0	0.0	0.6
G	Q1	12.4	14.0	4.9	9.2	5.5	3.8	5.2
	Q2	4.0	3.8	1.0	2.8	1.6	1.4	2.6
	Q3	2.9	1.2	1.0	0.2	0.0	0.2	0.8
	Q4	1.9	0.2	0.0	0.2	0.0	0.2	1.1

In addition, for the original randomization to treatment groups parameter, among the seven major events, only the estimate of the Log RR (-0.14) of cardiac endpoints is statistically significant—corresponding to an estimated risk reduction of 13%, and a 95% CI of 77% – 99%, for subjects originally randomized to the Gemfibrozil group as compared to subjects originally randomized to the Placebo group. The *P*-values and CIs for the RR of the other six major events are consistent with chance findings (Table 15.15).

It is interesting to note that the signs of the estimates of Log RR for the parameter reflecting the original randomization to treatment groups from the exposure/switching analyses performed are reasonable, in the sense that there is agreement between them and the observed data. A negative estimate implies that subjects originally randomized to the Gemfibrozil group were at less risk of experiencing a major event than subjects originally randomized to the Placebo group; whereas a positive estimate would imply that subjects originally randomized to the Gemfibrozil group were at greater risk of experiencing a major event than subjects originally randomized to the Placebo group. Table 15.18 shows the agreement between the direction of the estimated risk reduction and that observed in the original randomized groups for all events analyzed.

What analysis methodology one embraces depends on the trial objective and on the nature of the data. Since the objective of the Primary Helsinki Heart Study (HHS) was to assess how coronary endpoint risk reduction was correlated

TABLE 15.18

Observed Sign of the Difference between Gemfibrozil and Placebo Groups and the Sign of Group Parameter Estimate for Major Events

	CE	ACM	CR	NCR	NCRNCA	CAD	CA
Observed	−	+	−	+	+	+	−
Estimated	−	+	−	+	+	+	−

with the use of Gemfibrozil, exposure analyses may be more consistent with this objective. Exposure analyses as presented here utilize all subjects who were randomized to study medication. They are therefore also consistent with the "analyze what you randomize" interpretation of ITT analyses.

It is noted that the exposure analyses presented in this chapter assume that withdrawal is uninformative as to response. This means that (1) for subjects who withdrew, the decision regarding withdrawal was made without knowledge of their treatment group and (2) the reasons for withdrawal were unrelated to response. The study was double-blinded and monitored throughout to assure that blinding was maintained. Further, the treatment groups were comparable in terms of withdrawal rates and patterns. Therefore, the first condition reasonably holds. The reasons for withdrawal and the lag time between withdrawal and response support the second condition holding. Further, the data were analyzed assessing whether response and withdrawal status were correlated, and found not to be correlated ($P \gg 0.05$).

In summary, analyses of the Primary HHS [1,8] established that increases in HDL and decreases in LDL, due to Gemfibrozil over the 5-year double-blind study phase, were significantly correlated with a reduction of risk of cardiac endpoints, and provided no evidence that subjects were at significantly greater risk of dying or developing cancer. Based upon the analyses presented here, of 8-year data (the 5-year double-blind data plus data from 3 additional years of open-label follow-up) on these major events, which adjusted for subjects switching onto and off Gemfibrozil at the beginning of the open-label phase and differential exposure to study, there is no evidence to contradict the findings from the 5-year double-blind experience.

15.9 Concluding Remarks

It is customary for trials in CHD to covert the numerical difference between treatment and control in terms of cardiac endpoints or other major events into a ratio of treatment to control. For example, in the double-blind phase of the HHSPP trial 56/2046 (2.74%) in the Gemfibrozil group and 84/2035 (4.13%) subjects in the Placebo group experienced cardiac endpoints.

This reflects a numeric reduction (risk difference) of 1.39% among Gemfibrozil-treated subjects as compared to Placebo-treated subjects. An interpretation (frequentist) of this is that if 100,000 subjects were treated under study conditions with Gemfibrozil and 100,000 were "treated" with Placebo, 1390 fewer Gemfibrozil-treated subjects would be expected to experience cardiac endpoints than Placebo-treated subjects.

However, when the risk difference is converted $\{100(2.74 - 4.13)/4.13\}$ to a risk ratio and then expressed as a percentage, Gemfibrozil-treated subjects experienced a 33.7% (Table 15.1) reduction in cardiac endpoints as compared to Placebo-treated subjects—giving the appearance of a huge drug benefit. This does not mean that 1/3 fewer subjects would experience cardiac endpoints when treated with Gemfibrozil than when treated with Placebo.

Reported alone, the risk ratio hides the risk in the control group. In trials such as the HHSPP, the risk reduction, the risk ratio, and the risk of major events in the treatment and control groups should be reported.

Finally, this chapter concludes with a human interest story. The first author was head of Technical Operations at the Parke-Davis Pharmaceutical Research Division of Warner-Lambert Company during the late 1980s and was a consultant for several years thereafter. One of the development projects for which the first author had technical operations responsibility (biometrics, clinical data management, monitoring, and medical writing) was the HHSPP. The first author was one of a small group of company officials who frequently met with the FDA during their review of the Gemfibrozil SNDA for reduction in CHD. The FDA reviewing division, Metabolic and Endocrine Drug Products, called a meeting with company officials at 8:30 AM, December 22, 1988, to discuss issues raised in their review of the SNDA.

To attend and present at the FDA meeting, the first author had to cancel plans to attend a company clinical development meeting in Freiberg, Germany. In canceling, the first author gave up a seat on (the return) Pan AM Flight 103; the Boeing 747 that exploded over Lockerbie, Scotland on December 21, 1988 due to a terrorist's bomb [22].

References

1. Frick MH, Elo O, Haapa K, Heinonen OP, Heinsalmi P, Helo P, Huttunen JK, Kaitaniemi P, Koskinen P, Manninen V (1987): Helsinki heart study: Primary-prevention trial with gemfibrozil in middle-aged men with dyslipidemia. Safety of treatment, changes in risk factors, and incidence of coronary heart disease. *The New England Journal of Medicine*; 317(20): 1237–1245.
2. Frick MH, Heinonen OP, Huttunen JP, Koskinen P, Mänttäri M, Manninen V (1993): Efficacy of gemfibrozil in dyslipidaemic subjects with suspected heart disease; an ancillary study in the Helsinki heart study frame population. *Annals of Medicine*; 25(1): 41–45.
3. Peace KE, Carter WH Jr. (1993): Exposure analysis of dichotomous response measures in long term studies. *Journal of Biopharmaceutical Statistics*; 3(1): 129–140.
4. Huttunen JK, Heinonen OP, Manninen V, Koskinen P, Hakulinen T, Teppo L, Mänttäri M, Frick MH (1994): The Helsinki heart study: An 8.5-year safety and mortality follow-up. *Journal of Internal Medicine*; 235(1): 1–4.
5. Heinonen OP, Huttunen JK, Manninen V, Manttari M, Koskinen P, Tenkanen L, Frick MH (1994): The Helsinki heart study: Coronary heart disease incidence during an extended follow-up. *Journal of Internal Medicine*; 235(1): 41–49.

6. Haber H (1992): Interim analysis of the Helsinki heart study primary prevention trial. In: *Biopharmaceutical Sequential Statistical Applications*, Peace, KE (ed.), Marcel Dekker, Inc., New York, pp. 235–244.

7. Mänttäri M, Elo O, Frick MH, Haapa K, Heinonen OP, Heinsalmi P, Helo P, Huttunen JK, Kaitaniemi P, Koskinen P, Mäenpää H, Mälkönen M, Norola S, Pasternack A, Pikkarainen J, Romo M, Sjöblom T, Nikkilä EA (1987): The Helsinki heart study: Basic design and randomization procedure. *European Heart Journal*; **8**(Suppl I): 1–29.

8. Manninen V, Elo MO, Frick MH, Haapa K, Heinonen OP, Heinsalmi P, Helo P, Huttunen JK, Kaitaniemi P, Koskinen P, Mäenpää H, Mälkönen M, Mänttäri M, Norola S, Pasternack A, Pikkarainen J, Romo M, Sjöblom T, Nikkilä EA (1988): Lipid alterations and decline in the incidence of coronary heart disease in the Helsinki heart study. *Journal of the American Medical Association*; **260**: 641–651.

9. Mäenpää H, Manninen V, Heinonen OP (1992): Compliance with medication in the Helsinki heart study. *European Journal of Clinical Pharmacology*; **42**: 15–19.

10. Mantel N (1966): Evaluation of survival data and two new rank order statistics arising in its consideration. *Cancer Chemotherapy Reports*; **50**: 163–170.

11. Gehan EA (1965): A generalized Wilcoxon test for comparing arbitrarily singly-censored samples. *Biometrika*; **52**(1–2): 203–223.

12. Cox DR (1972): Regression models and life-tables (with discussion). *Journal of the Royal Statistical Society, Series B*; **34**: 187–220.

13. Stablein DM, Carter WH Jr., Wampler GL (1980): Survival analysis of drug combinations using a hazards model with time-dependent covariates. *Biometrics*; **36**: 537–546.

14. Zucker DM, Karr AF (1990): Nonparametric survival analysis with time-dependent covariate effects: A penalized partial likelihood approach. *Annals of Statistics*; **18**(1): 329–353.

15. Robins J, Tsiatis AA (1992): Semi-parametric estimation of an accelerated failure time model with time-dependent covariates. *Biometrika*; **79**(2): 311–319.

16. Fisher LD, Lin DY (1999): Time-dependent covariates in the Cox proportional-hazards regression model. *Annual Review of Public Health*; **20**: 145–157.

17. Peace KE, Carter HC (2006): Statistical analysis methods for providing inferences between primary response measures and exposure to study medication. *The Philippine Statistician*; **55**(1–2): 27–40.

18. Peace KE (1991): Exposure analysis of dichotomous data. In *Joint Statistical Meetings*, American Statistical Association, August, Atlanta, GA.

19. Peace KE (1992): Exposure analysis of time-to-event data in the ancillary Helsinki Heart Study. In: *Annual Meeting of the Drug Information Association*, June, San Diego, CA.

20. Peace KE (1993): Exposure analysis of time-to-event data in the primary Helsinki Heart Study. In: *Annual Meeting of the Drug Information Association*, July, Chicago, IL.

21. Peace KE (1991): Intention-to-treat: What is the question? In: *Joint Statistical Meetings of the American Statistical Association, Biometric Society and Institute of Mathematical Statistics*, American Statistical Association, Alexandria, VA, Abstract: 95.

22. Peace KE (2008): *Paid in Full*, Plowboy Press, Greensboro, GA; ISBN 978-0-615-19479-0 (www.plowboy-press.com).

16

Pivotal Proof-of-Efficacy Clinical Trials in the Treatment of Panic Disorder

16.1 Introduction

Patients with panic disorder experience sudden, unexpected episodes of intense apprehension or terror (a panic attack) with no apparent stimulus. Typical signs and symptoms include hyperventilation, tachycardia or palpitations, chest pain, sweating, trembling, and sensations of smothering or choking. Patients with the disorder may also experience blurred vision, weakness, or feelings of unbearable dread or terror. Many become so demoralized or incapacitated they are unable to leave their homes [1]. Panic disorder may occur with or without agoraphobia. Agoraphobia is a fear of places where help may not be available—such as crowded places (movie theaters, sports arenas, malls, etc.) or remote and isolated places.

Panic disorder with or without agoraphobia is common. The overall 12 month and lifetime prevalence rates are 2.1% and 5.1% [2]. It is a severe condition in those affected, often requiring visits to emergency rooms.

U.S. Federal Drug Regulations require at least two pivotal proof-of-efficacy clinical trials to support approval of a drug for a specific indication [3]. For drugs not yet approved, pivotal proof-of-efficacy trials occur in Phase III of the clinical development program. However, they may occur post marketing as Phase IV trials when a company develops evidence to support labeling for additional indications for an approved drug.

For example, Klonopin, a potent benzodiazepam, was originally U.S. FDA approved in the early 1970s for the treatment of Lennox–Gastaut syndrome (petit mal variant), akinetic and myoclonic seizures. Twenty years later, the parent company, Roche, initiated a clinical trials program that led to FDA approval of an SNDA that established Klonopin as effective in the treatment of patients with panic disorder with or without agoraphobia.

The SNDA clinical trials program consisted of two, pivotal proof-of-efficacy trials [4–6]. One incorporated a randomized, forced titration dose–response design while the other incorporated a flexible titration (according to response) design. Design aspects of these trials are detailed in Section 16.2.

Standard analysis approaches of efficacy data from such trials include treatment group comparisons at each follow-up visit in terms of variables, reflecting domains of the panic condition. These are discussed in Section 16.3. Results of the two Klonopin trials are reviewed in Section 16.4.

Analyses of efficacy data from such trials pose challenges as to (1) characterizing the dose–response profile across both studies, (2) characterizing duration of effect, (3) characterizing withdrawal effects, and (4) the choice of appropriate statistical analysis methods. Reasonable alternatives to the standard approaches are discussed in Section 16.5.

16.2 Design of Pivotal Proof-of-Efficacy Trials

The experimental, statistical design for both the forced titration dose–response trial (**FTDRT**, Figures 16.1 and 16.2) and the flexible titration according to response trial (**FTART**, Figure 16.3) is a completely randomized block design, with investigational centers as blocks. In addition, both are parallel, double blind, and placebo controlled. Both trials [4–6] consist of five consecutive phases: a 1-week placebo baseline run-in period, after which patients diagnosed with panic disorder [7] and who satisfy protocol eligibility criteria are randomized; then an upward titration dosing period of up to 3 weeks; then a fixed dosing period of 3–6 weeks; then a downward titration dosing period of variable length, depending on the patient's fixed dose; and finally a 1-week placebo washout period.

Both trials have approximately the same visit schedule: the initial screening visit, the baseline visit, weekly visits during the upward titration period, weekly or biweekly (depending on length) visits during the fixed dosing period, visits during the "middle" and at the end of the downward titration period, and a final visit at end of the placebo washout period.

	------- Forced titration -------	---------- Fixed dosing --------	Group
D_0	D_0	D_0	D_0	D_0 ---------------------------------|	D_0
D_1	D_1	D_1	D_1	D_1 ----------------------------------|	D_1
D_1	D_2	D_2	D_2	D_2 ---------------------------------|	D_2
D_1	D_2	D_3	D_3	D_3 ---------------------------------|	D_3
D_1	D_2	D_3	D_4	D_4 ---------------------------------|	D_4
D_1	D_2	D_3	D_4	D_5 ---------------------------------|	D_5

FIGURE 16.1
Randomized forced dosing schema for FTDRT.

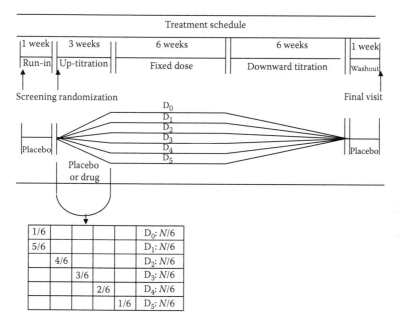

FIGURE 16.2
FTDRT schema.

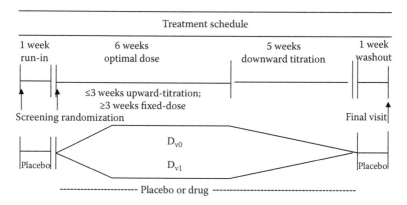

FIGURE 16.3
Titration according to response trial schema.

16.2.1 Forced Titration Dose–Response Trial: Experimental Design

For the FTDRT (Figures 16.1, 16.2), there may be up to six randomized dose groups: D_0, D_1, D_2, D_3, D_4, and D_5, where D_0 represents the placebo group, and D_i, $i = 1, \ldots, 5$ represent fixed doses of the drug under study. After randomization, $1/6$ of the patients are on D_0 for the duration of the trial, and $5/6$ are at D_1 for a fixed period of time, say T; then, $4/5$ of these move to D_2 for the period T and the other $1/5$ stay at D_1 until the end of the fixed dose period; then $3/4$ of those on D_2 move to D_3 for the period T and $1/4$ stay at D_2 until the end of the fixed dose period; then $2/3$ of those on D_3 move to D_4 for the period T and $1/3$ stay at D_3 until the end of the fixed dose period; then, $1/2$ of those on D_4 move to D_5 for the period T and $1/2$ stay at D_4 until the end of the fixed dose period, so that after a period of 5T (the upward titration period), all patients are at their randomized fixed dose, where they stay until the end of the fixed dosing period. It is noted that the randomization "forces" upward titration of dose regardless of response, and packaging ensures blindedness as to the identity of the dose.

16.2.2 Titration according to Response Trial: Experimental Design

For the FTART (Figure 16.3), there are two randomized groups (D_{v0}, D_{v1}), where D_{v0} represents the placebo group at variable "strengths," and D_{v1} represents the drug under study group (at variable strengths). The strengths available are usually the same as those used in the FTDRT: D_1, D_2, D_3, D_4, and D_5. After randomization, $1/2$ of the patients are on placebo throughout the trial dosing period (upward titration and fixed dose periods), and $1/2$ are on drug through the end of the trial dosing period. All patients (in the placebo and drug groups) are at strength D_1 for a period T (usually 2–4 days); those who respond (clinician's judgment) by the end of T stay at D_1 until the end of the trial dosing period, and those who do not are moved to strength D_2 for an additional period of T; those who respond to D_2 stay until the end of the trial dosing period, and those who do not are moved to strength D_3 for an additional period of T; those who respond to D_3 stay until the end of the trial dosing period, and those who do not are moved to strength D_4 for an additional period of T; those who respond to D_4 stay until the end of the trial dosing period, and those who do not are moved to strength D_5 for an additional period of T. After a period of 5T, all patients are at their "optimal" fixed dose, where they remain until the end of the fixed dosing period. If a patient has not responded by the end of the fixed dosing period, the investigator has the option to treat the patient outside the protocol. It is again noted that packaging ensures blindedness.

16.2.3 Efficacy Endpoints

Efficacy variables or endpoints collected in such trials are many and reflect domains of the panic condition. Primary efficacy measures are the number of panic attacks (**NPA**) between clinic visits and the clinician's global impression of severity (**CGIS**) (per a numeric rating scale) of the panic condition, both recorded at each visit to the end of the fixed dosing period.

Secondary efficacy measures include **CGIS** in the panic condition (recorded at post baseline office visits) and the patient's global impression of severity (**PGIS**) of his or her panic condition. There are many other secondary measures, including an assessment of activities of daily living, assessment of anxiety, items from the Hamilton Depression Scale, and data recorded on the patient's daily diary.

16.2.4 Trial Objectives

Obviously, the objective of each trial is to demonstrate efficacy of the drug in terms of primary endpoints reflecting the panic condition. Since each trial is placebo controlled, a directional alternative is appropriate [8] with a Type I error or false-positive rate of 5%.

16.2.4.1 Forced Titration Dose–Response Trial Objective

The objective of the FTDRT is formalized as the alternative hypothesis (H_a):

$$H_0: \mu_0 = \mu_1 = \mu_2 = \mu_3 = \mu_4 = \mu_5$$
$$H_a: \mu_0 \leq \mu_1 \leq \mu_2 \leq \mu_3 \leq \mu_4 \leq \mu_5,$$

where strict inequality ($<$) holds for at least one of the $\leq$, and where μ_i ($i = 0$, 1, 2, 3, 4, 5) represents the location parameter of the distribution of the efficacy variable or endpoint within each dose group D_i (with μ_0 being the location parameter in the placebo group D_0).

16.2.4.2 Titration according to Response Trial Objective

The objective of the titration according to response trial (TART) is formalized as the alternative hypothesis (H_a):

$$H_0: \mu_0 = \mu_D$$
$$H_a: \mu_0 \leq \mu_D,$$

where μ_0 and μ_D represent the location parameters of the distribution of the efficacy variable or endpoint within the placebo group and drug group, respectively.

16.2.5 Sample Size Determination

Although many choose a power of 80%, it is good practice for pivotal proof-of-efficacy trials to be designed with 95% power [9, Chapter 4]. The numbers of patients required to participate in each trial would then be determined using these error rates to detect a prespecified improvement (above placebo) in terms of the primary efficacy measures NPA and CGIS with a Type I error rate of 5%.

For the FTDRT, one has to decide how dose response should be characterized. One choice would be to detect a nonzero slope of the linear component of the dose–response curve. Another choice would be to detect a difference of δ (not greater than 20%) between a target dose group and the placebo group.

For the FTART, efficacy would be characterized as a prespecified difference of δ (>0) between the drug group and the placebo group.

16.3 Traditional Statistical Analysis Methods

Analysis of efficacy is restricted to efficacy data collected from baseline to the end of the fixed dosing period. Data collected past this point may be summarized and analyzed in an attempt to characterize withdrawal effects.

Traditional statistical analysis methods of efficacy measures are analysis of variance (ANOVA) or analysis of covariance (ANCOVA) methods. The choice of any particular analysis method should depend on whether the assumptions undergirding the validity of the method are appropriate for the behavior of the data [10, Chapter 9]. Since the distribution of the NPA is usually skewed, ANOVA or ANCOVA of ranks or nonparametric methods such as Cochran–Mantel–Haenszel [11] should be performed. Since change from baseline within an intervention group is an index of the effect of the intervention received, change from baseline (CNPA) in the NPA and change from baseline (CCGIS) in the CGIS may be preferred as primary measures of efficacy instead of NPA and CGIS, respectively.

There is a randomization basis for inferences as to dose response from the FTDRT. A statistically significant slope of the dose–response relationship over the six dose groups provides unequivocal evidence of a drug effect. This should be followed by step-down procedures to identify the minimally effective dose. This information will be helpful in the labeling of the drug once approved for marketing.

There is no randomization basis for inferences as to dose response from the FTART. The only valid randomization-based inference is the pairwise comparison of drug group to placebo group. In summarizing the results of this comparison, one would report the *P*-value, estimates of the mean and standard deviation of the efficacy response measure, and the distribution of the actual doses of drug used.

16.4 Overview of Efficacy Results of the Two Trials

The doses of Klonopin used in the two trials were 0, ½, 1, 2, 3, or 4 mg/day; i.e, $D_0 = 0$ mg/day (Placebo), $D_1 = ½$ mg/day, $D_2 = 1$ mg/day, $D_3 = 2$ mg/day, $D_4 = 3$ mg/day, and $D_5 = 4$ mg/day. The trials demonstrated that Klonopin was statistically significantly more effective than Placebo in treating panic disorder based upon change from baseline in the NPA and in the CGIS [12].

In the FTDRT, among the Klonopin dose groups, only the 1 mg/day group exhibited a consistently, statistically, significantly greater reduction in the NPA as compared to the Placebo group. Klonopin at 1 mg/day exhibited a reduction from baseline of approximately one panic attack per week as compared to Placebo. At the end of the fixed dosing period, nearly three quarters (74%) of 1 mg/day Klonopin patients were free of full panic attacks as compared to 56% of Placebo patients [12].

In the TART, the Klonopin group exhibited a reduction from baseline of approximately one panic attack per week as compared to the Placebo group. The mean dose of Klonopin over the optimal dosing period was 2.3 mg/day. At the end of the optimal dosing period, 62% of Klonopin patients were free of full panic attacks as compared to 37% of Placebo patients [12].

16.5 Alternative Design and Analysis Strategies

For the FTDRT, it is unlikely that there will be a clinic visit at each time $(T, 2T, \ldots, 5T)$ of forced upward titration and, consequently, there will be no efficacy data at some times of dose escalation. Were patients to return to the clinic at each time of such dose escalation and data recorded just prior to the escalation, it would be possible (provided T is sufficiently long) to assess the incremental benefit of the next dose level (for a period of T) as compared to remaining at the current dose level. (The de-escalation or withdrawal period suffers this same criticism.) Therefore, the utility of the forced upward titration period is to gradually get patients to their randomized fixed dose, rather than trying to separate out the effects of time and dose. Similarly, the utility of the withdrawal period is to gradually get patients completely off their fixed dose rather than trying to separate out the effects of time and dose reduction.

Another potential analysis issue may be: how best to deal with the problem of two primary efficacy endpoints? Should the overall Type I error be spread across each endpoint per Bonferroni or in an unequal manner to reflect one endpoint having greater weight than the other? Or should a bivariate analysis be performed? Or should the two endpoints be combined in some meaningful way and the result analyzed univariately?

In addition, since patients move to higher doses only if the clinician believes they are nonresponsive, there is the question of whether the FTART provides meaningful and interpretable dose–response information. At the end of the fixed dosing period, there will almost surely be subgroups of patients in both the drug and placebo groups who were titrated to a fixed dose of D_i, $i = 1, \ldots, 5$. However, a comparison of the drug group to the placebo group provides the only randomization-based inference. This comparison, based on data at the end of the fixed dosing period, would provide an inference as to the effectiveness of the drug at a dose equal to the average of the doses over the dosing period. Although it is a post-randomization stratified analysis, the comparison could be carried out by blocking on the fixed doses achieved.

Further, there is a desire to combine results across both the FTDRT and the FTART in a dose–response sense. Randomization ensures a valid inference base for pairwise comparisons of each dose to placebo from the FTDRT, but not so from the FTART. One way of combining results from both trials would be to estimate the effect of all dose groups combined (appropriately weighted) as compared to placebo from the FTDRT and combine this estimate with the estimate of the drug group compared to placebo from the TART using meta-analysis methods such as the Cochran–Dersimonian–Laird procedure [13]. This would then provide an overall estimate of the effectiveness of the drug over the range of doses $D_1, \ldots, D_5$ or at the average of the doses—simultaneously incorporating any heterogeneity across the trial estimates of effectiveness.

Efficacy analyses described are endpoint analyses; i.e., use the last observation available on patients in the fixed dosing period. As such, the inference reflects the degree to which the drug reduces the NPA or reduces the severity of the overall panic condition as reflected by the CGIS beyond such reductions in the placebo group. Typically, there is little or no interest in the duration of the effect. Whether duration of effect can be assessed will depend on the length of T over the upward titration period and/or on the length of the fixed dosing period. One definitional way to consider duration of effect is to define response as zero panic attacks or a prespecified reduction in the NPA. Once response is observed, particularly during the fixed dosing period, duration of response could be estimated using survival data analysis methods. These results would be interesting clinically, but would be difficult to interpret statistically as the group of responders is a subset of all randomized patients. In addition, survival data analysis methods could be used to provide a valid inference between drug and placebo groups in terms of time-to-response patterns. Yet another measure that may be of clinical interest is the proportion of the dosing period patients are in the response state. As nonresponders would have a value of zero for this measure, comparison of the drug and placebo groups would be based on all randomized patients.

Finally, modifications to the withdrawal phase of the trials could lead to better understanding of withdrawal effects as well as provide an inferential framework for conclusions. At the end of the fixed dosing period, patients could be re-randomized to a variety of de-escalation regimens to better characterize withdrawal effects. Good clinical judgment will be required in defining such de-escalation schemes so as to minimize severe withdrawal effects from abrupt reduction of the fixed dose. It is suggested that patients be seen at the clinic at more frequently scheduled visits (and NPA, CGIS, and any adverse experiences, recorded at such visits).

16.6 Concluding Remarks

Since the FTDRT and FTART are multicenter longitudinal with multiple endpoints, the usual issues inherent in such trials have to be adequately dealt with by the analyst. These include interactions (treatment group-by-center, treatment group-by-baseline factors such as disease severity or demographics, treatment group-by-time), how to handle missing data, and how to deal with the impact of multiplicities on overall conclusions.

References

1. Pary R, Lewis S (1992): Identifying and treating patients with panic attacks. *American Family Physician*; **46**(3): 841–848.
2. Grant BF, Hasin DS, Stinson FS, Dawson DA, Goldstein RB, Smith S, Huang B, Saha TD (2006): The epidemiology of DSM-IV panic disorder and agoraphobia in the United States: Results from the national epidemiologic survey on alcohol and related conditions. *Journal of Clinical Psychiatry*; **67**: 363–374.
3. Code of Federal Regulations (2005): Sec.314.126 Adequate and well-controlled studies. Title 21, Vol. 5 [21CFR314.126]; U.S. Government Printing Office via GPO Access; Revised as of April 1; 144–146.
4. Rosenbaum JF, Moroz G, Bowden CL (1997): Clonazepam in the treatment of panic disorder with or without agoraphobia: A dose-response study of efficacy, safety, and discontinuance. *Journal of Clinical Psychopharmacology*; **17**: 390–400.
5. Davidson JR, Moroz G (1998): Pivotal studies of clonazepam in panic disorder. *Psychopharmacology Bulletin*; **34**: 169–174.
6. Moroz G, Rosenbaum JF (1999): Efficacy, safety, and gradual discontinuation of clonazepam in panic disorder: A placebo-controlled, multi-center study using optimized dosages. *Journal of Clinical Psychiatry*; **60**(9): 604–612.
7. American Psychiatric Association (1994): *Diagnostic and Statistical Manual of Mental Disorders*, 4th edn., DSM-IV, Washington, DC.
8. Peace KE (1991): One-sided or two-sided p-values: Which most appropriately address the question of drug efficacy. *Journal of Biopharmaceutical Statistics*; **1**(1): 133–138.

9. Peace KE (2006): Sample size considerations in clinical trials pre-market approval. *The Philippine Statistician*; **55**(1, 2): 1–26.
10. Peace KE (2006): Validity of statistical inferences from medical experiments. *Philippine Statistical Association Newsletter*; **32**(2): 10–16.
11. Mantel N, Haenszel W (1959): Statistical aspects of the analysis of data from retrospective studies. *Journal of the National Cancer Institute*; **22**: 719–748.
12. Roche Product Information (2009): Klonopin tablets, Clinical pharmacology, clinical trials: Panic disorder; http://www.rocheusa.com/products/klonopin/; pp. 2–3.
13. DerSimonian R, Laird N (1986): Meta-analysis in clinical trials. *Controlled Clinical Trials*; **7**: 177–188.

17

Combination Clinical Trials

17.1 Introduction

The phrase combination clinical trial pertains to a clinical trial whose treatment or intervention groups include one that represents a combination of pharmaceutical products: two or more drugs, biologics, or medical devices. To date, most combination clinical trials involve two drugs, each at fixed doses.

One example is Arthrotec®, a fixed combination of the Diclofenac® and Misoprostol (Cytotec®). Diclofenac is a nonsteroidal anti-inflammatory drug (NSAID) similar to ibuprofen (e.g., Motrin® or Advil®) used to treat osteoarthritis symptoms. Misoprostol (see Chapter 13) is used to prevent gastric ulceration from developing due to chronic dosing with NSAIDs.

Another example is Dyazide®, a fixed combination of Hydrochlorothiazide and Triamterene, used to treat hypertension. Hydrochlorothiazide and Triamterene are diuretics that reduce blood pressure by ridding the body of excess water. Triamterene also has potassium-sparing properties.

Yet another example is Actifed®, a fixed combination of Triprolodine and Pseudoephedrine, used to treat seasonal allergic rhinitis (SAR) as well as other respiratory ailments. Triprolodine is an antihistamine that is used to treat hay fever–like symptoms. Pseudoephedrine is a sympathomimetic and is used to alleviate nasal congestion. Hay fever–like symptoms and nasal congestion are the hallmark symptoms of SAR.

The U.S. Food and Drug Administration's (FDA's) policy under the Federal Food, Drug, and Cosmetic Act regarding fixed-combination dosage form prescription drugs for humans is as follows [1]: "Two or more drugs may be combined in a single dosage form **when each component makes a contribution to the claimed effects** (of the combination) and the dosage of each component (amount, frequency, duration) is such that the combination is safe and effective for a significant patient population requiring such concurrent therapy as defined in the labeling for the drug."

Let A denote a drug at a fixed dose, and B denote a different drug at a fixed dose. Let AB denote the (fixed-dose) combination drug product of A and B. Some interpret the FDA policy requirement necessary for approval of the combination as the demonstration that it is better than each of its components; i.e., that AB > A and AB > B, and therefore that the design for clinical trials to establish the effectiveness of the combination only needs to contain three treatment groups—AB, A, and B.

A case may be made for this interpretation providing the effectiveness of both A and B has been established. However, if neither A nor B is known to be effective in treating the disease being studied, then a Placebo group is also needed [2]. The inclusion of a Placebo group enables not only the effectiveness of the combination to be established but also permits an assessment of the extent to which each component contributes to the effectiveness of the combination.

This chapter reviews the design of combination clinical trials, discusses the effectiveness of a combination, and illustrates the basis for estimating the contribution that each component makes to the combination. Three examples are also provided.

17.2 Two-by-Two Factorial Design

The inclusion of a Placebo group (P) leads to the full, two-by-two factorial design (Table 17.1):

where the 11 cell (AB) represents the combination of the fixed dose of A and the fixed dose of B, the 12 cell (A) represents the fixed dose of A without B (dose B = 0), the 21 cell (B) represents the fixed dose of B without A (dose A = 0), and the 22 cell represents Placebo (P)—0 dose of A and 0 dose of B.

TABLE 17.1

Two-by-Two Factorial Design Schema

AB	A
B	P

When this design is used in a clinical trial, subjects would be randomized to the four treatment groups: AB, A, B, and P. Further, to eliminate bias, investigational site personnel and subjects would be blinded as to the identity of the treatment subjects receive.

17.3 Effectiveness of the Combination

The combination AB is a drug product. In order for a drug product to gain market approval, the 1962 Kefauver–Harris Amendment requires that it must be shown to be effective; i.e., AB − P > 0. Consider the fundamental identity [2]

$$AB - P = (A - P) + (B - P) + \{(AB - A) - (B - P)\}, \qquad (17.1)$$

or

$$C(AB) = C(A) + C(B) + C(I), \qquad (17.2)$$

where
  C(AB) is the contrast (1, 0, 0, −1) on the treatment groups (AB, A, B, P) reflecting the effectiveness of the combination (as compared to Placebo)
  C(A) is the contrast (0, 1, 0, −1) reflecting the effectiveness of A alone
  C(B) is the contrast (0, 0, 1, −1) reflecting the effectiveness of B alone
  C(I) is the contrast (1, −1, −1, 1) reflecting the interaction between A and B

Note that C(I) may be positive, negative, or zero.
  It follows that

$$C(AB) > C(A) + C(B), \quad \text{if } C(I) > 0. \qquad (17.3)$$

C(I) is positive if the effect of B in the presence of A is greater than the effect of B in the absence of A. In this case, we have **synergism** between A and B; i.e., the effectiveness of the combination is greater than the sum of its parts.
  Further,

$$C(AB) < C(A) + C(B), \quad \text{if } C(I) < 0. \qquad (17.4)$$

C(I) is negative if the effect of B in the presence of A is less than the effect of B in the absence of A. In this case, we have **antagonism** between A and B; i.e., the effectiveness of the combination is less than the sum of its parts.
  Finally,

$$C(AB) = C(A) + C(B), \quad \text{if } C(I) = 0. \qquad (17.5)$$

C(I) is zero if the effect of B in the presence of A is equal to the effect of B in the absence of A. In this case, we have **additivity** between A and B; i.e., the effectiveness of the combination is the same as the sum of its parts.
  The FDA policy requirement for combination drugs seems to call for a three-arm clinical trial (AB, A, and B) and the demonstration that AB > A and AB > B. The latter would require controlling the Type I error rate across the two pairwise comparisons via Bonferonni or in some other manner. However, the effectiveness of the combination should be addressed by comparing it to Placebo, which can only happen if a Placebo arm is also included. One could compare AB to A and AB to B. Both could be statistically significant, but one could not conclude that the combination was effective unless A and B were known to be effective via extra-trial data or results.

17.4 Contribution of Components to the Effectiveness of the Combination

Now, replace the contrasts in Equation 17.2 with their estimates (e.g., MLEs or least squares) and form the percentages:

$$P(A) = 100 \left[\frac{E(A)}{E(AB)} \right], \tag{17.6}$$

$$P(B) = 100 \left[\frac{E(B)}{E(AB)} \right], \tag{17.7}$$

and

$$P(I) = 100 \left[\frac{E(I)}{E(AB)} \right], \tag{17.8}$$

where E now reflects that the contrasts have been replaced with their estimates. Upon dividing both sides of the resulting equation by E(AB), we obtain

$$100\% = P(A) + P(B) + P(I). \tag{17.9}$$

Equation 17.9 permits one to quantitatively estimate and report the contribution of A to the combination, the contribution of B to the combination, and the contribution of their interaction to the combination, which is required by the fixed-dose combination drug regulation.

Note from this design, it is possible for the combination to be effective if both A and B are effective, if either A or B is effective, or if neither A nor B is effective. In the last case, the effectiveness of the combination would be due to synergism of the components.

17.5 Factorial Designs in Other Clinical Development Areas

The two-by-two factorial design has a place in the development of combination drugs in many areas—including oncologic drugs in an adjuvant setting (e.g., to surgery). For example, suppose A is one chemotherapy drug at a specified dose, B is another chemotherapy drug at a specified dose. Then a clinical trial could be conducted using the two-by-two factorial design in Table 17.1, and the methods in Sections 17.3 and 17.4 could be used to assess the contribution of each chemotherapy drug to the effectiveness of the combination AB. As another example, A could be a chemotherapy drug at a specified dose and B could be some immunotherapy at a specified dose. For these two examples to be amenable to the fixed-dose combination drug regulation, one would theoretically administer A and B simultaneously IV (or orally if such formulations exist). One could study the effect of spacing (schedule) between A and B by going to a larger factorial design, say a two-by-two-by S, where S is the distinct number of schedules or spacing.

In addition, one could study several doses of A (say a), several doses of B (say b), and several schedules (say S) in the Phase II program. A full factorial would require the product of a, b, and S, drug-dose–schedule combinations, and patients would be randomized to these combinations. However, one would not have to use a full factorial. One could use fractional factorials, or central composite designs, and use response surface methodology and be guided to a region of the factor space (doses of A by doses of B by schedules) that would correspond to predictions of clinically optimal response (in some defined sense). Such information could be useful in improving the design of Phase III confirmatory trials of efficacy.

Larger factorial designs studying the effect of several doses of each of two drugs have been used in the development of combination drugs to treat hypertension [3–5]. Response surface methodology is helpful in determining the doses of the two drugs or a region of doses for which lowering of blood pressure would be predicted to be clinically optimal (in some defined sense).

17.6 Example 1: Actifed® in the Treatment of SAR Following DESI Review

Actifed is a fixed-combination drug product of Triprolodine and Pseudoephedrine. Both were widely marketed individually; e.g., Triprolodine as Actidil® and Pseudoephedrine as Sudafed®. Triprolodine is an antihistamine and is used to treat hay fever–like symptoms. Pseudoephedrine is a sympathomimetic and used to alleviate nasal congestion. Hay fever–like symptoms and congestion are the hallmark of SAR. Therefore, there was a rationale for marketing the combination; i.e., it is more convenient for a patient to take one dose of the combination than to take one dose of each component.

Actifed was developed and approved for the treatment of SAR by Burroughs Wellcome (now a part of GlaxoSmithKline) Pharmaceutical Research in 1958. It was therefore marketed prior to the 1962 Kefauver–Harris Amendment. As is indicated in Chapter 2, many drugs on the market at that time underwent review by the Drug Efficacy Study Implementation (DESI) committee to determine whether new clinical trials would be needed to confirm their efficacy. The review deemed that a clinical trial would have to be conducted to demonstrate the effectiveness of Actifed for the treatment of SAR.

17.6.1 Design and Randomized Treatment Groups

A parallel clinical trial was conducted [6] using a two-by-two factorial design with fixed, parallel, treatment groups: the combination (**TP**) product, Triprolodine alone (**T**), Pseudoephedrine alone (**P**), and Placebo (**0**). Approximately 160 patients with SAR were randomized in balanced and double-blind fashion to the four treatment groups.

17.6.2 Objective

The **primary objective** of the trial was to demonstrate the effectiveness of the combination **TP** in the treatment of SAR. The **secondary objective** was to illustrate how each component contributes to the claimed effects of the combination.

17.6.3 Efficacy Endpoints

The efficacy endpoints were nasal airway resistance (**NAR**) and the frequency and severity of hay fever–like symptoms: sneezing, rhinorrhea, lacrimation, or itching of the eyes, nose, or throat. NAR ranged from 1 to 6 in order of increasing severity. Each hay fever symptom was rated individually according to frequency and severity. The individual ratings were then totaled across symptoms producing a hay fever symptom complex score (**HFSCS**), ranging from 0 to 44. Endpoint assessments were made at baseline (hour 0), and at each hour thereafter through 8 h post-baseline dose. Patients received three doses: the first just after baseline and the second and third at 3 and 6 h, respectively, thereafter.

17.6.4 Sample Size Requirements

Approximately 160 patients with SAR were randomized in balanced and double-blind fashion to the four parallel treatment groups. Forty patients per treatment group would provide a power of 80% to detect a between-treatment-group difference of 20% in mean NAR (or HFSCS) with a relative standard deviation of 36% and a one-sided Type I error to 5%.

17.6.5 Statistical Analysis Methods

Sections 17.3 and 17.4 present arguments that support (1) demonstrating the effectiveness of the combination (as compared to Placebo), and (2) estimating the extent to which each component contributes to the effectiveness of the combination, as a more logical alternative to satisfy the combination policy. However, when we conducted the trial, we also addressed the stricter interpretation that TP must be shown to be better than each component alone; i.e., that $TP > T$ and $TP > P$.

On the surface, it may appear that the combination must be shown to be better than each component alone for both NAR and HFSCS. If so, two endpoints and two pairwise comparisons could be interpreted as allocating the 0.05 Type I error as 0.0125 for each pairwise comparison and each endpoint. Since T is not expected to affect NAR, adding T to P should produce a combination that is better than T for NAR; i.e., $TP > T$ for NAR. Similarly, since P is not expected to affect HFSCS, adding P to T should produce a combination that is better than P for HFSCS; i.e., $TP > P$ for HFSCS.

Therefore, the combination policy requirement would be addressed by showing that $TP > T$ for NAR and $TP > P$ for HFSCS each at the 0.025 Type I error level. However, combining both T and P into a single dosage form should not detract from the effectiveness of P for NAR, nor should it detract from the effectiveness of T for HFSCS. Consequently, it is desirable to demonstrate that the combination is better than Placebo $(TP > 0)$ for both NAR and HFSCS. Inference on the effectiveness contrast $(TP > 0)$ for NAR and for HFSCS was provided using 95% confidence intervals.

Separate analyses of covariance methods were applied to NAR and HFSCS using their baseline values as the covariates. These analyses were facilitated using the Statistical Analysis System (SAS) with a linear model that included the covariate and treatment group as fixed effects. Treatment group sums of squares were partitioned to provide estimates of $(T - 0)$, $(P - 0)$, and the interaction (I) between T and P. Additional analyses were performed to assess the generalizability of treatment group differences across time of assessment and across levels of the covariates.

Examination of the endpoint data from the trial revealed that both NAR and HFSCS had to undergo logarithmic transformations to induce normality. Since the lower limit of the range of HFSCS could be 0, the number 1 was added prior to transformation.

Plots of the individual endpoints across hour of assessment and by treatment group were generated. Figure 17.1 reflects mean Log (NAR) for each treatment group and hour of assessment. Figure 17.2 reflects mean of Log $(HFSCS + 1)$ for each treatment group and hour of assessment.

To get an idea of how NAR and HFSCS vary jointly, bivariate plots of both endpoints were generated [7]. Figure 17.3 provides plots of mean pairs of each transformed endpoint by treatment group and hour of assessment. To generate the data for plotting, the NAR and HFSCS data for each subject at each time of assessment is averaged over subjects in each treatment group. This provides coordinates {Log $(HFSCS + 1)$, Log (NAR)} at each time of assessment for each treatment group. The numbers 0, 1, 2, 3, 4, 5, 6, 7, and 8 along each treatment group plot represent the hour of assessment, with 0 representing baseline.

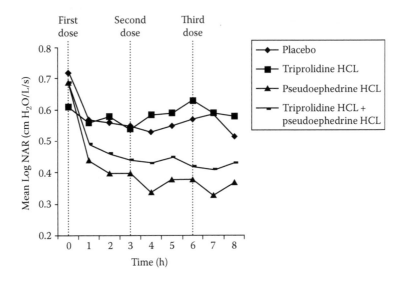

FIGURE 17.1
Plot of mean Log NAR by treatment group and time of assessment. Baseline values are shown at time zero.

The treatment group graphs in each Figures 17.1 through 17.3 reflect what one expects for Pseudoephedrine (decongestant with little or no effect on HFSCS) alone, Triprolodine (antihistamine with little or no effect on NAR) alone, the combination, and Placebo.

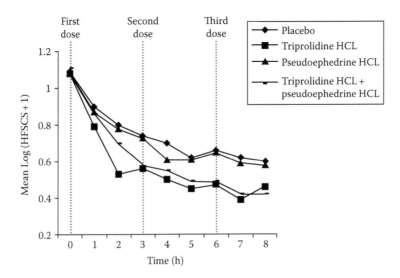

FIGURE 17.2
Plot of mean Log (HFSCS + 1) by treatment group and time of assessment. Baseline values are shown at time zero.

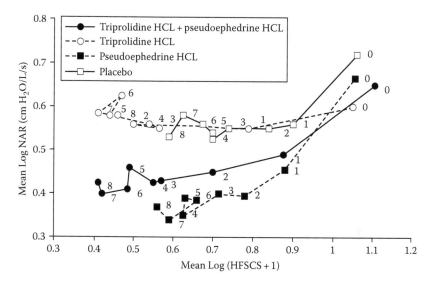

FIGURE 17.3

Plot of mean Log (HFSCS + 1) and mean Log (NAR) by group and hour of assessment. Baseline values are at zero.

17.7 Example 2: Crossover Trial of Actifed in the Treatment of SAR

An earlier crossover trial in SAR was conducted [8,9]. This trial was conducted over five consecutive 2-week treatment periods. All patients who qualified for entry received the combination treatment in the first 2-week period. Forty patients in whom the combination was deemed suitable were then randomized in double-blind manner to the four treatment groups: TP, T, P, and 0, for the second 2-week treatment period. The order of the remaining three treatments received in the third, fourth, and fifth 2-week treatment periods was determined randomly.

SAR symptoms were rated according to -2, -1, 0, $+1$, and $+2$, where

$-2 =$ for each day deemed to be very bad

$-1 =$ for each day worse than usual

$0 =$ for each average day

$+1 =$ for each day better than usual

$+2 =$ for each day free of symptoms

A total score was then obtained by adding the ratings across symptoms. Table 17.2 summarizes the distribution of mean scores by treatment group.

TABLE 17.2

Total Mean Score Distribution by Treatment

	Treatment			
Response	TP	T	P	0
Mean score	16.25	11.15	11.13	7.95
N	40	40	40	40

These data may be used to illustrate the contribution each component makes to the effectiveness of the combination.

The estimate of the effectiveness of the combination (TP) contrast is

$$TP - 0 = 16.25 - 7.95 = 8.3.$$

The estimate of the effectiveness of the Triprolidine (T) contrast is

$$T - 0 = 11.15 - 7.95 = 3.2.$$

The estimate of the effectiveness of the Pseudoephedrine (P) contrast is

$$P - 0 = 11.13 - 7.95 = 3.18.$$

The estimate of the interaction (I) contrast is

$$I = (16.25 - 11.15) - (11.13 - 7.95) = 5.1 - 3.18 = 1.92.$$

Note that since $I > 0$, T and P contribute in a synergistic manner to the effectiveness of TP.

From Equation 17.9,

$$100\% = \frac{3.2}{8.3} + \frac{3.18}{8.3} + \frac{1.92}{8.3} = 38.55\% + 38.31\% + 23.13\%.$$

Therefore, T alone contributes 38.55%, P alone contributes 38.31%, and I contributes (in a synergistic manner) 23.13%, respectively, to the effectiveness of TP.

17.8 Example 3: Parallel Trial of Actifed in the Treatment of the Common Cold

Another parallel, double-blind, randomized, Placebo (0)-controlled clinical trial was conducted to assess the effectiveness of Triprolidine (T) and Pseudoephedrine (P) alone and in combination (TP) in treating symptoms (12) of

TABLE 17.3

Response Distribution by Treatment

Response	Treatment			
	TP	T	P	0
Improved	28 (58%)[a]	27 (48%)	29 (53%)[a]	14 (25%)
Unchanged	12 (25%)	18 (32%)	17 (31%)	30 (55%)
Worsened	8 (17%)	11 (20%)	9 (16%)	11 (29%)
Ambiguous	5	8	8	8
N	53	64	63	63

[a] $P < 0.01$ versus 0.

the common cold [9,10]. This trial was conducted in four different regions of England. Four-hundred and sixty-six subjects who were otherwise healthy were randomized to the four treatment groups. One-hundred and ninety-nine (199) subjects reported a total of 243 colds.

For each cold, subjects were asked to rate how they felt after treatment compared to when they started taking trial medication according to whether they were improved, unchanged, or worse. Table 17.3 summarizes the percentages of colds in each treatment group rated as improved, unchanged, or worsened. These data may be used to illustrate the contribution each component makes to the effectiveness of the combination.

The estimate of the effectiveness of the combination (TP) contrast is

$$TP - 0 = 58\% - 25\% = 33\%.$$

The estimate of the effectiveness of the Pseudoephedrine (P) contrast is

$$P - 0 = 53\% - 25\% = 28\%.$$

The estimate of the interaction (I) contrast is

$$I = (58\% - 48\%) - (53\% - 25\%) = 10\% - 28\% = -18\% \text{ (Antagonism)}.$$

Note that since $I < 0$, T and P contribute in an antagonistic manner to the effectiveness of TP.

From Equation 17.9,

$$100\% = \frac{23\%}{33\%} + \frac{28\%}{33\%} = \frac{18\%}{33\%} = 69.7\% + 84.8\% - 54.5\%.$$

Therefore, T alone contributes 69.7%, P alone contributes 84.8%, and I contributes (in an antagonistic way) −54.5%, respectively, to the effectiveness of TP.

17.9 Concluding Remarks

Another argument that supports the need to include a Placebo group in addition to the AB, A, and B groups in a clinical trial whose aim is to satisfy the combination policy is consistency of efficacy requirements. For example, suppose that both A and B are the same doses of drug A. Then AB equals AA, which equals twice the dose of A. If a three-group (AA, A, A) trial was conducted with N patients per group, it is doubtful that efficacy could be concluded by demonstrating that $AA > A$ and $AA > A$. If a two-group (AA, A) trial was conducted where the two A groups were combined (so that the number of patients on A is twice the number on AA), it is doubtful that efficacy could be concluded by demonstrating that $AA > A$. Although section 314.126 of the IND/NDA regulations permit a low dose (no effect) of A as a control, twice the low dose would probably not be significantly better than the low dose.

References

1. CITE: 21CFR300.50. Code of Federal Regulations: Title 21, Vol. 5; Revised April 1, 2005.
2. Peace KE (1986): Some thoughts on combination drug development. In: *Proceedings of the Biopharmaceutical Section*, The American Statistical Association, Las Vegas, NV.
3. Canter D, Frank GJ, Knapp LE, Phelps M, Quade M, Texter M (1994): Quinapril and hydrochlorothiazide combination for control of hypertension: Assessment by factorial design. *Journal of Human Hypertension*; **8**(3): 155–162.
4. Frishman WH, Bryzinski BS, Coulson LR, DeQuattro VL, Vlachakis ND, Mroczek WJ, Dukart G, Goldberg JD, Alemayehu D, Koury K (1994): A multifactorial trial design to assess combination therapy in hypertension: Treatment with bisoprolol and hydrochlorothiazide. *Archives of Internal Medicine*; **154**(13): 1461–1468.
5. Pool JL, Cushman WC, Saini RK, Nwachuku CE, Battikha JP (1997): Use of the factorial design and quadratic response surface models to evaluate the fosinopril and hydrochlorothiazide combination therapy in hypertension. *American Journal of Hypertension*; **10**: 117–123.
6. Diamond L, Gerson K, Cato A, Peace KE, Perkins JG (1981): An evaluation of triprolidine and pseudoephedrine in the treatment of allergic rhinitis. *Annals of Allergy*; **47**(2): 87–91.
7. Peace KE, Tsai K-T (2009): Bivariate or composite plots of endpoints. *Journal of Biopharmaceutical Statistics*; **19**: 324–331.
8. Empey DW, Bye C, Hodder M, Hughes DT (1975): A double-blind crossover trial of pseudoephedrine and triprolidine, alone and in combination, for the treatment of allergenic rhinitis. *Annals of Allergy*; **34**(1): 41–46.

9. Medical Officer's Review of Safety Data (1982): *RX to OTC Marketing of Actifed, NDAs 11–935 and 11–936*, Department of Health & Human Services, Food and Drug Administration, Rockville, MD, pp. 1–10.
10. Bye CE, Cooper J, Empey DW, Fowle AS, Hughes DT, Letley E, O'Grady E (1980): Effects of pseudoephedrine and triprolidine, alone and in combination, on symptoms of the common cold. *British Medical Journal*; **281**: 189–190.

18

Monitoring Clinical Trials for Adverse Events

18.1 Introduction

In the clinical development of a new drug it is rare that clinical trials are designed to provide definitive evidence that the drug is safe, particularly in terms of its side effect or adverse event (AE) profile. It is possible (and statutorily required for pivotal proof of efficacy) to design Phase III trials to provide definitive evidence that the drug is effective. Clinical trials of efficacy of new drugs should therefore be monitored for safety and the safety profile described within and across trials in an ongoing cumulative manner. Confidence intervals are recommended as the appropriate statistical inferential methodology for doing this. Such intervals provide an interval estimate on the unknown incidences of AEs among patients who could be treated with each regimen, as well as permit a conclusion that two regimens are different.

There is little argument that for drugs for which it is possible to design clinical trials to provide definitive information on aspects of safety, there are few issues. One would develop a protocol (see Chapter 6) in a manner similar to developing a protocol for a clinical trial of efficacy. There have been a few occasions where it has been possible to design trials to provide definitive information on questions about the safety of drugs [1,2].

18.2 Designing for Safety: Antibiotic Rash Example

As a first example, in the clinical development of a new antibiotic, a skin rash was observed among several patients at the top dose of a Phase II dose comparison trial of an antibiotic. Since the top dose appeared to be more efficacious, a trial was subsequently designed and executed to confirm the rash experience before deciding to terminate the top dose from further clinical development. In designing the follow-up trial, the Phase II dose comparison trial provided estimates for sample size determination. The follow-up trial consisted of a single arm of the top dose, incorporated sequential procedures as discussed by Armitage [3], and required 47 patients to confirm the skin rash. The decision was subsequently made to terminate the top dose from further clinical development.

18.3 Designing for Safety: Hypokalemia Example

A second example is of a clinical trial that was designed and conducted to assess the hypokalemia potential of two doses of hydrochlorothiazide: 25 mg (H_{25}) and 50 mg (H_{50}), and 25 mg of hydrochlorothiazide plus 50 mg of triamterene ($H_{25}T$). Hypokalemia was defined as serum potassium concentration less than or equal to 3.5 meq/L. The protocol required patients with mild to moderate hypertension to be treated for up to 6 months. Data analyses were to be performed sequentially in time after patients completed 6, 12, 18, and 24 (6 months) weeks of treatment. Approximately 171 patients per group were needed to detect a 10% (8% versus 18%) difference in the incidences of hypokalemia among any two regimens with a Type 1 error rate of 5% and a power of 80%. The outcome of the trial at the first analysis is reflected by the ordering: $H_{25}T < H_{25} < H_{50}$. That is, the combination exhibited a lower incidence of hypokalemia than did 25 mg of hydrochlorothiazide alone—which exhibited a lower incidence than the 50 mg dose of hydrochlorothiazide alone.

18.4 Designing for Safety: Hypertensive Rebound Example

As a third example, the Phase III clinical development plan for a new antihypertensive compound included two definitive proof-of-efficacy clinical trials. Both trials were randomized and double blinded. One was a forced titration, placebo-controlled dose comparison trial, that included 0 (Placebo) and low (D_1), middle (D_2) and high (D_3) doses of the compound. The other was a positive controlled trial in which once versus twice daily administration of the target dose (D_2) was compared to a marketed antihypertensive (positive control) drug.

A medical concern in the use of some antihypertensive drugs was their potential to exhibit *hypertensive rebound* or *blood pressure overshoot* if the patient stops taking the drug. *Hypertensive rebound* or *blood pressure overshoot* is characterized by a fairly rapid rise in blood pressure to levels above those at baseline when the patient began taking the drug. There was reason to believe that patients taking the new drug were less likely to experience "hypertensive rebound" or "blood pressure overshoot" upon withdrawing the drug than among patients treated with the marketed compound.

Although the latter trial furnished antihypertensive efficacy information on the target dose of the new drug (given both once and twice daily) relative to the positive control, another objective of trial was to compare the new drug to the marketed drug in terms of *hypertensive rebound* or *blood pressure overshoot*; thus addressing an important medical concern in the clinical use of the new drug. Demonstrating that the risk of hypertensive rebound of the new drug was less than that of the marketed drug would also enable the new drug to be more successfully marketed.

Briefly, design considerations consisted of an initial phase representing 6 months of treatment to control blood pressure, followed by a phase where both drugs were withdrawn and blood pressure subsequently monitored for up to 7 days for overshoot. The number of patients required qualitatively was the number necessary to discriminate between the two regimens in terms of overshoot inflated to account for the proportions expected to become normotensive over the first (treatment) phase.

18.5 Premarket Approval Trials: Designed for Efficacy

The previous three examples illustrate instances where it was possible to design clinical trials to provide definitive information on aspects of safety. However, for most drugs, particularly premarket approval ones, it is not possible to do so. Some reasons are (1) inadequate information to formulate the objective or question; (2) inadequate information to specify the primary safety endpoints; and (3) inadequate information to characterize the target population. Even if the endpoints are specified, the question formulated and the target population identified, there is usually inadequate information on estimates of endpoints for sample size determination. In addition, if the endpoints are specified, the question formulated, the target population identified, and sufficient information existed to determine adequate sample sizes, logistical difficulties and/or financial constraints may preclude conducting a trial that large.

Therefore, a rational position in the development of new drugs is to design (Phase III) trials to provide definitive information about efficacy, monitor safety, and describe the safety profile in each trial, and accumulate and describe the safety profile across trials. This position is consistent with the statutory requirement for regulatory approval of a new drug in the United States; i.e., provide both clinical and statistical evidence of efficacy and adequately describe the safety profile. It is thus reasonable to expect that a new drug application (NDA), which contains clinical and statistical evidence of the claimed efficacy effects and an adequate description of the safety profile, which in itself represents no unacceptable safety concerns (acceptable benefit to risk), would be given regulatory approval to be marketed.

Regulatory requirements for new drug development allow the sponsor to proceed along the lines indicated by two axioms of drug development [1,2]: (1) drugs in development are considered nonefficacious until proven otherwise; and (2) drugs in development are considered safe until proven otherwise. From the biostatistician's point of view, axiom 1 implies that the null hypothesis (H_{0E}) is the drug is nonefficacious and that the alternative hypothesis (H_{aE}) is the drug is efficacious. Axiom 2 implies that the null hypothesis (H_{0S}) is the drug is safe whereas the alternative hypothesis (H_{aS}) is the drug is not safe.

For a sponsor's drug to be approved as being efficacious, enough information must be accumulated to contradict the null hypothesis (H_{0E}). This implies that the Type I error is synonymous with the regulatory decision risk regarding approval for efficacy and that the Type II error is synonymous with the sponsor's risk of failing to detect a truly efficacious drug. For the drug to be approved with a decision as to safety, the null hypothesis (H_{0S}) must not be contradicted by the available safety information. This implies that the Type II error is synonymous with regulatory decision risk regarding approval whereas the Type I error is synonymous with the sponsor's risk.

18.6 Premarket Approval Trials: Quality of Adverse Event Information

If clinical trials in the development of new drugs are designed to provide definitive information about efficacy rather than safety, it is important to consider the quality of safety information from such trials. As a definition, a trial will be regarded as being designed to provide definitive evidence of efficacy if it has a power of 95% to detect a clinically important difference (δ) between the target and reference (e.g., control) regimens in terms of the primary response measure, with a false positive rate of 5%. For discussion purposes, the clinically important difference is assumed to be 20% and the response variable is assumed to be dichotomous. A dichotomous response variable for efficacy assessment allows a natural connection between the efficacy endpoint and safety endpoints such as the proportion of patients who experience AEs.

The number of patients required per regimen for a clinical trial defined in terms of these characteristics will range anywhere from 125 to 164 patients, depending on whether one takes the viewpoint that the alternative hypothesis is one or two sided and also whether one adopts the worst case of the binomial variance or adopts a position less conservative. It is important to note that a trial designed in the manner described above to detect a (δ) percent difference between two regimens will permit the statistical detection (at the 0.05 nominal significance level) of a difference as small as one-half (δ) percent at the analysis stage. However, a trial designed definitively in this manner is unlikely to provide any information about a rare event.

For example, if the fraction of a population who would develop an AE upon treatment with a drug at a given dose were 0.1%, one would require 4604 (Table 18.1) patients to be treated with the drug at the given dose in order to have 99% confidence of observing at least one patient with the AE. If one required a greater degree of certainty, say 99.99%, about 10,000 patients would require treatment. In fact, the definitively designed efficacy trial would not enable one to detect any AEs with near certainty if they occurred less frequently than in 6% of the treated population.

Taking a trial with 150 patients per arm as representative of the definitively designed efficacy trial, one is unlikely to observe in such a trial any patients with rare AEs. For example, the probability of observing no patient with an AE among 150 treated patients given that the true incidence in the

TABLE 18.1

Number of Patients Requiring Treatment with a Dose of a Drug in order to Have $100(1 - \alpha)$% Confidence of Observing at Least 1 AE Given the True AE Rate in the Population is P

$P\backslash\alpha$	0.90	0.95	0.99	0.999	0.9999
0.001	2302	2995	4604	6906	9208
0.005	460	599	920	1380	1840
0.01	230	300	460	690	920
0.015	**153**	200	306	459	612
0.02	114	**149**	228	342	456
0.03	76	99	**152**	218	304
0.04	57	75	114	171	228
0.05	45	59	90	**135**	180
0.06	38	50	76	114	**152**
0.07	32	42	64	96	128
0.08	28	37	56	88	112
0.09	25	33	50	75	100
0.10	22	29	44	66	88
0.15	15	20	30	45	60
0.20	11	15	22	33	44
0.30	07	10	14	21	28
0.40	05	07	10	15	20
0.50	04	06	08	12	16

population is 0.1% is 0.861. It is therefore highly likely that the outcome of such a trial will be 0 divided by 150; i.e., an incidence of 0% among 150 patients treated. An exact 95% confidence interval based on 0/150 ranges from 0% to 2.4%. If what was known about the mechanism of action, the pharmacology and/or toxicology of the drug suggested certain untoward AEs were possible, and one monitored specifically for such events in a definitively designed efficacy trial, the fact that no such events were observed among 150 treated patients should be insufficient for regulatory approval in view of the upper limit of the 95% confidence interval being 2.4%. As Dr. Paul Leber (former head of the CNS medical Review Division at FDA) often said "Absence of proof is not proof of absence."

For AEs occurring in 6% or greater of the population, the typical definitively designed trial for efficacy would permit discrimination between two arms of approximately a 20% difference in the incidences of AEs with a power of 95% and a nominal false positive rate of 5% or, alternatively, discrimination between two arms of approximately a 10% difference with a power of 50% and a nominal false positive rate of 5%. The latter quantifies the smallest observed difference at the analysis stage, which would be indicative of a real difference.

18.7 Monitoring for Safety

Since a trial designed to provide definitive efficacy information is unlikely to provide much information about safety, it is therefore important to monitor all trials of new drugs for safety. Some reasons are (1) it is in the patient's best interest, ideally one would want to know as early as possible when anything untoward began to happen to the patient so that appropriate medical procedures could be initiated; (2) it is in the primary investigator's best interest; and (3) it is in the sponsors best interest in terms of credibility, prompt reporting to the regulatory agency, and minimizing potential litigation consequences.

However, there are logistical hurdles in monitoring trials for safety (or efficacy) information. These may depend on (1) the frequency of patient follow-up visits; (2) the rate of patient accession; (3) the data-collection instrument; (4) the quality of the data collected; (5) the field monitoring staff; (6) the ability to rapidly generate a quality-assured data base in an ongoing manner; (7) the ability to rapidly generate appropriate displays, summaries, or analyses; (8) the identification of personnel to review such displays or summaries; (9) the identification of who will make decisions based upon such reviews; and (10) the formulation of other committees such as data safety monitoring boards [4,5]. Although not very recent, Kamm et al. [6] provide an excellent reference on organizational structure reflecting the logistics of being able to rapidly monitor a trial (TASS) for safety. Briefly, the TASS (Ticlopidine Aspirin Stroke Study) trial was quadruple blind and parallel with patients stratified by sex, cardiovascular history, and previous stroke, prior to randomization. Over 3000 patients with transient ischemic attacks (TIA) or minor stroke participated in the trial and were followed for up to 6 years. Organizational structure consisted of an operations committee, a randomization center, a drug-distribution center, clinical centers, a central laboratory, an endpoint review committee, an interim statistical analysis group, and a safety committee that interacted with the FDA and the IRB and a policy committee.

18.8 Statistical Methodology: Individual Trial

Given that the logistics for monitoring a trial for safety are put in place, what should be the appropriate analysis or summarization methodology for generating information to be reviewed? First, one should distinguish between methodologies that might be used for rare events versus methodology that might be used for common events. For rare events, each event is important, especially if untoward. Procedures aimed at comparing treatment regimens may not be appropriate, particularly from individual trials designed for efficacy. Therefore, a simple descriptor such as the number of patients experiencing the event to the number of patients exposed to treatment may be sufficient. As more information accumulates, time-to-event methods may be applied as well as meta-analytic methods to descriptively and inferentially (if an adequate control exists) combine information across trials.

For common events, statistical methodology should be based on confidence intervals. Confidence intervals are statistically more appropriate than hypothesis testing in the absence of design considerations for safety. They also utilize the observed incidence as well as the estimate of the variability of the observed incidence. Confidence intervals should also better facilitate a decision by an informed reviewer. For a two-sided confidence interval with a large confidence coefficient, the lower limit being greater than 0 may indicate that the drug is not safe, whereas the upper limit, if small enough, may be interpreted as evidence of safety. This would be particularly true if one were able to set an acceptable safety limit. If the upper limit of the confidence interval with a large confidence coefficient were, in fact, less than the acceptable safety limit, then proof of safety (according to that criterion) would be indicated. Whereas the lower confidence limit exceeding the acceptable safety limit would be indicative of proof of being unsafe. In the utilization of confidence intervals, the confidence level (the compliment of the Type I error) should be chosen. In addition, statistical rigor requires that the confidence level be preserved or adjusted if multiple or interim analyses are performed. However, it may not be so important to preserve the confidence level or the Type I error, particularly if *absolute safety* of the sponsor's compound alone is of interest. Presumably, one would want to know the first moment when the accumulated information on an untoward event was different from that of untreated or control patients at *some* level of confidence. If, however, it is important to preserve the Type I error, there are procedures for doing so [7].

18.8.1 Direct Comparison Methodology

In using confidence intervals to display and to help monitor AEs in clinical trials of new drugs, the more traditional approach would be to directly compare two regimens. The aim of the comparison would be to provide estimates of the *difference* between regimen incidences. To construct a two-sided $100(1 - 2\alpha)\%$ confidence interval on the true difference in incidences of AEs between two regimens, one would proceed as follows: Let p_i and p_j denote the true incidences of some AE in the populations to be treated with the ith and jth regimens, respectively; let P_i and P_j denote the corresponding observed incidences among N_i and N_j treated patients, respectively; then the difference $\delta_{ij} = P_i - P_j$ in observed incidences is an unbiased estimate of the difference in true incidences; the estimate of the variance of the observed difference is given by $V_i + V_j$ where V_i is the estimate of the variance of the observed incidence in the ith regimen given by $P_i(1 - P_i)/N_i$. The confidence interval may be represented as

$$L_{ij} \leq p_i - p_j \leq U_{ij}, \tag{18.1}$$

where
  L_{ij} is the lower limit
  U_{ij} is the upper limit

and are given by

$$L_{ij} = P_i - P_j - Z_\alpha (V_i + V_j)^{1/2} \tag{18.2}$$

$$U_{ij} = P_i - P_j + Z_\alpha (V_i + V_j)^{1/2} \tag{18.3}$$

where Z_α is the upper percentile of the distribution of $P_i - P_j$ under the assumption of no difference in true incidences.

The direct comparison of two regimens via $100(1 - 2\alpha)\%$ confidence intervals also permits concluding that two regimens are different. If the lower limit L_{ij} were positive (presuming that the observed incidence in the ith regimen exceeded the observed incidence in the jth regimen), one would conclude that the two regimens were different at the nominal significance level α.

18.8.2 Indirect Comparison Methodology

A nonstandard, indirect approach for comparing two regimens follows. The primary or initial aim of this approach is to provide estimates of the true incidences for each regimen. Let p_i, p_j; P_i, P_j; N_i, N_j; and V_i, V_j be as identified before. A two-sided $100(1 - 2\alpha_1)\%$ confidence interval on the true incidence p_i in the ith regimen is

$$L_i \leq p_i \leq U_i \tag{18.4}$$

where
   L_i is the lower limit
   U_i is the upper limit

and are given by

$$L_i = P_i - Z_{\alpha 1}(V_i)^{1/2} \tag{18.5}$$

$$U_i = P_i + Z_{\alpha 1}(V_i)^{1/2} \tag{18.6}$$

where $Z_{\alpha 1}$ is the $100(1 - \alpha_1)$ percentile of the distribution of P_i.

In addition to such confidence intervals furnishing information on the true incidence in each regimen, they also permit two regimens to be indirectly compared. One could infer that regimens i and j are statistically different at the nominal significance level α_1 if the lower limit of the $100(1 - 2\alpha_1)\%$ confidence interval on the true incidence of regimen i was greater than the upper limit of regimen j; i.e., if $L_i > U_j$ where again the observed incidence in the ith regimen is greater than the observed incidence in the jth regimen.

Using the per group (indirect) confidence intervals should make it easier to monitor the emerging AE rate as there would be no need to know the identity of each arm as long as one was looking for the earliest signal that any two groups were statistically different. Further, it is similar to what one usually does in profiling crude response rates in time; i.e., crude response rates $\pm$ one standard error units are displayed. For observed response rates and sample sizes sufficient for the binomial distribution to be well approximated by the normal distribution, one would conclude that $p_i > p_j$ if $\{P_i - (V_i)^{1/2}\} > \{P_j + (V_j)^{1/2}\}$ at the 15.87% one-sided Type I error level. Instead of displaying crude response rates $\pm$ one standard error units $\{P_i \pm (V_i)^{1/2}\}$, one displays crude response rates $\pm CR_{\alpha 1}$ standard error units $\{P_i \pm CR_{\alpha 1}(V_i)^{1/2}\}$ and concludes that $p_i > p_j$ if $\{P_i - CR_{\alpha 1}(V_i)^{1/2}\} > \{P_j + CR_{\alpha 1}(V_j)^{1/2}\}$ at the Type I error level α_1, where $CR_{\alpha 1}$ is such that

$$CR_{\alpha 1} < \left\{ \frac{(P_i - P_j)}{\left[(V_i)^{1/2} + (V_j)^{1/2}\right]} \right\}, \tag{18.7}$$

and α_1 is determined as the lower bound of the area under the distribution of P_i (or P_j) to the right of $\{(P_i - P_j)/[(V_i)^{1/2} + (V_j)^{1/2}]\}$. This method is implemented and computations illustrated with an example in Section 18.9.

18.8.3 Connection between Direct and Indirect Comparison Methods

The direct comparison and the indirect comparison methods connect. To illustrate, think of the null hypothesis as no difference in true incidences (H_0: $p_i = p_j$) among the regimens, and the alternative hypothesis as there is a difference (H_a: $p_i > p_j$). The rejection rule for the direct comparison method is the incidence of regimen i statistically exceeds that of regimen j at the significance level α if $L_{ij} > 0$. The rejection rule for the indirect comparison method is the incidence of regimen i statistically exceeds that of regimen j at the significance level α_1 if $L_i > U_j$, presuming that $P_i > P_j$. The equivalence of the rejection rules is expressed as

$$Z_{\alpha 1} = \left[\frac{\left\{ (V_i)^{1/2} + (V_j)^{1/2} \right\}}{(V_i + V_j)^{1/2}} \right]^{-1} Z_\alpha \qquad (18.8)$$

That is, they are equivalent if the relationship between the critical point for the indirect comparison is proportional to the critical point for the direct comparison where the proportionality constant is the ratio of the variances given in Equation 18.8.

As an example, under the assumption of homogeneous variances of the two groups, the critical point corresponding to the indirect comparison would be $2^{1/2}/2 = 0.7071$ times the critical point for the direct comparison. For response rates and sample sizes large enough for the binomial distribution to be well approximated by the normal distribution, if α equals 5%, α_1 would be 12.24%. That is, if one were using a nominal 90% two-sided confidence interval to directly compare two regimens and the lower limit of that confidence interval exceeded 0, one would say with a confidence level of 95% or a Type I error rate of 5% that the two regimens were in fact different. To reach the same decision using the indirect comparison, one would construct two-sided 75.52% confidence intervals on the true incidence in each regimen and require that the lower limit of one be greater than the upper limit of the other.

For trials with several arms using the (direct) two-sided confidence interval on the difference in crude response rates between two arms would require displays of not only per group profiles but also of the possible pairwise differences among the arms. For five groups, the number of pairwise comparisons is 10.

18.9 Example

18.9.1 Adverse Event Data from a Clinical Trial

Data on an AE from a parallel, randomized, double-blind clinical trial of two doses (D_1, D_2) of a new drug compared to a control (C) appear in Table 18.2. The trial was designed to detect a 20% difference in efficacy between a dose group ($n = 150$) and the control with 95% power and a 5% Type I error rate. Entry of patients into a clinical trial is staggered; i.e., occurs in stages (intervals of time). The data consist of the number of patients entered and the number having the AE in each group totaled sequentially across stages.

These data are used retrospectively to illustrate the methods discussed in this chapter. The notation for columns two through seven is as follows: N_{iD2} is the total number of patients in D_2; f_{iD2} is the total number of AEs in D_2; N_{iD1} is the total number of patients in D_1; f_{iD1} is the total number of AEs in D_1; N_{iC} is the total number of patients in the control group; and f_{iC} is the total number of AEs in the control group by ith stage, respectively. Note that the time of AE is not recorded, so that the AE rate through the ith stage is the crude rate. Therefore, when these rates are plotted (Figure 18.1) by treatment group and stage, they may oscillate across stages.

Figure 18.1 illustrates the AE rates by accrual stage for the three treatment groups. It may be observed that the AE rates for dose group D_1 and the control group C are quite similar and lower than those of dose group D_2. However, the AE rates for D_2 are substantially higher than those in the control group. Therefore, analyses are consistent with monitoring focus on comparing these two groups. In Figure 18.1, the solid vertical lines from D_2 represent the lower one standard deviation (SD), $P_{D2} - SD_{D2}$, and the dashed

TABLE 18.2

Cumulative Entry and AEs in a CT of Two Doses (D_1, D_2) of Drug D against Control C

Stage	N_{iD2}	f_{iD2}	N_{iD1}	f_{iD1}	N_{iC}	f_{iC}
1	15	1	15	0	15	0
2	30	2	31	0	29	0
3	50	4	48	1	49	0
4	70	4	68	3	72	2
5	95	6	94	4	95	3
6	120	9	119	5	120	4
7	140	11	138	5	141	6
8	150	12	150	6	150	7

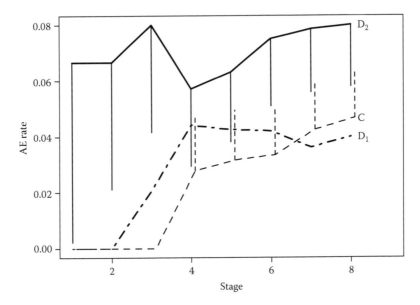

FIGURE 18.1

Crude AE rates of treatment groups: $-(D_2)$ or $+$ (C) one standard deviation.

lines represent the upper one standard deviation, $P_C - SD_C$, which are shifted slightly to the right for easier visualization. Due to overlapping, it is clear that D_2 and C are not statistically different from stages 4 through 8. However, the two groups may be statistically different at some level of significance at earlier stages (although unlikely at stage 1).

18.9.2 The Classical Direct Comparison Confidence Interval Method

In monitoring the AE rate in this trial, the CIs for the direct comparison are summarized in Table 18.3. This table lists all statistics associated with the direct comparison of D_1 to C as well as for D_2 to C based on the methodology in Section 18.8.1. It may be observed that there is no positive lower limit for the comparison from D_1 to C indicating that D_1 and C are not statistically significant at any stage, whereas the positive lower limit is achieved at stage 3 (bolded in the table) indicating D_2 and C are statistically different at this stage.

To more directly reflect the methodology in Section 18.8.1, the 95% confidence limits in Table 18.3 are based on the normal approximation of the binomial distribution. For small frequencies of AE occurrence, the analyst may want to compute exact confidence limits. Since variability is 0 when frequencies of occurrence is 0 in both groups, confidence limits are not presented for these stages.

TABLE 18.3

Summary Statistics for Direct Comparison

Stage	f_{D1}	f_C	$f_{D1} > f_C$	N_1	N_2	P_1	P_2	$P_1 - P_2$	L	U
D_1 *versus control*										
1	0	0	No	15	15	0.000	0.000	0.000		
2	0	0	No	31	29	0.000	0.000	0.000		
3	1	0	Yes	48	49	0.021	0.000	0.021	−0.020	0.061
4	3	2	Yes	68	72	0.044	0.028	0.016	−0.045	0.078
5	4	3	Yes	94	95	0.043	0.032	0.011	−0.043	0.065
6	5	4	Yes	119	120	0.042	0.033	0.009	−0.040	0.057
7	5	6	No	138	141	0.036	0.043	−0.006	−0.052	0.039
8	6	7	No	150	150	0.040	0.047	−0.007	−0.053	0.039
D_2 *versus control*										
1	1	0	Yes	15	15	0.067	0.000	0.067	−0.060	0.193
2	2	0	Yes	30	29	0.067	0.000	0.067	−0.023	0.156
3	**4**	**0**	**Yes**	**50**	**49**	**0.080**	**0.000**	**0.080**	**0.005**	**0.155**
4	4	2	Yes	70	72	0.057	0.028	0.029	−0.037	0.096
5	6	3	Yes	95	95	0.063	0.032	0.032	−0.029	0.092
6	9	4	Yes	120	120	0.075	0.033	0.042	−0.015	0.099
7	11	6	Yes	140	141	0.079	0.043	0.036	−0.020	0.092
8	12	7	Yes	150	150	0.080	0.047	0.033	−0.022	0.088

18.9.3 The Indirect Comparison Confidence Interval Method

Summary statistics based on Equations 18.5 and 18. 6 for the indirect comparison method of Section 18.8.2 are given in Table 18.4. In search for a specific stage where the lower limit L_i in group i is greater than the upper limit U_j in group j, we can identify that at stage 3, the lower limit ($L_{D2} = 0.005$) for D_2 is greater than the upper limit of control ($U_C = 0$). This again confirms the conclusion from the direct comparison.

To more directly reflect the methodology in Section 18.8.2 one set of 95% confidence limits in Table 18.4 are based on the normal approximation of the binomial distribution. Since frequencies are small, confidence limits were also computed using the empirical binomial distribution. The analyst may want to compute exact confidence limits. Since variability is 0 when the frequency of occurrence is 0 in any group, confidence limits are not presented for the first two stages. Although the frequency of occurrence is 0 in the control (C) group at stage 3, confidence limits of 0 are provided at this stage to connect to the results from the direct comparison methodology. Further, the upper limits for the control and the lower limits for dose 2 (D_2) group appear in bold to draw attention to the indirect comparison methodology. It is noted that the indirect comparison results lead to the same statistical inferences as did the direct comparison methodology results.

TABLE 18.4

Summary Statistics for Indirect Comparison

	Stage	N	f	P	Normal Approximation		Binomial	
					L	U	L	U
	1	15	0	0.0000				
	2	29	0	0.0000				
	3	49	0	0.0000	0.0000	**0.0000**	0.0000	**0.0000**
	4	72	2	0.0278	−0.0102	0.0657	0.0000	0.0694
Control	5	95	3	0.0316	−0.0036	0.0667	0.0000	0.0737
	6	120	4	0.0333	0.0012	0.0655	0.0083	0.0667
	7	141	6	0.0426	0.0092	0.0759	0.0142	0.0780
	8	150	7	0.0467	0.0129	0.0804	0.0133	0.0800
	1	15	0	0.0000				
	2	31	0	0.0000				
	3	48	1	0.0208	−0.0196	0.0612	0.0000	0.0625
	4	68	3	0.0441	−0.0047	0.0929	0.0000	0.1029
D_1	5	94	4	0.0426	0.0017	0.0834	0.0106	0.0851
	6	119	5	0.0420	0.0060	0.0781	0.0084	0.0840
	7	138	5	0.0362	0.0051	0.0674	0.0072	0.0725
	8	150	6	0.0400	0.0086	0.0714	0.0133	0.0733
	1	15	1	0.0667	−0.0596	0.1929	0.0000	0.2000
	2	30	2	0.0667	−0.0226	0.1559	0.0000	0.1667
	3	50	4	0.0800	**0.0048**	0.1552	**0.0200**	0.1600
	4	70	4	0.0571	0.0028	0.1115	0.0143	0.1143
D_2	5	95	6	0.0632	0.0142	0.1121	0.0211	0.1158
	6	120	9	0.0750	0.0279	0.1221	0.0333	0.1250
	7	140	11	0.0786	0.0340	0.1231	0.0357	0.1286
	8	150	12	0.0800	0.0366	0.1234	0.0400	0.1267

18.9.4 Computing Significance or Confidence Levels for the Indirect Method

As proposed in Section 18.8.2, a novel confidence or significance level method *alpha* (denoted as α_1 in that section) has to be determined so that the lower confidence bound on the true AE rate of D_2 is greater than the upper confidence bound of C. There are two ways to determine this significance level, which are based on different distributional assumptions leading to $CR_{\alpha 1}$. One is to use an iterative approach based on the exact empirical binomial distribution and another is based on the normal approximation.

The binomial approach is based on the well-known fact that if f is binomially distributed with binomial(N, p), then the exact $(1 - 2\alpha_1)$% confidence interval can be obtained by finding L and U such that $\sum_{k=0}^{L}$ binomial(k, N, p) $\leq \alpha_1$ and $\sum_{k=U}^{N}$ binomial(k, N, p) $\geq \alpha_1$. Therefore, we can find α_1 such that $L_{D2} \geq U_C$

TABLE 18.5

Alpha Levels Determined from Binomial Distribution and Normal Approximation

Distribution	Stage	1	2	3	4	5	6	7	8
Binomial	α_1	0.353	0.099	0.011	0.230	0.199	0.186	0.148	0.198
Normal approximation	α_1	0.150	0.072	0.019	0.267	0.231	0.151	0.182	0.199

where L_{D2} is determined from $\sum_{k=0}^{L_{D2}} \text{binomial}(k, N_2, \hat{p}_2) \leq \alpha_1$ and U_C is determined from $\sum_{k=U_C}^{N} \text{binomial}(k, N_C, \hat{p}_C) \geq \alpha_1$. Note that $\hat{p}_2 = f_{D2}/N_{D2}$ and $\hat{p}_C = f_C/N_C$, and α_1 may be determined iteratively from the two previous inequalities in which α_1 appears both as an upper bound and a lower bound. The α_1 are listed in Table 18.5 and graphically illustrated in Figure 18.2.

The normal approximation approach is based on the indirect comparison methodology in Section 18.8.2. Here α_1 is such that $L_i \geq U_j$ (e.g., $L_{D2} \geq U_C$); i.e., $\hat{p}_i - z_{\alpha_1}^* \sqrt{v_i} \geq \hat{p}_j + z_{\alpha_1}^* \sqrt{v_j}$. The latter inequality may be rearranged as

$$z_{\alpha 1} \leq \frac{\hat{p}_i - \hat{p}_j}{\sqrt{v_i} + \sqrt{v_j}}.$$

Therefore, α_1 is given by

$$\alpha_1 \geq pnorm\left(\frac{\hat{p}_i - \hat{p}_j}{\sqrt{v_i} + \sqrt{v_j}}\right)$$

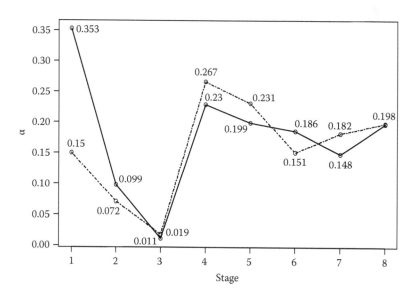

FIGURE 18.2

Alphas determined from the binomial distribution (solid line) and the normal approximation (dashed line) for data in Table 18.1. Numerical values are listed in Table 18.5.

where *pnorm* is the cumulative normal probability function. These alphas are also summarized in Table 18.5 and illustrated graphically in Figure 18.2. This method also leads to the same statistical inference as did the direct and the indirect confidence interval methods. The R program that details the implementation of these methods appears in Appendix 18.A.1. Readers may wish to check analysis results and/or apply the methods to their own trial data.

The methods presented in this chapter are intended to serve as an *alerting mechanism* in the usual monitoring of AEs in clinical trials. Their attractiveness is their simplicity and the fact that they represent little effort beyond what is usually done in monitoring AEs as they accumulate. The methods were applied to AE data from a completed clinical trial. Therefore, they were applied to the crude-rate AE data across all stages of entry for illustration. Had they been applied prospectively as the trial was ongoing and the AE was serious, the significant excess of the AE in the highest dose group as compared to control (if placebo) at stage 3 would have led to serious discussions about possibly stopping the trial or at least dropping the high dose group.

18.10 Statistical Methodology: Across Trials

The methodology presented in this chapter could be used to monitor AEs as they accumulate in individual clinical trials of a new drug. If there are several trials being conducted under the clinical development plan of the drug, the AE rates from individual trials could be combined across trials using an appropriate weighted estimate of the individual rates. The fact that individual trials were designed to address different efficacy objectives is not necessarily a constraint to combining AE rates, as the mechanism of action of the drug leading to AEs may be independent of the mechanism of action with respect to efficacy. Emerging AE rates although signaling no alarm in individual trials might be compelling when combined across trials.

18.11 Concluding Remarks

To summarize the points made, it was recognized that it may be possible to design some trials to provide definitive safety information. Three occasions were presented where indeed that was the case. However, for most new drugs in clinical development it is not possible. Therefore, a rational approach is to design definitively for efficacy and monitor and describe safety. This position is in fact consistent with the statutory requirement for approval to market new drugs in the United States. Statistical procedures involving confidence intervals were also suggested for monitoring trials for safety. Further, confidence intervals on the true AE rate for each treatment group are suggested as being preferable confidence intervals that directly compare two groups.

In addition, the following suggestions/observations are made. (1) Since open trials do not permit unbiased comparisons of groups and positive controlled trials may reflect an upward bias, the primary assessment of safety should come from double-blind, placebo-controlled trials. (2) Ideally, the clinical development plan for a new compound should address plans for assessing efficacy *and* safety as characteristics of the drug. This should include developing how the null hypothesis that the drug is not efficacious (HOE) and the drug is safe (HOS) would be contradicted. The ideal development plan would also include procedures for monitoring each trial for safety as well as for monitoring the development plan as data accumulate across trials. (3) If rare AEs are of interest, development plans should be designed to have a high probability of observing one or more events in each dose regimen; this includes post-marketing surveillance trials as well. (4) The preferred statistical methodology for monitoring and analyzing AE data is per regimen confidence intervals with large coefficients. This approach allows one to provide interval estimates on the true incidence of each regimen; permits sequential procedures such as those of Jennison and Turnbull [7] to be incorporated; also permits sequential procedures such as those of Schultz et al. [8] or Fleming [9] to be incorporated regarding a decision to terminate any arm independent of other arms; and would minimize breaking the blind of studies. (5) The impact on ideal clinical development plans if a Hauck and Anderson [10] approach were taken to reverse the null and alternative hypotheses regarding safety should be investigated [11]. That is, consider the null hypothesis to be "the drug is not safe" and the alternative hypothesis to be "the drug is safe." Such an approach would provide consistency between the regulatory risks for approval based on efficacy as well as on safety. (6) The impact on ideal clinical development plans, if efficacy and safety are viewed as compound hypotheses, should be investigated. That is, view the null hypothesis as "the drug is not efficacious and the drug is not safe" and the alternative hypothesis as "the drug is efficacious and the drug is safe." Other alternative hypotheses less stringent may also be proposed. (7) If we continue to design only for efficacy, the quality of safety information per trial and across trials provided by the total sample size for each clinical development plan should be explored. If this is sufficiently uninformative, then larger sample sizes may be needed. (8) In addition to requiring a safety review committee of impartial observers, such as an independent safety monitoring board for each trial, pharmaceutical companies should have a chief safety information officer [12]. (9) Finally, and ideally, each patient in each clinical trial conducted in the development of new drugs should be monitored for safety. When changes are noted that would give the physician concern, one should care for the patient and then assess whether such changes are different from those among untreated comparable patients. This in itself argues for accumulating large *experimental* data bases on placebo-treated patients from placebo-controlled trials.

The focus here has been to stress the importance of monitoring clinical trials of new drugs individually and across the clinical development plan for safety. In addition, methods were suggested for doing so. Once the NDA has been filed and the FDA approves the drug for marketing, the responsibility of the drug sponsor does not end there. Safety of drugs is a life-cycle exercise [13,14] and requires the sponsor to develop and put in place risk management [15] procedures for monitoring safety post market approval.

Appendix 18.A R Program to Analyze the Data in Table 18.2

```
##= = = = = = = = = = = = = = = = = = = = = = = = = = = = = = = = = = =
# Title: R for AE: Chapter 18
##= = = = = = = = = = = = = = = = = = = = = = = = = = = = = = = = = = =

#
# 1. get the data from Table 18.2
#
dat         = read.table ("data.txt", header = T)
dat$p2      = dat$fD2/dat$ND2
dat$p1      = dat$fD1/dat$ND1
dat$pC      = dat$fC/dat$NC
dat$V2      = dat$p2* (1-dat$p2) /dat$ND2
dat$V1      = dat$p1* (1-dat$p1) /dat$ND1
dat$VC      = dat$pC* (1-dat$pC) /dat$NC
len         = length (dat [,1])
dat$stage = 1:len

#
# 2. make plot
#

# 2.1. plot just the ps
plot (p2~stage, type = "n",dat,xlim = c (1,9) ,ylim = c (0,max (dat$p1, dat$p2, dat$pC) ),
xlab = "Stage", las = 1, ylab = "AE Rate")
lines (pC~stage, dat, lty = 8)
lines (p1~stage, dat, lty = 4)
lines (p2~stage, dat, lty = 1)
text (8.3,dat$pC [8] , "C")
text (8.3,dat$p1 [8] , "D1")
text (8.3,dat$p2 [8] , "D2")

# 2.2. plot with CI
shift = 0.1 # shife a little bit for Control
plot (p2~stage,type = "n",dat,xlim = c (1,9) ,ylim = c (0,0.08) ,xlab = "Stage", las = 1,
   ylab = "AE Rate")
```

```
lines(p2~stage, dat, lty=1,lwd=3)
lines(pC~I(stage+shift), dat, lty=8, lwd=3)
lines(p1~stage, dat, lty=4,lwd=4)
text(8.3,dat$pC[8], "C")
text(8.3,dat$p1[8], "D1")
text(8.3,dat$p2[8], "D2")
segments(dat$stage, dat$p2,dat$stage, dat$p2-sqrt(dat$V2),
  lwd=2, lty=1) # low half of D2
segments(I(dat$stage+shift),dat$pC,I(dat$stage+shift),dat$pC+sqrt(dat$VC),
  lwd=2, lty=8) # upper half of C


#
# 3. function for direct comparison
#
direct.CI=function(N1,f1,N2,f2, alpha){
p1=f1/N1; p2=f2/N2
v1=p1*(1-p1)/N1;v2=p2*(1-p2)/N2

z.alpha=qnorm(1-alpha)

low=(p1-p2)-z.alpha*sqrt(v1+v2)
up=(p1-p2)+z.alpha*sqrt(v1+v2)

data.frame(f1=f1,f2=f2,testf=f1>f2,N1=N1,N2=N2,p1=p1,p2=p2,diff=p1-p2,
  testp=p1>p2,low=low, up=up)
}

CI1toC=direct.CI(dat$ND1, dat$fD1, dat$NC, dat$fC, 0.025)
(CI1toC)
CI2toC=direct.CI(dat$ND2, dat$fD2, dat$NC, dat$fC, 0.025)
CI2toC


#
# 4. function for indirect comparison:
#

# 4.1. using normal approximation
indirect.CI=function(N,f,alpha){
p=f/N
v=p*(1-p)/N
z.alpha=qnorm(1-alpha)
low     =p-z.alpha*sqrt(v)
up      =p+z.alpha*sqrt(v)
data.frame(N=N,f=f,p=p,low=low,up=up)
}

CIC=indirect.CI(dat$NC, dat$fC, 0.025)
CIC
CI1=indirect.CI(dat$ND1, dat$fD1, 0.025)
CI1
CI2=indirect.CI(dat$ND2, dat$fD2, 0.025)
CI2

cat("make decision on stage to see Low_D1 > up_C","\n\n")
out=data.frame(stage= dat$stage, direct.test=CI1$low>CIC$up,
low1=CI1$low, upC =CIC$up)
print(out)

cat("make decision on stage to see Low_D2 > up_C","\n\n")
out=data.frame(stage= dat$stage, direct.test=CI2$low>CIC$up,
```

```
low2 = CI2$low, upC = CIC$up)
print(out)

# 4.2. exact CI with binomial
exact.CI = function(N,f, alpha){
p   = f/N
low = qbinom(alpha, N, p)
up  = qbinom(1-alpha,N,p)
data.frame(N=N,p=p,f=f,low=low,up=up, plow = low/N, pup=up/N)
}

CIC = exact.CI(dat$NC, dat$fC, 0.025)
CIC
CI1 = exact.CI(dat$ND1, dat$fD1, 0.025)
CI1
CI2 = exact.CI(dat$ND2, dat$fD2, 0.025)
CI2

cat("make decision on stage to see Low_D2 > up_C","\n\n")
out = data.frame(stage= dat$stage, direct.test = CI2$plow > CIC$pup,
low2 = CI2$plow, upC = CIC$pup)
print(out)

out = data.frame(stage= dat$stage, direct.test = CI1$plow > CIC$pup,
low1 = CI1$plow, upC = CIC$pup)
print(out)

#
# 5. the significance level methods
#

# 5.1. the binomail approach
fn = function(alpha, stage)
exact.CI(dat$ND2,dat$fD2,alpha)$plow[stage]-exact.CI(dat$NC,dat$fC,alpha)$pup[stage]

binom.alpha = NULL
for(s in 1:len) binom.alpha[s] =uniroot(fn, c(0,0.8), stage=s)$root # 1-2*alpha interval
binom.alpha

# 5.2. alpha from normal approximation
bound.CI = function(N1,f1,N2,f2){
p1 = f1/N1; p2 = f2/N2
v1 = p1*(1-p1)/N1;v2 = p2*(1-p2)/N2
data.frame(N1=N1,f1=f1,p1=p1,N2=N2,f2=f2,p2=p2,bound= (p2-p1)/(sqrt(v1)+
  sqrt(v2)))
}

d0 = bound.CI(dat$NC,dat$fC,dat$ND2,dat$fD2)
d0$alpha = 1-pnorm(d0$bound)
d0

# 5.3. make the plot
plot(dat$stage,binom.alpha,type="o",xlab="Stage",ylab=expression(alpha),las=1,
  main="")
text(dat$stage, est.alpha,round(est.alpha,3))

points(dat$stage, d0$alpha)
lines(dat$stage, d0$alpha, lty=4)
text(dat$stage, d0$alpha,round(d0$alpha,3))
```

References

1. Peace KE (1988): Design, monitoring and analysis issues relative to adverse events. *Drug Information Journal*; **21**: 21–28.
2. Peace KE (1993): Design and analysis considerations for safety data, particularly adverse events. In: *Drug Safety Assessment in Clinical Trials*, Gilbert, GS (ed.), Marcel Dekker, Inc., New York, pp. 305–316.
3. Armitage P (1954): Sequential tests in prophylactic and therapeutic trials. *Quality Journal of Medicine*; **91**: 255–274.
4. Ellenberg SS, Fleming TR, DeMets DL (2003): *Data Monitoring Committees in Clinical Trials: A Practical Perspective*, John Wiley & Sons, Chichester, West Sussex, England.
5. Herson J (2009): *Data and Safety Monitoring Committees in Clinical Trials*, Chapman & Hall/CRC, Boca Raton, FL.
6. Kamm B, Maloney B, Cranston B, Roc R, Hassy W (1984): Ticlopidine aspirin stroke study organizational structure. In: *Presented at Society for Controlled Clinical Trials*, Miami, FL.
7. Jennison C, Turnbull BW (1984): Repeated confidence intervals for group sequential trials. *Controlled Clinical Trials*; **5**: 33–45.
8. Schultz TR, Nichol FR, Elfring GL, Weed SD (1973): Multiple stage procedures for drug screening. *Biometrics*; **29**: 293–300.
9. Fleming TR (1982): One-sample multiple testing procedure for phase II clinical trials. *Biometrics*; **38**: 143–151.
10. Hauck WW, Anderson S (1983): A new procedure for testing equivalence in comparative bioavailability and other clinical trials. *Communications in Statistics: Theory and Methods*; **12**: 2663–2692.
11. Peace KE (1985): *Design, Monitoring and Analysis Issues Relative to Adverse Events*, DIA Workshop, December, Arlington, VA.
12. Peace KE (2007): Summarization and analysis of pharmaceutical safety data. In: *Fourteenth Annual Biopharmaceutical Applied Statistics Symposium*, November 4, Savannah, GA.
13. Peace KE (1989): Some thoughts on the biopharmaceutical section and statistics. In: *ASA Proceedings Sesquicentennial Invited Paper Session*, Alexandria, VA, pp. 98–105.
14. Peace KE (2008): Commentary: Safety of drugs is indeed a lifecycle exercise. *Bio-IT-World*, July 21.
15. Robinson M, Cook S (2006): *Clinical Trials Risk Management*, Taylor & Francis Group, Boca Raton, FL.

Index

Printed and bound by CPI Group (UK) Ltd, Croydon, CR0 4YY

24/10/2024

01778278-0019